# Lung Cancer

Edited by
Anne-Marie C. Dingemans, Martin Reck
and Virginie Westeel

Editor in Chief
Tobias Welte

This book is one in a series of *ERS Monographs*. Each individual issue provides a comprehensive overview of one specific clinical area of respiratory health, communicating information about the most advanced techniques and systems required for its investigation. It provides factual and useful scientific detail, drawing on specific case studies and looking into the diagnosis and management of individual patients. Previously published titles in this series are listed at the back of this *Monograph*.

*ERS Monographs* are available online at www.erspublications.com and print copies are available from www.ersbookshop.com

Continuing medical education (CME) credits are available through many issues of the *ERS Monograph*. Following evaluation, successful *Monographs* are accredited by the European Board for Accreditation in Pneumology (EBAP) for 5 CME credits. To earn CME credits, read the book of your choice (it is clearly indicated on the online table of contents whether CME credits are available) then complete the CME question form that is available at www.ers-education.org/e-learning/cme-tests.aspx



Managing Editor: Rachel White
European Respiratory Society, 442 Glossop Road, Sheffield, S10 2PX, UK
Tel: 44 114 2672860 | E-mail: Monograph@ersj.org.uk

Published by European Respiratory Society ©2015
June 2015
Print ISBN: 978-1-84984-061-3
Online ISBN: 978-1-84984-062-0
Print ISSN: 2312-508X
Online ISSN: 2312-5098
Printed by Charlesworth Press, Wakefield, UK



C | O | P | E COMMITTEE ON PUBLICATION ETHICS

This journal is a member of and subscribes to the principles of the Committee on Publication Ethics.

MIX Paper from responsible sources FSC® C016379

THOMSON REUTERS BOOK CITATION INDEX INDEXED

ERS | monograph

# Contents

Lung Cancer

Number 68
June 2015

# Preface

Tobias Welte, Editor in Chief

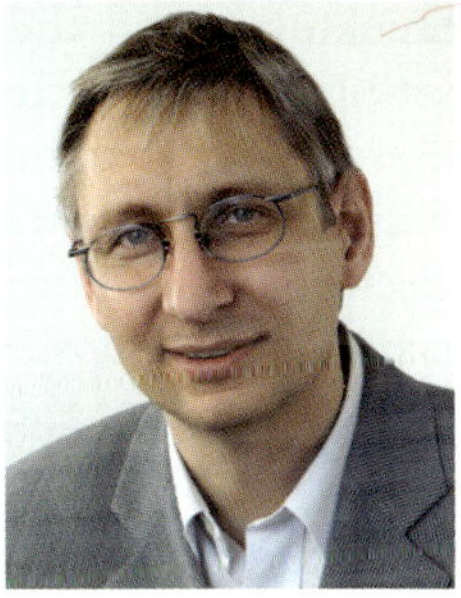

The GLOBOCAN project (http://www.globocan.iarc.fr) is a comprehensive cancer surveillance database managed by the International Association of Cancer Registries (IACR) and supported by the World Health Organization (WHO). The project aims to provide up-to-date estimates of the incidence, mortality and prevalence of major cancer types, at a national level, for 184 countries. GLOBOCAN estimate that ~14.1 million new cancer cases and 8.2 million deaths occurred in 2012 worldwide [1]. There were estimated to be 1.8 million new lung cancer cases in 2012 (12.9% of the total), 57% (65% of cancer deaths worldwide) of which occurred in the less developed regions, making lung cancer the most common cancer in the world. In both more and less developed countries, lung cancer is the leading cause of cancer death among males, with the highest estimated age-standardised incidence rates occurring in Central and Eastern Europe (53.5 per 100 000) and Eastern Asia (50.4 per 100 000). In more developed countries, lung cancer has surpassed breast cancer as the leading cause of cancer death among females. The highest estimated rates in females are in northern America (33.8) and northern Europe (23.7), with a relatively high rate in Eastern Asia (19.2) and the lowest rates in Western and Middle Africa (1.1 and 0.8 per 100 000, respectively) [1].

Lung cancer is the most common cause of death from cancer worldwide; it is estimated that it causes nearly one in five deaths (1.59 million deaths, 19.4% of the total). Its high fatality (it has an overall the overall mortality to incidence ratio of 0.87) and the relative lack of variability in survival in different regions of the world, mean that the geographical patterns of mortality closely follow those of incidence. Even so, most lung cancer patients are diagnosed late, with the majority of them at an advanced disease stage. There are currently no curative therapy options available and long-term survival amongst lung cancer patients is still low.

Nevertheless, enormous progress has been made during the last decade. Multimodal therapies have improved the prognosis as has the development of new surgical techniques, the optimisation of

 Print ISBN: 978-1-84984-061-3. Online ISBN: 978-1-84984-062-0. Print ISSN: 2312-508X. Online ISSN: 2312-5098.

radiation therapy and the introduction of new chemotherapeutic agents. However, the decisive breakthrough has been the development of new immunopathological techniques, which allow for the detection of special genetic mutations and initiate individualised therapy according to this finding. The number of patients who benefit is still small; however, the quality of life and survival rates of those who respond to this treatment are impressive. The pharmaceutical industry invests heavily in the development of new diagnostic tools and effective treatment modalities, so expectations for the future are great.

Smoking is still the most important risk factor worldwide. The set-up of preventive measures to reduce the smoking rate is therefore of paramount importance. However, some measures must be viewed with a critical distance. The dissemination of electronic cigarettes all over the world is viewed critically by experts and most of the lung societies [2]. The long-term consequences of these devices must be carefully examined before a final assessment is possible.

Thoracic oncology plays an increasingly important role in respiratory medicine, as well as in the European Respiratory Society (ERS). Knowledge about oncology must make up a substantial part of a respiratory physician's training, not only for those working in a hospital, but also for those in an outpatient setting.

This issue of the *ERS Monograph* provides a comprehensive overview of the current knowledge of lung cancer in clinical practice and research. The Guest Editors have done great job of ensuring that all aspects of this complex disease are represented, meaning this book will be of interest to a very broad readership.

## References

1. Torre LA, Bray F, Siegel RL, *et al.* Global cancer statistics, 2012. *CA Cancer J Clin* 2015; 65: 87–108.
2. Brandon TH, Goniewicz ML, Hanna NH, *et al.* Electronic nicotine delivery systems: a policy statement from the American Association for Cancer Research and the American Society of Clinical Oncology. *Clin Cancer Res* 2015; 21: 514–525.

# Guest Editors

## Anne-Marie C. Dingemans

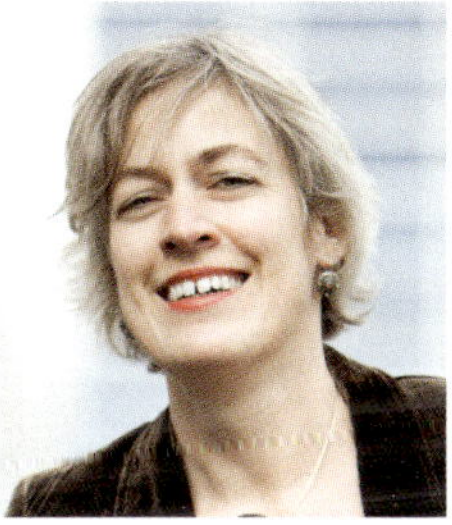

Anne-Marie C. Dingemans has been associate professor of pulmonology at the Maastricht University Medical Center (Maastricht, the Netherlands) since 2004, where she currently she coordinates clinical lung cancer trials and is involved in translational research on lung cancer.

Anne-Marie Dingemans received her medical degree at Maastricht University (Maastricht) in 1994 and subsequently her PhD at VU Medical Center (Amsterdam, the Netherlands) in 2000 for laboratory research on resistance to chemotherapy in lung cancer. She performed her training as a pulmonologist at VU Medical Center and at Leiden University Medical Center (Leiden, the Netherlands).

Anne-Marie is a board member of the Netherlands Respiratory Society (NRS) and the secretary of the NVALT studies foundation. She is also a member of the Lung and Other Thoracic Tumours faculty of the European Society for Medical Oncology (ESMO), and of the Harmonised Education in Respiratory Medicine for European Specialists (HERMES) Thoracic Oncology task force. Anne-Marie is a member of the American Association of Cancer Research (AACR), the American Society of Clinical Oncology (ASCO), the International Association for the Study of Lung Cancer (IASLC) and the European Thoracic Oncology Platform (ETOP). She has (co)-authored more than 80 publications and book chapters.

## Martin Reck

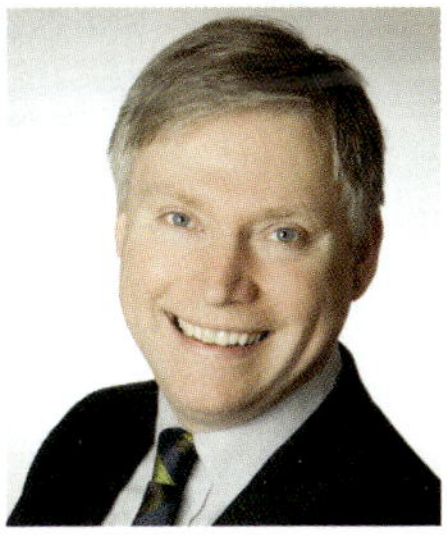

Martin Reck is head of the Department of Thoracic Oncology and head of the Clinical Trial Department in the Department of Thoracic Oncology at the Lung Clinic Grosshansdorf (Grosshansdorf, Germany). He is also Principal Investigator at the Airway Research Center North (ARCN) (Lung Clinic Grosshansdorf), which is a member of the German Centre for Lung Research (DZL).

 Print ISBN: 978-1-84984-061-3. Online ISBN: 978-1-84984-062-0. Print ISSN: 2312-508X. Online ISSN: 2312-5098.

Martin Reck underwent medical training at the University of Hamburg (Hamburg, Germany) from 1986–1993. He completed his doctorate at the General Hospital Wandsbek, Hamburg, in 1995, and received post-graduate training at the Hospital Grosshansdorf. He was appointed as a specialist in internal medicine in 2001 and as a specialist in pulmonology in 2002. In 2008, he was awarded a post-doctoral lecturing qualification by the University of Schleswig-Holstein (Kiel, Germany).

Martin Reck has acted as a Principal Investigator or Co-Principal Investigator in various clinical trials since 1993. His main interests are new medical treatments for thoracic malignancies and translational research related to predictive markers. A particular focus of his work is the clinical development of antiangiogenic compounds, such as bevacizumab, nintedanib and other compounds. Recently, he also has been deeply involved in several key trials with immunotherapies, including ipilimumab, programmed cell death protein-1 and programmed cell death ligand-1 antibodies and other agents.

In addition to the International Association for the Study of Lung Cancer (IASLC), Martin Reck is also a member of the European Society for Medical Oncology (ESMO), the American Society of Clinical Oncology (ASCO), the German Working Group for Lung Cancer, the German Cancer Society (DKG) and the German Respiratory Society (DGP). He has published papers in numerous peer-reviewed journals and is member of the Editorial Boards of the *Journal of Thoracic Oncology*, *Annals of Oncology* and *Lung Cancer*.

## Virginie Westeel

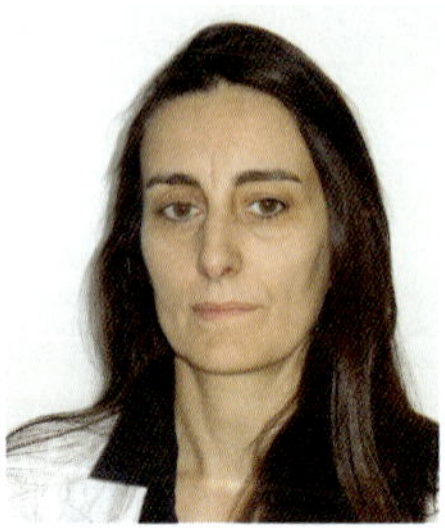

Virginie Westeel is professor of pulmonology at the University of Franche-Comté (Besançon, France) and head of the Thoracic Oncology unit at the University Hospital of Besançon (Besançon).

She is a graduate of the University of Franche-Comté. Her clinical and research activities are exclusively dedicated to lung cancer and her research interests include lung cancer therapeutics, follow-up and evidence-based medicine.

Virginie Westeel is currently the Principal Investigator of the only large multicentre randomised trial that has been conducted to date on follow-up after lung cancer surgery. Her 93 publications mostly include the results of clinical trials in both early stage and advanced lung cancer.

Virginie Westeel took on the role of Joint Coordinating Editor of the Cochrane Lung Cancer Review Group in 2013. She led the development of the French guidelines for lung cancer staging. She has been a member of the scientific committee of the French research group, the Intergroupe Francophone de Cancérologie Thoracique (IFCT), from 2009 to 2013, and she is currently a member of the executive committee of IFCT. Virginie was also a member of the scientific committee of IASLC between 2005 and 2009, and of the scientific committee of several World Conference on Lung Cancer (WCLC). She is a member of the American Society of Clinical Oncology (ASCO) and the International Association for the Study of Lung Cancer (IASLC).

# Introduction

Martin Reck[1], Anne-Marie C. Dingemans[2] and Virginie Westeel[3]

Lung cancer still represents one of the most frequent solid tumours with the highest tumour-associated mortality and increasing global incidence rates.

Relevant changes have been seen in epidemiology and there have been substantial improvements in all disciplines of lung cancer treatment. However, the picture of lung cancer treatment has become quite complex, and treatment strategies are moving more and more from global treatment algorithms to individualised treatment.

Standardised and adequate histological, as well as molecular classification (as it is reflected in the recommendations for ADC classification), have become crucial in order to give the individual patient the chance of optimal treatment.

As well as relevant steps in surgery and radiotherapy, new impressive opportunities in systemic treatment have opened up through the identification of treatable oncogenic driver alterations and the appropriate targeted therapies. Furthermore, in 2015, after decades of negative trials, we are experiencing a fascinating phase of immunotherapy with a completely new class of agents.

Of all the solid tumours, lung cancer has really demonstrated rapid and substantial progress in treatment efficacy based on major progress in diagnostics. Therefore, it is of paramount importance that the pulmonologist as key member of the interdisciplinary team is familiar with the current state of the art in lung cancer care.

We hope that this issue will be of interest to all researchers, clinicians and surgeons in the respiratory field and that it will help to improve understanding about lung cancer, answering all the questions encountered in everyday practice.

[1]Dept of Thoracic Oncology, Lung Clinic, Airway Research Center North (ARCN), Grosshansdorf, Germany. [2]Pulmonology, Maastricht University Medical Centre, Maastricht, The Netherlands. [3]Service de Pneumologie, CHRU Hôpital Jean Minjoz, Besançon cedex, France. [4]Université de Franche-Comté, Besançon, France.

Correspondence: Dept of Thoracic Oncology, Lung Clinic, Airway Research Center North (ARCN), Woehrendamm 80, Grosshansdorf 22927, Germany. E-mail: m.reck@lungenclinic.de

 Print ISBN: 978-1-84984-061-3. Online ISBN: 978-1-84984-062-0. Print ISSN: 2312-508X. Online ISSN: 2312-5098.

# List of abbreviations

| | |
|---|---|
| ADC | Adenocarcinoma |
| ALK | Anaplastic lymphoma kinase |
| COPD | Chronic obstructive pulmonary disease |
| CT | Computed tomography |
| CTLA4 | Cytotoxic T-lymphocyte antigen 4 |
| $D_{LCO}$ | Diffusing capacity of the lung for carbon monoxide |
| EBUS | Endobronchial ultrasound |
| EGF | Epidermal growth factor |
| EGFR | Epidermal growth factor receptor |
| EGFR-TKI | Epidermal growth factor receptor tyrosine kinase inhibitor |
| EUS | Endoscopic ultrasound |
| FEV1 | Forced expiratory volume in 1 s |
| FGFR | Fibroblast growth factor receptor |
| FISH | Fluorescence *in situ* hybridisation |
| FVC | Forced vital capacity |
| HER2 | Human epidermal growth factor receptor 2 |
| HGF | Hepatocyte growth factor |
| IHC | Immunohistochemistry |
| LCNEC | Large cell neuroendocrine carcinoma |
| NGS | Next-generation sequencing |
| NSCLC | Nonsmall cell lung cancer |
| PET | Positron emission tomography |
| PFS | Progression-free survival |
| SCC | Squamous cell carcinoma |
| SCLC | Small cell lung cancer |
| TGF | Transforming growth factor |
| TKI | Tyrosine kinase inhibitor |
| VATS | Video-assisted thoracoscopic surgery |
| VEGF | Vascular endothelial growth factor |
| VEGFR | Vascular endothelial growth factor receptor |

Chapter 1

# Epidemiology: development and perspectives

Georgia Hardavella[1,2] and Tariq Sethi[1,2]

This chapter aims to offer a brief overview of the epidemiology of lung cancer worldwide and particularly in Europe. It presents important epidemiological data in terms of incidence, mortality and 5-year survival, identifies developing epidemiological trends based on published data, and at the same time tries to highlight the needs and areas of potential interest for future epidemiological studies in lung cancer.

The epidemiology of lung cancer has evolved impressively. Lung cancer was a rare disease at the start of the 20th century; however, since the mid-1980s it has been the most common cancer worldwide, in terms of incidence. Today, it is considered to be a pandemic with major financial and social consequences. The wide social acceptance of tobacco consumption during the past century together with diverse environmental exposures are a few of the factors contributing to this pandemic.

Today, several sources provide comprehensive epidemiological data for lung cancer; they include the World Health Organization (WHO), the American Cancer Society, the National Cancer Institute, Cancer Research UK, the International Agency for Research on Cancer (IARC), the European Network of Cancer Registries, and the Organisation for Economic Co-operation and Development, among others. The development of national lung cancer registries is still a work in progress in many European countries and the development of national registries is expected to streamline the reporting of all lung cancer cases in Europe.

In this chapter, we present recent epidemiological data for lung cancer, and highlight changes, trends and future perspectives in an attempt to identify where the bigger picture will move in the next few years.

## Incidence

Lung cancer accounts for ~13% of all cancer diagnoses in both Europe and the USA [1, 2]. Recent GLOBOCAN data have shown that Northern America and Europe have the highest incidence of lung cancer, while the lowest incidence is in Africa, Latin America and the Caribbean [3].

[1]Dept of Respiratory Medicine, King's College Hospital, London, UK. [2]Dept of Respiratory Medicine and Allergy, King's College, London, UK.

Correspondence: Georgia Hardavella, King's College Hospital London, Dept of Respiratory Medicine, 2nd Floor Cheyne Wing, Denmark Hill, London, SE5 9RS, UK. E-mail: g.hardavella@nhs.net

 Print ISBN: 978-1-84984-061-3. Online ISBN: 978-1-84984-062-0. Print ISSN: 2312-508X. Online ISSN: 2312-5098.

Lung cancer is the fourth most common cancer in Europe, with more than 410 000 new cases diagnosed in 2012. In the USA it appears that the incidence rate has been declining since the 1980s in males and since the mid-2000s in females. However, the actual numbers remain appalling as an estimated 224 210 new cases of lung cancer are expected in the USA in 2014, accounting for ~13% of all cancer diagnoses [2].

In Europe, there is variation in incidence between different countries. Table 1 summarises the highest and lowest incidence and mortality rates, by sex, in Europe. The highest incidence rates for lung cancer among males are seen in Hungary (109 cases per 100 000 males) and the former Yugoslav Republic of Macedonia (102 cases per 100 000); among females, the highest incidence rates are seen in Denmark (54.9 cases per 100 000 females), Hungary (46.4 cases per 100 000) and the UK (38.7 cases per 100 000) [3–5]. The lowest incidence rates in males have been reported by Finland and Sweden (45 and 29 cases per 100 000, respectively), and by Ukraine and Belarus (9 cases per 100 000). However, there are several questions to be answered regarding the contingency of reporting lung cancer cases in the latter countries [4, 5].

Underreporting of lung cancer has been a matter of concern for several countries worldwide, and has resulted in significantly low incidence rates or new cases rates being reported. This contributes to the ongoing discussion about the lack of uniformly accredited and standardised national lung cancer registries and processes that would entail the prompt and accurate reporting of lung cancer cases, and at the same time provide accurate and easily usable information about the actual burden and implication of the disease, which could potentially identify areas meriting future targeted interventions for improvement. The ERS Thoracic Oncology Assembly and the Lung Cancer Working Group have acknowledged the importance of this issue and there is work in progress addressing this.

This concerning issue is not limited to lung cancer in Europe, but extends to all types of cancer worldwide. Therefore, IARC/WHO have created the Global Initiative for Cancer Registry Development (http://gicr.iarc.fr), which is an international partnership that combines technical support, training and advocacy to facilitate the development of cancer registry systems worldwide to inform national cancer control.

Table 1. Europe in the spotlight. Highest and lowest estimated age standardised rates (European standard) for lung cancer incidence and mortality in Europe, by sex

| | **Incidence (cases per 100 000 population)** | | **Mortality (cases per 100 000 population)** | |
|---|---|---|---|---|
| | **Highest** | **Lowest** | **Highest** | **Lowest** |
| **Males** | Hungary (109)<br>Former Yugoslav Republic of Macedonia (102) | Finland (45)<br>Sweden (29) | Hungary (96.4)<br>Former Yugoslav Republic of Macedonia (91.6) | Cyprus (36.8)<br>Sweden (26.4) |
| **Females** | Denmark (54.9)<br>Hungary (46.5) | Russian Federation (10)<br>Ukraine and Belarus (9) | Denmark (42.3)<br>Hungary (37.7) | Ukraine (6.6)<br>Belarus (5.4) |

Data from [3].

## Histology

The incidence of SCLC is often quoted as ~20% of all lung cancers and its incidence is reportedly decreasing over time [4].

The National Cancer Intelligence Network analysed the incidence trends of SCLC and compared them with the overall trends in all lung cancer in both sexes in south-east England during the period 1970–2007. Incidence rates of SCLC and all lung cancer were higher in males than in females, and in particular the proportion of SCLC in males increased from 9% in 1972 to 10% in 2007. In contrast, the percentage of females with SCLC decreased from 13% in 1972 to 11% in 2007. When the analysis was limited to lung cancer with specified histology only, it was reported that the proportion of SCLC decreased in both sexes (males: 21% in 1972 to 15% in 2007, females: 32% in 1972 to 17% in 2007). SCLC incidence decreased over time in males and remained relatively stable in females. The slightly more rapid decrease in SCLC incidence rates compared with all lung cancer probably reflects the reduction in smoking rate over the study period as well as the change in the types of cigarettes smoked [6].

In NSCLC, ADC is more frequent in females than males regardless of smoking status and ADC rates have been increasing in both sexes in many developed countries [7]. Specifically in females, ADC has been rising steadily in most countries, irrespective of trends in the other subtypes of lung cancer. In males, SCC has been the most frequent subtype of NSCLC with incidence rates decreasing over the years. Large cell carcinoma is the least frequent subtype in both males and females [8].

The shifting trend from SCC to ADC can be linked with the changes in cigarette manufacturing, composition and design. There has been a rise in filtered, lower nicotine- and tar-containing cigarettes, which has presumably led to smokers inhaling deeper to meet their nicotine needs resulting in a more peripheral distribution of tobacco smoke in the lung. This promotes a shift from central tumours (SCC and small cell carcinomas) to peripheral tumours (ADCs). In addition, the decrease in SCCs can also be attributed to the reduction in polycyclic aromatic hydrocarbons and increase in tobacco-specific *N*-nitrosamines as the former induce SCC and the latter induce ADCs [8].

## Common risk factors for lung cancer

European incidence rates of lung cancer seem to be linked to European patterns of incidence of smoking. In the GLOBOCAN 2012 data [3], Hungary has the biggest incidence of lung cancer in Europe and 2010 data show that 26.5% of the adult population aged >15 years old smokes daily. This is one of the highest smoking rates in Europe, which has been maintained for years, and it could explain the increased incidence of lung cancer in the country. By contrast, Sweden has one of the lowest incidences of lung cancer in males in Europe and in a similar vein only 14% of the adult population >15 years old smokes daily. This is the lowest smoking rate in Europe and can be used to justify the comparatively lower incidence of the disease in the country [3, 9].

Variations in incidence are also present within the same country. The historical UK example is the higher lung cancer incidence in Scotland and northern England, which are among the highest in the world, reflecting the higher smoking rates in these areas [1].

However, recent data from the Welsh Cancer Intelligence and Surveillance Unit show that lung cancer incidence in Welsh females has increased by more than a third in the past decade (from 825 in 2003 to 1121 in 2012) making it one of the highest in Europe, although it is still lower than that of Scotland [10]. This has been attributed to the increase in female smokers in the 1970s, 1980s and early 1990s, with numbers peaking in the 1980s. In contrast, the figures for males have remained consistent over the past 10 years with 1294 cases in 2003 and 1249 in 2012 [10]. On a national level, in 1975, for every 10 lung cancer cases diagnosed in females in the UK there were 39 cases in males, whereas today for every 10 cases in females there are 12 cases in males [1].

Overall, around the world trends in lung cancer incidence in different countries reflect the maturity of the smoking epidemic.

It is interesting how lung cancer incidence rates in males increased significantly in the late 1970s and since then have decreased by ~48%. This corresponds with the increased smoking habits of males during the Second World War and subsequent decline after the war ended. However, females behaved differently during that time. Consequently from the mid-1970s to the late 1980s, lung cancer rates in females increased by ~45% as there was an increase in smoking habit among females between the Second World War and the 1970s, while since then the increase in lung cancer rate has been merely 19% [1, 3].

Interestingly, the proportion of lung cancer cases in female never-smokers is particularly high in East and South Asia (61% and 83%, respectively), reflecting that this cancer is a separate entity that is currently under investigation [11].

Air pollution (both indoor and outdoor) is equally considered to be a risk factor for lung cancer [4]. The ESCAPE (European Study of Cohorts for Air Pollution Effects) study used data from 17 cohort studies based in nine European countries and showed that particulate matter air pollution contributes to lung cancer incidence in Europe [12].

Overall, the risk depends on the level of air pollution people are regularly exposed to, but due to variability of air pollution levels it is hard to specify how the risk is affected for the people living in a certain area. The general consensus is that the risk for lung cancer increases with the extent of exposure to air pollution [1]. Therefore, it will be interesting to assess how the incidence of lung cancer in various countries is affected in the long term when the national thresholds for pollution are exceeded. For example, Finland has a very low incidence of lung cancer in males and low smoking rates, but was one of the very few countries to exceed the national emission ceiling for percentage $SO_2$ in 2011 [1], hence it would be interesting to assess the long-term impact of this on the future incidence of lung cancer in the country.

Indoor pollution also plays significant role and affects the incidence of lung cancer in various countries [4]. About half of the world's population (~3 billion people) have little or no access to modern forms of energy and use biomass fuels for cooking, heating and lighting, which are usually burned indoors in fireplaces or unmodernised stoves [4]. LISSOWSKA *et al.* [13] studied 2861 cases with exposure to indoor pollution and 3118 controls recruited during 1998–2002 in the Czech Republic, Hungary, Poland, Romania, Russia, Slovakia and the UK, and noticed a modest increased risk of lung cancer related to solid-fuel use for cooking rather than heating. It would be interesting to know how this has affected the incidence of lung cancer in each one of the European countries.

Radon is another acknowledged risk factor for lung cancer. Darby *et al.* [14] published an interesting collaborative analysis of individual data from 13 case–control studies of residential radon and lung cancer from nine European countries and concluded that hazards from residential radon are appreciable, particularly for smokers and recent ex-smokers, while radon is responsible for ~2% of all deaths from cancer in Europe. However, this study did not include information about how much radon *per se* affects the incidence of lung cancer in any of the countries included in the study. Cancer Research UK scientists have found that exposure to radon accounts for only 3% of all UK cases of lung cancer, however, there are no specific data as to how radon affects incidence of lung cancer in the UK [1].

Like radon, asbestos is another known risk factor for lung cancer [4]. However, it is really difficult to tell asbestos-related cancers apart from those due to other causes such as smoking. Therefore, there are no precise data reporting the overall scale of asbestos-related lung cancer incidence and the number of asbestos-related deaths has to be estimated rather than counted. Current estimates indicate in excess of 2000 deaths each year in Great Britain are due to asbestos-related lung cancer [15].

The asbestos-related cancer burden today is predominantly found in Europe, North America, Australia, Japan, South Africa and parts of South America. However, China, Russia, India, Kazakhstan, Ukraine, Thailand, Brazil and Iran have the highest current consumption of and exposure to asbestos, and thus the future burden is expected to grow significantly in these areas. For countries with the highest percentage of deaths from mesothelioma in males, estimates of the lung cancer population attributable fraction due to asbestos were between 3% and 8% for 2001–2005 [16]. In almost all of these countries, lung cancer made up 20–30% of cancer deaths, thus even 3–8% of this is a considerable contribution to the most common cause of cancer mortality in males in these settings [16].

## Mortality

Lung cancer is estimated to be responsible for nearly 1.59 million deaths worldwide, which accounts for 19.4% of all cancers in total [1, 2]. The US mortality is 48.4 per 100 000 males and females per year [17] and the European Union (EU) average mortality is 35.2 deaths per 100 000 person-years as reported by the European Network of Cancer Registries [18].

The European countries with the highest and lowest estimated mortality rates for 2012, using the GLOBOCAN 2012 data [3], are shown in table 1. Hungary has the highest mortality rates for males and Denmark has the highest mortality rates for females.

It will be interesting to see how the epidemiological map of lung cancer mortality in the EU will evolve in the next few years following the two EU enlargements, in 2004 and 2007, and the movement of populations. The EU countries that have joined the EU during these recent enlargements had a higher average mortality and tobacco consumption for both females and males than the pre-existing EU member states [1, 3].

Bray *et al.* [19] published a comprehensive analysis of the different phases of the lung cancer epidemic in different European countries and the disparities involved between the sexes. Between 1970 and 2007, lung cancer mortality rates among females reached a plateau or had even begun to decline in a number of Eastern European countries and in Northern Europe, particularly in countries that had been in the epidemiological spotlight like

Hungary and Denmark. This is reflected in successive declines in risk among females born predominantly after 1950 in these regions.

These observations reflect the smoking habits of generations of males and females born from the late 19th century onwards, but also point to the relative successes or failures of smoking prevention and cessation efforts over the continent in the past few decades [2, 3, 18–20].

In the UK, lung cancer mortality rates for males have more than halved since the 1970s, while for females the mortality rate increased by 60% between the early 1970s and the late 1980s and since then rates have increased more slowly [1]. In the UK, the age specific mortality rates per 100 000 population for 2010–2012 were 62.6 for males and 48.8 for females (all ages) [1].

Lung cancer screening is thought to play a promising role in reducing lung cancer mortality and the results of the NLST (National Lung Screening Trial) trial supported this [20], while the results of a large Dutch study of lung cancer screening, the NELSON trial, are anticipated.

The NLST has set the foundation for plans to implement screening in various countries. Heavy smokers (>30 pack-years) aged 55–74 years old were recruited and randomly assigned to undergo three annual screenings with either low-dose chest CT scan or posteroanterior chest radiography. There were 247 deaths from lung cancer per 100 000 person-years in the low-dose CT group and 309 deaths per 100 000 person-years in the radiography group, which represented an overall reduction of 20% in the mortality from lung cancer [20]. It is of note that a total of 96.4% of the positive screening results in the low-dose CT group and 94.5% in the radiography group were false positive results, which instigated a cascade of investigations.

The potential implementation of lung cancer screening programmes in Europe is expected to further change the epidemiological pattern of mortality and it would be an interesting area to assess in the long term. However, the false positive results and the cost effectiveness of investigations that are derived from incidental findings need to be thoroughly thought through.

## Survival

Worldwide data for lung cancer confirm that it still remains lethal in the majority of geographical areas, although there are some countries reporting more encouraging survival rates.

The CONCORD II study collected information from 279 tumour registries in 67 countries and reported a typically low age-standardised 5-year net survival from lung cancer (10–20%) for the majority of geographical areas in the developed and developing world [21]. However, Japan and Israel presented more encouraging 5-year survival rates (30% and 24%, respectively) for patients diagnosed during 2005–2009, while Mauritius presented a promising 37% survival rate (this was, however, based on only 84 cases diagnosed in 2005–2007). It should be noted that almost half of ADCs in Asian people have an EGFR mutation and, therefore, more patients are eligible for TKIs, which give a favourable prognosis [22].

Bulgaria, Lithuania, Mongolia and Thailand presented survival rates <10% and Libya 2%. Between 2005 and 2009, Israel and Japan reported 5-year survival rates of 24% and 30%, respectively, a 7% rise in comparison with the earlier period 1995–1999. During the same time period, China reported a rise from 8% to 18% and South Korea from 10% to 19%. Smaller rises (2–4%) were noted in Colombia, North America and Europe. Decreases in lung cancer survival were noted in Turkey (from 19% to 10%), but this could be attributed to improvements in data quality and collection. Smaller decreases (2–4%) were seen in Cyprus, Croatia, Malaysia and Lithuania [21].

The EUROCARE-4 study is another excellent example of a large collaboration that reported survival data for patients diagnosed with cancer in 2000–2002, collected from 47 European cancer registries. The European mean age-adjusted 5-year survival calculated using the period method for 2000–2002 was low for lung cancer (10.9%, 95% CI 10.5–11.4%) [23].

It is of note that the Argentinian registries reported a decrease in 5-year survival from 20.8% (cases diagnosed during 2000–2004) to 11.9% (cases diagnosed during 2005–2009), which coincides with the national debt crisis, whereas Iceland presented a stable rate of 15% from 1995 until 2009 despite a similar financial situation.

Table 2 presents an overview of the highest and lowest 5-year survival rates within the EU for cases diagnosed during 2005–2009. The UK, quite surprisingly, presents one of the lowest 5-year survival rates in Europe. It is one of the few European countries that has a robust system in place to tackle waiting times for patients that are referred to lung cancer services for investigations and treatment, and also uses a multidisciplinary approach in the decision making process for diagnosis, treatment and follow-up of these patients. However, the drawbacks seem to be due to a number of reasons such as delayed diagnosis as only one in seven people seem to present with early stage disease [24], underuse of successful treatments and unequal access to treatment, particularly among elderly people. However, one should also take into account patient factors such as the level of smoking, alcohol misuse and poor diet in the UK.

Late diagnosis seems to be the overwhelming factor as the vast majority of lung cancer patients (67.6%) are already in stages III and IV of the disease at the time of diagnosis, with only 14.5% and 7.3% in stages I and II, respectively [1]. The 1-year survival rates are significantly lower as the lung cancer stage progresses as the two are strongly related. People presenting at stage I have the highest 1-year survival (71%) while those diagnosed with stage IV disease have the lowest (14%) [1].

## Perspectives and future needs

The era of personalised medicine and targeted therapies, refined radiotherapy techniques and novel staging tools is anticipated to improve lung cancer survival and outcomes.

Table 2. European Union countries at a glance: the highest and lowest 5-year survival rates for lung cancer cases diagnosed during 2005–2009

| Highest | Lowest |
|---|---|
| Austria (17.9%) | Bulgaria (6.7%) |
| Belgium (16.6%) | Lithuania (7.7%) |
| Sweden (15.6%) | UK (9.6%) |

Data from [3].

However, equal access of all patients to these novel diagnostic and therapeutic modalities as well as to equal quality of care still remains an issue in many countries, especially on the grounds of financial austerity that has arisen mainly in Southern Europe. All lung cancer patients should ideally have same access to modern diagnostic tools (*e.g.* PET-CT and EBUS) and advanced therapies (stereotactic radiotherapy, targeted chemotherapy *etc.*). It will be interesting to assess the impact of this difficult economic era on the quality of lung cancer care, epidemiological trends and overall public health. In this background, the ERS Thoracic Oncology Assembly addressed the quality of care that lung cancer patients receive throughout Europe by proposing "The European Initiative for Quality Management in Lung Cancer Care (EIQMLCC)" in 2009. The initiative aimed to evaluate the provision of lung cancer care across Europe, to survey the resources available, and to establish a platform of lung cancer physicians with which to promote region-specific improvements in lung cancer care and improve the quality of care [25].

Asbestos is a known risk factor for lung cancer and the EU has taken a firm position and banned the extraction of asbestos as well as the manufacture and processing of asbestos products (Directive 2003/18/EC), this was followed by a ban of all types of utilisation of asbestos from January 1, 2005 (Directive 1999/77/EC). The impact of these significant measures on national/local/professional epidemics would be an interesting area to assess, with the aim to prove that the circle of deaths caused by this epidemic has closed (table 3).

Lung cancer screening is another new promising area of research that is anticipated to change the field of lung cancer epidemiology by improving lung cancer stage at diagnosis, outcomes and survival. The first promising data came in 2011 from the NLST in the USA [20], which demonstrated that screening with low-dose CT reduces mortality from lung cancer by 20%. The ongoing lung cancer screening trials in the Netherlands (NELSON trial) [26] and the UK (UK Lung Cancer Screening Trial) [27] will assess the reproducibility of the US results in Europe as well as the cost efficiency. With the possible implementation of lung cancer screening, it would be interesting to study its long-term effects on lung cancer epidemiology in Europe and worldwide. Screening detected abnormalities are statistically significantly associated with smoking cessation [28]. Therefore, integration of smoking cessation programmes within screening programmes would be expected to lead to further reductions in smoking-related morbidity and mortality, and this is an area that would merit further study.

Table 3. Suggested areas for epidemiological development/research in lung cancer

1) Impact of austerity measures on lung cancer epidemiology, quality of care and access to healthcare services
2) Differences in access in molecular analysis and targeted therapies throughout Europe
3) EU implementation of the WHO Tobacco Free Initiative and its impact on smoking habits and incidence of lung cancer in EU member states
4) Asbestos ban within the EU and the completion of the circle for related local/professional epidemics
5) Implementation of lung cancer screening and lung cancer epidemiology
6) Integration of smoking cessation services into screening programmes
7) Epidemiological databases of lung cancer and national registries
8) Mapping of lung cancer healthcare in Europe and its relation to lung cancer outcomes
9) Lung cancer in nonsmokers
10) Early detection of lung cancer

Early detection of lung cancer is another area that needs further investigation and appears very attractive on a clinical and public health level. The National Health Service in Scotland is currently funding a multicentre study (EarlyCDT Lung Cancer Scotland) that aims to use a simple blood test (earlyCDT) to aid in the risk assessment and early detection of lung cancer. Recruitment closes on June 30, 2015 and the results will be anticipated a few years later [29].

Uniform epidemiological databases across Europe and reporting of the disease are a vital component of all epidemiological studies in lung cancer. They would allow a prompt recognition of all trends and provide space for public health interventions where required. Mapping the status of lung cancer healthcare in Europe and providing evidence of how that affects lung cancer epidemiology (incidence, mortality, survival, *etc.*) would be of great interest, as it would provide new insights into the epidemiological profile of the disease. It would also highlight areas for change that could potentially improve the long-term burden of the disease.

Currently, 17 EU countries have implemented smoke-free laws and among these the UK, Ireland, Spain, Greece, Malta, Hungary and Bulgaria have the strictest smoke free provisions as smoking is completely banned in enclosed public places, on public transport and in workplaces, with only limited exceptions allowed [30]. Recent data indicate that the actual smoke exposure rates for EU citizens dropped from 2009 to 2012, for example for citizens visiting bars and pubs the smoke exposure rate dropped from 46% to 28% [30]. However this is not representative for the whole EU as enforcement of the law seems to be challenging in some member states.

On these grounds it will be interesting to assess the long-term impact of the WHO Tobacco Free Initiative (www.who.int/tobacco/en) and its EU implementation on the incidence of lung cancer in EU member states. Although one would expect smoking habits and consequently lung cancer incidence rates to decrease in the long term, there seems to be an important confounding factor. The EU legislation was implemented at the dawn of the European financial crisis and austerity measures, which have affected social behaviours and hence smoking habits. It was only a year after the implementation of the Tobacco Free Initiative when Southern EU countries (Greece, Spain and Portugal) adopted strict austerity measures, which increased the pressure on their health systems, and together with budget cuts resulted in decreased funding and limited access to healthcare services. In addition, increased financial austerity is thought to impact on mental health and the latter is linked with the onset of smoking [31, 32].

It would be interesting to study how all these public health features will impact on the epidemiology of lung cancer in EU over the next decades. The picture will become clearer in the next few years when there will be a straightforward answer as to where smoking habit has indeed increased or decreased, and how much austerity has affected implementation of EU law around smoking bans. Further studies could also be directed towards the rising rates of lung cancer in nonsmokers and may identify new pathways for relevant translational research.

## Conclusion

Lung cancer epidemiology presents a number of challenging perspectives for the future as it will need to assess and investigate big conflicting changes and their impact on lung cancer incidence, mortality and survival. First, there are the changing trends of the disease and the predominantly late stage at presentation. Secondly, there is the new era of socioeconomic changes and austerity measures in Europe and the potential impact of health cuts and accessibility to healthcare services. Finally, there are the technological advances in the diagnosis and treatment of lung cancer as well as the potential implementation of lung cancer screening. The epidemiological map of lung cancer in Europe is anticipated to present interesting changes in the future.

## References

1. Cancer Research UK. Lung cancer incidence statistics. www.cancerresearchuk.org/cancer-info/cancerstats/types/lung/incidence/uk-lung-cancer-incidence-statistics Date last accessed: January 3, 2015. Date last updated: May 29, 2014.
2. American Cancer Society. Cancer Facts & Figures 2014. Atlanta, American Cancer Society, 2014.
3. International Agency for Research on Cancer. GLOBOCAN 2012: Estimated Incidence, Mortality and Prevalence Worldwide in 2012. http://globocan.iarc.fr/Pages/fact_sheets_cancer.aspx Date last accessed: December 31, 2014.
4. Lung Cancer. *In*: Gibson J, Loddenkemper R, Sibille Y, *et al.*, eds. The European Lung White Book. Sheffield, European Respiratory Society, 2013.
5. Ferlay J, Steliarova-Foucher E, Lortet-Tieulent J, *et al.* Cancer incidence and mortality patterns in Europe: estimates for 40 countries in 2012. *Eur J Cancer* 2013; 49: 1374–1403.
6. Riaz SP, Lüchtenborg M, Coupland VH, *et al.* Trends in incidence of small cell lung cancer and all lung cancer. *Lung Cancer* 2012; 75: 280–284.
7. Devesa SS, Bray F, Vizcaino AP, *et al.* International lung cancer trends by histologic type: male:female differences diminishing and adenocarcinoma rates rising. *Int J Cancer* 2005; 117: 294–299.
8. Lortet-Tieulent J, Soerjomatarama I, Ferlay J, *et al.* International trends in lung cancer incidence by histological subtype: adenocarcinoma stabilizing in males but still increasing in women. *Lung Cancer* 2014; 84: 13–22.
9. OECD Health Data 2012, Eurostat Statistics Database, WHO Global Infobase. 2.5.1 Adult population smoking daily, 2010 and change in smoking rates, 2000-2010 (or nearest year). *In:* Health at a Glance: Europe 2012. OECD, 2012. www.oecd-ilibrary.org/sites/9789264183896-en/02/05/g2-05-01.html?itemId=/content/chapter/9789264183896-24-en&_csp_=bc3da9a79108c2160f7cb21300faa0fe Date last accessed: March 1, 2015.
10. Welsh Cancer Intelligence and Surveillance Unit Health Intelligence Division, Public Health Wales. Lung Cancer in Wales, a detailed analysis of population trends of incidence and stage of diagnosis up to and including 2012. Cardiff, Welsh Cancer Intelligence and Surveillance Unit, 2014.
11. Sun S, Schiller JH, Gazdar AF. Lung cancer in never smokers – a different disease. *Nat Rev Cancer* 2007; 7: 778–790.
12. Raaschou-Nielsen O, Andersen ZJ, Beelen R, *et al.* Air pollution and lung cancer incidence in 17 European cohorts: prospective analyses from the European Study of Cohorts for Air Pollution Effects (ESCAPE). *Lancet Oncol* 2013; 14: 813–822.
13. Lissowska J, Bardin-Mikolajczak A, Fletcher T, *et al.* Lung cancer and indoor pollution from heating and cooking with solid fuels: the IARC international multicentre case-control study in Eastern/Central Europe and the United Kingdom. *Am J Epidemiol* 2005; 162: 326–333.
14. Darby S, Hill D, Auvinen A, *et al.* Radon in homes and risk of lung cancer: collaborative analysis of individual data from 13 European case-control studies. *BMJ* 2005; 330: 223.
15. Health and Safety Executive. Asbestos related lung cancer. www.hse.gov.uk/Statistics/causdis/lungcancer/index.htm Date last accessed: February 28, 2015.
16. McCormack V, Peto J, Byrnes G. Estimating the asbestos-related lung cancer burden from mesothelioma mortality. *Br J Cancer* 2012; 106: 575–584.
17. National Cancer Institute. SEER Stat Fact Sheets: Lung and Bronchus Cancer. http://seer.cancer.gov/statfacts/html/lungb.html Date last accessed: December 30, 2014.
18. European Network of Cancer Registries. Lung Including Trachea and Bronchus (LUNGC) Cancer Factsheet. www.encr.eu/images/docs/factsheets/ENCR_Factsheet_Lung_2014.pdf Date last accessed: December 29, 2014. Date last updated: June, 2014.
19. Bray FI, Weiderpass E. Lung cancer mortality trends in 36 European countries: secular trends and birth cohort patterns by sex and region 1970–2007. *Int J Cancer* 2010; 126: 1454–1466.
20. National Lung Screening Trial Research Team, Aberle DR, Adams AM, *et al.* Reduced lung-cancer mortality with low-dose computed tomographic screening. *N Engl J Med* 2011; 365: 395–409.
21. Allemani C, Weir HK, Carreira H, *et al.* Global surveillance of cancer survival 1995–2009: analysis of individual data for 25,676,887 patients from 279 population-based registries in 67 countries (CONCORD-2). *Lancet* 2015; 385: 977–1010.

22. Shi Y, Au JS, Thongprasert S, *et al.* A prospective, molecular epidemiology study of EGFR mutations in Asian patients with advanced non-small-cell lung cancer of adenocarcinoma histology (PIONEER). *J Thorac Oncol* 2014; 9: 154–162.
23. Verdecchia A, Francisci S, Brenner H. Recent cancer survival in Europe: a 2000–02 period analysis of EUROCARE-4 data. *Lancet Oncol* 2007; 8: 784–796.
24. Walters S, Maringe C, Coleman MP, *et al.* Lung cancer survival and stage at diagnosis in Australia, Canada, Denmark, Norway, Sweden and the UK: a population-based study, 2004–2007. *Thorax* 2013; 68: 551–564.
25. Blum TG, Rich A, Baldwin D, *et al.* The European initiative for quality management in lung cancer care. *Eur Respir J* 2014; 43: 1254–1277.
26. Ru Zhao Y, Xie X, de Koning HJ, *et al.* NELSON lung cancer screening study. *Cancer Imaging* 2011; 11: S79–S84.
27. UK Lung Cancer Screening Trial (UKLS). www.ukls.org/index.html Date last accessed: December 15, 2014.
28. Tammemägi MC, Berg CD, Riley TL, *et al.* Impact of lung cancer screening results on smoking cessation. *J Natl Cancer Inst* 2014; 106: dju084.
29. UK Clinical Research Network Study Portfolio. ECLS: EarlyCDT Lung Cancer Scotland (ECLS) Study. http://public.ukcrn.org.uk/search/StudyDetail.aspx?StudyID=14532 Date last accessed: March 20, 2015.
30. European Commission Public Health. Smoke-free environments. http://ec.europa.eu/health/tobacco/smoke-free_environments/index_en.htm Date last accessed: December 15, 2014. Date last updated: April 8, 2015.
31. Karanikolos M, Mladovsky P, Cylus J, *et al.* Financial crisis, austerity, and health in Europe. *Lancet* 2013; 381: 1323–1331.
32. Hockenberry JM, Timmons EJ, Vander Weg MW. Adolescent mental health as a risk factor for adolescent smoking onset. *Adolesc Health Med Ther* 2011; 2: 27–35.

Disclosures: None declared

Chapter 2

# Screening

John K. Field[1], Anand Devaraj[2], Stephen W. Duffy[3] and David R. Baldwin[4]

Lung cancer CT screening has the potential to save many lives if implemented in Europe. The National Lung Screening Trial (NLST) found a 20% reduction in lung cancer mortality following three annual CT screenings, with a cost per quality-adjusted life year of US$81 000 in the USA. The European trials have provided evidence for: 1) the use of a risk prediction model to select high-risk individuals; 2) the use of volumetric analysis and volume doubling time to determine the care pathway for CT-detected nodules; 3) the potential for undertaking biennial screening after 2 years of scans with no evidence of disease; 4) the importance of integrated smoking cessation, which uses the CT screen as a way to augment quit rates. The NELSON (Dutch–Belgian Randomised Lung Cancer Screening Trial) and the pooled European trial data will be available in 2016, so it is imperative we start planning for the implementation of lung cancer screening now.

There were 310 000 new cases of lung cancer and 268 000 lung cancer deaths in the European Union (EU) in 2012; this represents more than one in five of all cancer deaths (www.globocan.iarc.fr). The primary control for lung cancer is through the reduction of tobacco smoking, which is responsible for ~90% of lung cancer cases in men and 80% in women [1]. The lifetime risk of lung cancer among former smokers remains high [2] and in populations where the large majority of smokers have quit smoking, ~40% of lung cancer cases now occur among ex-and never-smokers [3]. However, smoking rates remain significant in many European countries. The EU conducts regular surveys that include the prevalence of smoking in EU countries. For each survey, called the "Eurobarometer", ~1000 people in each country are interviewed. The survey reported that in 2012, 28% of European adults were current smokers, 21% were ex-smokers and 51% had never smoked; these rates were similar to those in 2009, although smoking rates in some countries had declined since 2006 [4].

These statistics highlight the need for early detection of lung cancer that complements public health efforts to curb tobacco smoking.

## US National Lung Screening Trial

The results of the US National Lung Screening Trial (NLST) were published in 2011 and are considered a landmark event in lung cancer research. This randomised trial of >55 000

[1]Roy Castle Lung Cancer Research Programme, The University of Liverpool Cancer Research Centre, Liverpool, UK. [2]Dept of Radiology, Royal Brompton Hospital, London, UK. [3]Wolfson Institute of Preventive Medicine, Barts and The London School of Medicine and Dentistry, Queen Mary University of London, London, UK. [4]Respiratory Medicine Unit, David Evans Research Centre, Nottingham University Hospitals, Nottingham, UK.

Correspondence: John K. Field, Roy Castle Lung Cancer Research Programme, The University of Liverpool Cancer Research Centre, Roy Castle Building, 200 London Road, Liverpool, L3 9TA, UK. E-mail: J.K.Field@liv.ac.uk

 Print ISBN: 978-1-84984-061-3. Online ISBN: 978-1-84984-062-0. Print ISSN: 2312-508X. Online ISSN: 2312-5098.

current and former smokers of 55–75 years of age was stopped 1 year earlier than planned when the stop criteria of a 20% decrease in lung cancer mortality was achieved in the CT arm, compared to the chest X-ray [5]. An International workshop reported shortly after this on the further need for research into CT screening and implementation [6]. The recommendations from this workshop represent the only truly international view on screening, involving >75 international experts. Their recommendations were: 1) optimisation of the identification of high-risk individuals; 2) development of radiological guidelines; 3) development of guidelines for the clinical work-up of indeterminate nodules; 4) development of guidelines for pathology reporting; 5) definition of the criteria for surgical and therapeutic interventions of suspicious nodules identified through lung cancer CT screening programmes; and 6) development of recommendations for the integration of smoking cessation practices into future national lung cancer CT screening programmes. Resolution of these issues is important to ensure that future national lung cancer screening programmes target a population at a high enough risk of developing lung cancer, while minimising the potential for harm, in a cost-effective manner [7].

However, five clinical and professional groups in the USA over the past 4 years have also provided in-depth recommendations, which are naturally focussed on USA clinical practice [7]. They all supported the implementation of CT screening with varying details on the definition of risk groups and methodology. More recently, following a commissioned independent analysis of the evidence, the US Preventive Services Task Force (USPSTF) recommended that lung cancer screening should be offered to individuals of comparable risk to NLST, but with extension of the upper age limit to 80 years [8]. The USPSTF recommended that screening should be discontinued once a person has not smoked for 15 years, develops a health problem that substantially limits life expectancy or is willing to have curative lung surgery. Recently, Medicare, has agreed to cover the costs of screening; it is of note that it has specified a number of stringent requirements (table 1) [9].

The NLST is the only fully powered randomised controlled trial (RCT) to date that provides evidence of a mortality advantage in CT-screened individuals and has to be considered a landmark trial in lung cancer screening [4]. However, one still has to be cognisant of the fact that if lung cancer screening is not implemented in centres of excellence, it is unlikely that we will still see the same mortality advantage and the possibility of a higher morbidity associated with CT screening programmes. Furthermore, we still need the evidence to continue screening annually until 80 years of age, which will have a cumulative radiation exposure, with possible adverse events. There is a control intervention in the NLST: chest X-ray. This may mean that the effect of low-dose CT screening would be larger than observed in NLST in comparison with usual care in most settings.

## Cost-effectiveness

The situation in Europe is complex, as it has been uniformly agreed to await the outcome of the NELSON (Dutch–Belgian Randomised Lung Cancer Screening Trial) and the pooling of the EU smaller trials in approximately 2016, which will provide European mortality and cost-effectiveness data [7]. Clearly the major stumbling block at present is the cost-effectiveness of lung cancer screening, as there is no published estimate from a randomised trial in a European healthcare setting. The cost per quality-adjusted life year (QALY) in the NLST has recently been shown to be US$81 000, an acceptable figure in the US at least [10]. However, the risk profile used by the NLST trial has been analysed by a

Table 1. Centers for Medicare and Medicaid Services (CMS) decision to cover lung cancer screening costs

| CMS beneficiary eligibility criteria |
|---|
| Age 55–77 years |
| Asymptomatic (no signs or symptoms of lung cancer) |
| Tobacco smoking history of ⩾30 pack-years (1 pack-year = smoking one pack per day for 1 year; 1 pack = 20 cigarettes) |
| Current smoker or one who has quit smoking within the last 15 years |
| Receives a written order for low-dose CT lung cancer screening that meets the following criteria: |
| A lung cancer screening counselling and shared decision-making visit includes the following elements: |
| Determination of the beneficiary's eligibility, including age, absence of signs or symptoms of lung cancer, a specific calculation of cigarette-smoking pack-years, and if a former smoker, the number of years since quitting |
| Counselling on the importance of the adherence to annual lung cancer low-dose CT screening, the impact of comorbidities and the ability or willingness to undergo diagnosis and treatment |
| Counselling on the importance of maintaining cigarette-smoking abstinence if a former smoker, or the importance of smoking cessation if a current smoker and, if appropriate, furnishing of information about tobacco-cessation interventions |

Reproduced and modified from [9].

number of groups, especially when applying the PLCO (prostate, lung, colorectal and ovarian) risk model, which was found to be more sensitive than the NLST criteria for lung cancer detection [11]. Indeed the 5-year lung cancer death model developed by KOVALCHIK *et al.* [12] demonstrated that there were extremes in the range of lung cancer risk for the five quintiles, and showed that screening with low-dose CT prevented the greatest number of deaths from lung cancer among participants who were at highest risk, and prevented very few deaths among those at lowest risk. Thus, it is evident from the NLST's cost-effectiveness calculations that their cost per QALY incremental cost-effectiveness ratio (ICER) would have been at least halved had screening been confined only to those in the two highest-risk quintiles (combining the 4th and 5th quintiles; US$42 000 per QALY) [10].

However, the USA has a very different healthcare system to that of Europe. Recent estimates from the USA indicate that the annual costs of a comprehensive screening programme would be in excess of US$1 billion [13]. Modelling cost-effectiveness in the UK, prior to the UK Lung Cancer Screening (UKLS) trial, provided an estimate of ~£14 000 per QALY gained, which is within the current National Institute for Health and Care Excellence (NICE) threshold for recommending funding of new health interventions [14].

## European CT screening trials

There are currently eight ongoing European randomised trials comparing lung cancer CT screening with no screening: the Multicentric Italian Lung Detection (MILD) trial [15]; the Detection and Screening of Early Lung Cancer by Novel Imaging Technology and Molecular Essays (DANTE) trial [16]; the Depiscan study (a French randomised pilot trial of lung cancer screening comparing low-dose CT scan and chest X-ray) [17]; ITALUNG [18];

the NELSON trial [19]; the Danish Lung Cancer Screening Trial (DLCST) [20]; the German LUng cancer Screening Intervention (LUSI) study [21]; and the UKLS trial [22]. To date, three of these studies have published results showing no mortality benefit of lung cancer CT screening (table 2); however, none of them were powered to observe a significant mortality benefit [20, 23, 24]. The NELSON trial [19] is the largest of all the European trials and we await the results, which are anticipated to be published in 2016. Following this, an analysis of the pooled data from European RCTs will be performed to look at both mortality and cost-effectiveness from the more mature data [25]. This will mean further questions can be addressed regarding screening frequency and the evaluation of abnormal screens.

## Selection of high-risk populations for screening programmes

Future implementation of lung cancer screening requires accurate identification of the population that will benefit the most from future screening programmes; this is essential in order to ensure that the benefits of screening outweigh the harms. Current recommendations based on the NLST include screening all individuals between the ages of 55–80 years with a smoking history of ⩾30 pack-years (1 pack-year is 20 cigarettes per day for 1 year or 10 cigarettes per day for 2 years, *etc.*) [8]. However, in-depth analysis of the NLST showed that there were significant differences in the number of lung cancer cases detected based on underlying risk, even though all participants had satisfied the criteria for participation in the study and were considered at high risk. 60% of participants at highest risk for lung cancer death (quintiles 3–5) accounted for 88% of the prevented deaths, whereas the 20% of participants at lowest risk (quintile 1) accounted for only 1% of prevented lung cancer deaths [11]. This definition of high risk based on age and smoking history needs to be substantially improved if screening programmes are to maximise their positive impact on the early detection of lung cancer. The US study has shown that, even if screening reduces lung cancer mortality by 20%, the drawback is false-positive results. The data reported by Kovalchik *et al.* [12] clearly demonstrate this point (table 3). Kovalchik *et al.* [12] calculated the 5-year cause-of-death model and divided the NLST data into quintiles; screening 5276 individuals at the lowest risk prevented only one cancer death and produced the greatest

Table 2. Low-dose CT trials reporting effects on lung cancer mortality

| Trial [ref.] | Subjects/ controls n | Screening rounds | Average follow-up years | Intervention regimen | Control regimen | Lung cancer mortality RR (95% CI) |
|---|---|---|---|---|---|---|
| **DLCST [20]** | 2052/2052 | 5 | 4.8 | Annual CT | Usual care | 1.37 (0.62–2.99) |
| **DANTE [16]** | 1276/1196 | 5 | 3.0 | Annual CT | Baseline chest X-ray | 0.94 (0.50–1.79) |
| **NLST** | 26 722/ 26 732 | 3 | 6.2 | Annual CT | Annual chest X-ray | 0.80 (0.73–0.93) |
| **MILD [15]** | 2376/1723 | 5 or 3 biennial | 4.4 | Annual or biennial CT, plus smoking cessation advice and spirometry | Smoking cessation advice, spirometry | 1.50 (0.62–3.60) |

The combined lung cancer mortality is 0.81 (0.70–0.92). RR: risk ratio; DLCST: Danish Lung Cancer Screening Trial; DANTE: Detection and Screening of Early Lung Cancer by Novel Imaging Technology and Molecular Essays; NLST: National Lung Screening Trial; MILD: Multicentric Italian Lung Detection. Reproduced and modified from [7] with permission from the publisher.

Table 3. 5-year risk of lung cancer death applied to the National Lung Screening Trial (NLST) data

| Quintile | 5-year risk of death % | Deaths n (%) | False-positives per prevented death n | Number needed to screen |
|---|---|---|---|---|
| 1 | 0.15–0.55 | 1 (5) | 1648 | 5276 |
| 2 | 0.56–0.84 | 10 (28.6) | 181 | 531 |
| 3 | 0.85–1.23 | 13 (28.9) | 147 | 415 |
| 4 | 1.24–2.00 | 31 (42.5) | 64 | 171 |
| 5 | >2.00 | 33 (18.2) | 65 | 161 |

Reproduced and modified from [12] with permission from the publisher.

number of false-positives, whereas the highest quintile screened 161 individuals and identified 33 lung cancer deaths. These data argue for a reassessment of the lung cancer risk criteria.

The study by Tammemagi *et al.* [26] used the $PLCO_{M2012}$ risk model to evaluate the risk threshold for selecting individuals for screening and compared its efficiency with the USPSTF criteria. By analysing NLST data using the $PLCO_{M2012}$ model, the 65th percentile in PLCO smokers represents a risk of 0.0151. The mortality rates among NLST participants screened with CT were found to be consistently lower than the mortality rates in the chest X-ray arm; 255 people with a $PLCO_{M2012}$ risk of ⩾0.015 would need to be screened to prevent one lung cancer death. The study demonstrated that 8.8% fewer people had a $PLCO_{M2012}$ risk of ⩾0.051 than the USPSTF criteria for screening, but 12.4% more lung cancers were identified. The $PLCO_{M2012}$ risk model improved the sensitivity and specificity of the selection of individuals for lung cancer screening in comparison with the UPSTF criteria; however, a major limitation of the $PLCO_{M2012}$ risk ⩾0.015 threshold for the selection of individuals for screening is that the evaluation was not based on cost-effectiveness.

The only risk-prediction model that has so far been used in the recruitment of participants into a CT Lung Cancer Screening RCT, is the Liverpool Lung Project (LLP)v2 risk model in the pilot UKLS trial [22].

The LLP risk model was based on a case–control study [27]. The LLPv1 model utilised conditional logistic regression to develop a model based on factors that were significantly associated with lung cancer (smoking duration, prior diagnosis of pneumonia, occupational exposure to asbestos, prior diagnosis of malignant tumour and early onset (<60 years), and family history of lung cancer) [27]. The multivariable model was combined with age-standardised incident data to estimate the absolute risk of developing lung cancer. The discrimination of the LLP risk model was evaluated and its predicted benefit for stratifying patients for CT screening was demonstrated using data from three independent European and North American studies [28]. In this study, the LLP risk model performed better than smoking duration or family history alone in stratifying high-risk patients for lung cancer CT screening. The LLPv2 model included all respiratory diseases and all smokers (cigarette, pipe and cigar) and was used to select high-risk individuals from the UKLS [29]. UKLS randomised subjects were selected on the basis of their ⩾5% risk of developing lung cancer in the next 5 years. Using this selection criterion may show that a screening programme will be more cost-effective if it is limited to the high-risk individuals. Overall, there was a

1.7% prevalence of lung cancer at baseline, which is higher than that reported by the NLST [5] or NELSON [19, 30].

## CT-detected lung nodules: controversies around indeterminate nodules

The management of indeterminate pulmonary nodules has varied between US and European trials [7]. In Europe, the NELSON, the UKLS trial, the DLCST, LUSI and MILD have used nodule volume analysis software (volumetry) [31]. However, the current evidence of a mortality benefit for CT radiological decisions is based on nodule diameter measurements using manually placed electronic callipers in the NLST. The proportion of pathological stage I disease detected was 70.8% in the NELSON and 61.6% in the NLST. An important component of the work-up of nodules is growth in the interval between two scans. In the EU trials using volumetry, growth is uniformly defined as a change in volume of ⩾25% between the first and the second scan. The NLST defined growth as a 10% increase in diameter.

The nodule growth definition and care pathway used within in the UKLS trial is shown in figure 1 [22]; it has many similarities to the NELSON methodology. In the NELSON trial, nodules <50 $mm^3$ were classified as negative, nodules >500 $mm^3$ were classified as positive, and nodules 50–500 $mm^3$ were classified as indeterminate [19]. Indeterminate nodules underwent a 3-month follow-up low-density CT to assess growth. Volume-doubling times (VDTs) [32] were then used to distinguish between positive screens (VDT <400 days) requiring additional diagnostic procedures and negative screens.

The NLST defined screen positivity as the largest nodule diameter of 4 mm. 24% of first CT screens in the NLST were positive and received further diagnostic investigation [7]. The Early Lung Cancer Action Program (ELCAP) investigators analysed the effect of nodule size detection thresholds on positive test results and showed that in their study, a threshold increase from 5 mm to 9 mm diameter would decrease test positives from 16% to 10% whilst delaying diagnosis ⩽9 months in 6.7% of cancer cases [33]. However, these data should be interpreted with care, as it may not be possible to generalise this conclusion between risk populations [34].

Published data from the NLST, the ELCAP and the NELSON were used to develop a consensus for the Lung Imaging Reporting and Data System (Lung-RADS) criteria published by the American College of Radiology in 2014 [35]. The main finding of the Lung-RADS criteria when compared with the NLST criteria is that it raised the baseline from a 4 mm to a 6 mm greatest transverse diameter [36]. The conclusion from this analysis was that Lung-RADS may reduce the false positives but sensitivity was decreased; however, the potential effect of reduced sensitivity on mortality is unknown.

Recently, the NELSON investigators quantified lung cancer probability on the basis of nodule diameter, volume and VDT using data from 9681 nodules in 7155 individuals. Lung cancer had a low probability in participants with a nodule volume of 100 $mm^3$ or <5 mm diameter (0.6%), which was not significantly different from individuals with no nodules. Lung cancer probability in indeterminate nodules 100–300 $mm^3$ or 5–10 mm diameter was 2.4%. However, when VDT was also taken into account, the risk was 0.8% in those with a VDT of ⩾600 days, 4.0% in those with a VDT of 400–600 days and 9.6% in those with a VDT of ⩽400 days [37]. These data provided further evidence that nodules with a diameter of <5 mm or a volume of <100 $mm^3$ are not predictive of cancer, and may be considered the most appropriate methodology for any future lung cancer screening programme.

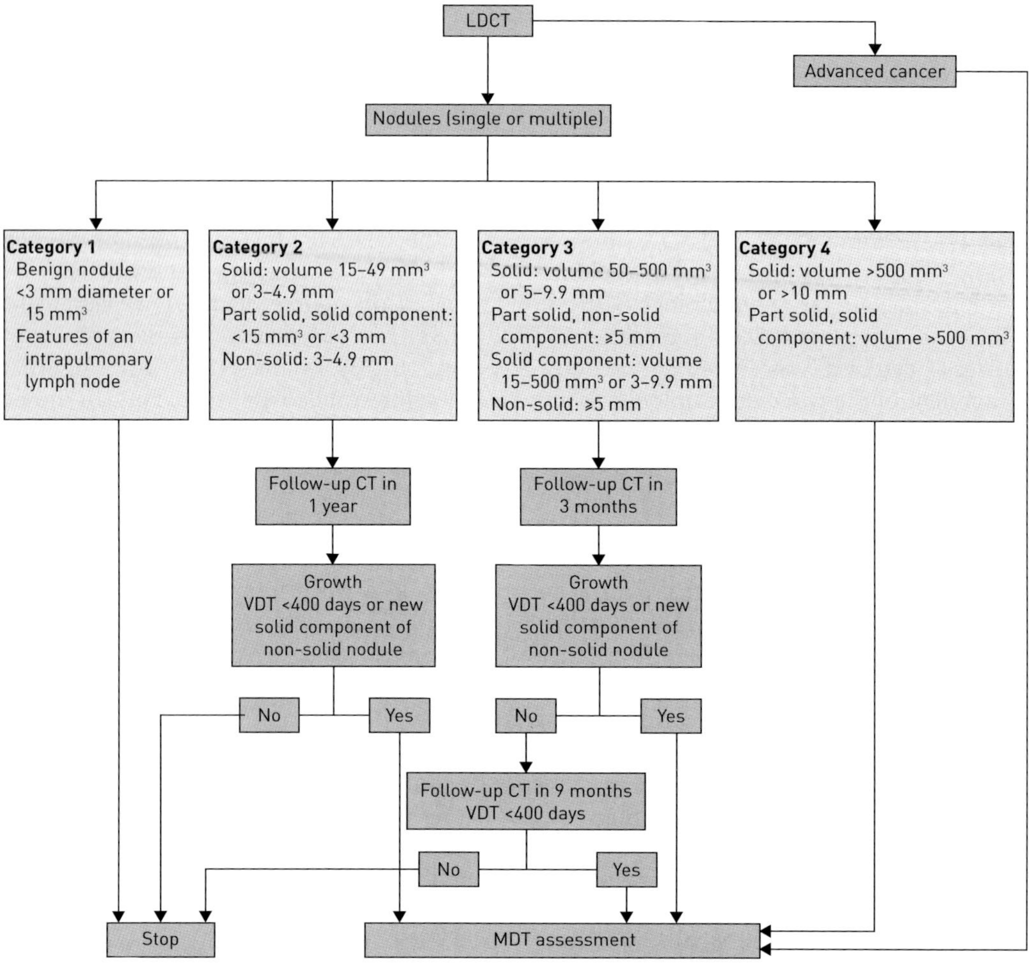


Figure 1. UK Lung Cancer Screening (UKLS) nodule care pathway management protocol. LDCT: low-dose CT; VDT: volume-doubling time; MDT: multidisciplinary team. Reproduced and modified from [22] with permission from the publisher.

One of the issues of the implementation of lung cancer CT screening programmes is the availability of radiologists. It has not yet been resolved whether radiographers can be used as sole readers or be part of a dual-read methodology, whereby they read the CT prior to evaluation by a radiologist. The cost-effectiveness of various approaches needs further investigation but preliminary experience from the UKLS pilot study suggests that routine reading of all CTs by two independent observers is unnecessary and that volumetric assessment of CT scans could potentially be undertaken jointly between radiographers and radiologists [38].

## Annual *versus* biennial screening: what is the evidence?

Currently, there are no RCT cost-effectiveness data available in the European community; however, a judgement call may eventually have to be made between providing an affordable biannual screening programme, which saves a substantial proportion of lung cancer patients, or potentially no screening programme. However, there has to be a balance between the number of lives that can be saved and the cost of implementing a yearly screening programme.

Duffy *et al.* [39] have modelled the impact of an inter-screening interval based on a high-risk group for annual and biennial screening with a 4 mm threshold, as used by the NLST, which would save lives (100–240 cancer deaths prevented for 90000 CT screening episodes) (tables 4 and 5). The absolute impact of screening is very dependent on baseline risk, which is in turn dependent on age, smoking and other risk factors [39]. Although the NLST has a more relaxed risk criterion, the eligible UKLS population will include some individuals who would not qualify for NLST, as the UKLS criteria are based on additional risk factors besides smoking and age [39].

Their findings suggested that 2-yearly screening is less effective in absolute terms but will cause substantially fewer harms than annual screening, such as overdiagnosis, radiation-related deaths from lung cancer, false-positive results and a reduced number of screening examinations per individual [39]. It is also more cost-effective.

In support of the recommendation to consider biennial screening, the NELSON group have provided strong evidence for this approach, based on their study of lung cancer probability

Table 4. Estimated outcomes per million UK population in the target age range (55–75 years), for 10 years of annual or biennial low-dose CT

| Screening frequency | Outcome | UKLS incidence compliance | |
|---|---|---|---|
| | | 30% | 60% |
| **Annual** | Eligible and participating | 30000 | 50000 |
| | Prevalence screens | 30000 | 50000 |
| | Prevalence screen cancers | 839 | 1399 |
| | Incidence screens | 300000 | 500000 |
| | Incidence screen cancers | 3318 | 5530 |
| | Interval cancers | 882 | 1470 |
| | Further investigations | 46200 | 77000 |
| | Deaths prevented ITT | 857 (291–1144) | 1428 (486–1906) |
| | Deaths prevented PP | 956 (325–1276) | 1594 (542–2128) |
| | Overdiagnosed cancers | 457 (0–748) | 733 (0–1247) |
| **Biennial** | Eligible and participating | 30000 | 50000 |
| | Prevalence screens | 30000 | 50000 |
| | Prevalence screen cancers | 839 | 1399 |
| | Incidence screens | 150000 | 250000 |
| | Incidence screen cancers | 2646 | 4410 |
| | Interval cancers | 1554 | 2590 |
| | Further investigations | 43200 | 72000 |
| | Deaths prevented ITT | 685 (233–914) | 1142 (388–1525) |
| | Deaths prevented PP | 802 (273–1071) | 1336 (454–1784) |
| | Overdiagnosed cancers | 383 (0–627) | 639 (0–1046) |

Data are presented as n and n (95% CI). Based on the parameters in Duffy *et al.* [39], with uncertainty intervals on the deaths prevented and overdiagnosed cancers. UKLS: UK Lung Cancer Screening; ITT: intention to treat; PP: per protocol. Reproduced and modified from [39] with permission from the author.

Table 5. Estimated outcomes and uncertainty intervals expressed as screening activity and undesired outcomes per lung cancer death prevented

| Frequency | Benefit estimate | Outcome per death prevented | UKLS incidence |
|---|---|---|---|
| **Annual** | ITT | Persons screened for 10 years | 35 (26–103) |
| | | Screening episodes | 385 (288–1132) |
| | | Further investigations | 54 (40–159) |
| | | Overdiagnosed cases | 0.5 (0.0–0.9) |
| **Annual** | PP | Persons screened for 10 years | 32 (24–94) |
| | | Screening episodes | 345 (258–1015) |
| | | Further investigations | 48 (36–141) |
| | | Overdiagnosed cases | 0.4 (0.0–0.8) |
| **Biennial** | ITT | Persons screened for 10 years | 44 (33–129) |
| | | Screening episodes | 263 (197–774) |
| | | Further investigations | 63 (47–185) |
| | | Overdiagnosed cases | 0.6 (0.0–1.0) |
| **Biennial** | PP | Persons screened for 10 years | 38 (28–112) |
| | | Screening episodes | 224 (168–659) |
| | | Further investigations | 54 (40–159) |
| | | Overdiagnosed cases | 0.4 (0.0–0.8) |

Data are presented as n and n (95% CI). Stratified by incidence of target population, screening frequency and benefit estimate (intention to treat (ITT) or per protocol (PP)). UKLS: UK Lung Cancer Screening. Reproduced and modified from [39] with permission from the author.

in CT-detected nodules [37]. No pulmonary nodules were detected in more than half of the NELSON participants in the CT arm of the trial. The 2-year probability of developing lung cancer was 0.4%, which suggests that a screening interval of ⩾2 years might be safe to apply in these individuals. This will reduce both the radiation exposure of a long-term CT-screening programme and the cost.

## Integration of smoking cessation into future CT screening programmes

In addition to the public health message that smoking cessation is the primary method by which lung cancer incidence should be prevented, there is evidence that the integration of smoking cessation into screening programmes has a synergistic effect in particular subgroups.

In the NELSON trial, 14.5% in the screened arm and 19.1% in the control arm quit smoking compared with a background population quit rate of 6–7% [40]. This would suggest that certain individuals are reassured by a negative screening, so cessation advice might need to be tailored to mitigate this effect. Effective smoking cessation has the potential to improve the cost-effectiveness of screening but in one study, it did not alter costs sufficiently to meet the threshold set by NICE [41, 42].

The impact of lung cancer CT screening has been assessed in a subgroup of the NLST patients to ascertain the participants' response to smoking cessation during the trial [43]. The NLST was a collaborative study between the Lung Screening Study (LSS) and the American College of Radiology Imaging Network (ACRIN). There were 16 265 (47%)

baseline smokers amongst the LSS participants, of which 788 developed lung cancer and were excluded from the analysis. It is of particular note that smoking cessation was strongly associated with the level of abnormality identified in the previous year's screening ($p>0.0001$). The smoking intensity was inversely associated with the severity of the screening result. The authors found that there was an increased risk of continuing to smoke in individuals with a lower age, with a lower education, who were spouseless, who had a lower BMI, who had a history of heavy smoking and who were exposed to second-hand smoke, thus demonstrating the major challenges in implementing good smoking cessation programmes in CT screening trials.

## The potential for implementation of lung cancer screening outside the USA

The advent of lung cancer screening, particularly in Europe, is still at least 2 years away, as we await the results from the NELSON trial and the pooling of the European trials thereafter. However, this is not the time for European health services to await events; it is very important that planning is put in place immediately [44]. Within the UK, the recommendation is that we start to plan for the impact of services, particularly the provision of CT facilities and the preparation of a reporting practice, which may use trained radiographers working alongside CT screening radiologists, akin to mammographic breast screening practices in some EU countries [44].

Depending on the forthcoming data from the NELSON trial, and if it demonstrates a mortality advantage in the CT screen arm and also cost-effectiveness with the pooled NELSON/UKLS data, one would argue that CT screening should be implemented within the UK [44]. The data from the UKLS trial indicate that we should use a risk prediction model, such as the LLPv2 (www.MyLungRisk.org), in order to focus on the highest-risk group [29]. The optimal screen interval has yet to be determined and will be influenced by financial considerations. Although annual screening may save more lives and will do that within an acceptable cost per QALY, the overall cost may mean biennial screening is a more pragmatic solution, at least initially. It may also be that an interval tailored according to risk will be adopted, with shorter intervals for older people or according to the calculated risk. It is imperative that all screening programmes capitalise on the opportunity to prevent lung cancer by incorporating strong smoking cessation interventions to maximise the benefit to the population screened. There remain many potential ways to deliver screening programmes that will need to adapt to the national healthcare landscape. It is essential to start planning now.

## References

1. Jha P, Peto R, Zatonski W, *et al.* Social inequalities in male mortality, and in male mortality from smoking: indirect estimation from national death rates in England and Wales, Poland, and North America. *Lancet* 2006; 368: 367–370.
2. Peto R, Darby S, Deo H, *et al.* Smoking, smoking cessation, and lung cancer in the UK since 1950: combination of national statistics with two case-control studies. *BMJ* 2000; 321: 323–329.
3. OECD. Health at a Glance: Europe 2014. Paris, OECD Publishing, 2014.
4. European Commission. Attitudes of Europeans towards tobacco. Special Eurobarometer 385/Wave EB77.1 – TNS Opinion & Social. European Commission, 2012.
5. Aberle DR, Adams AM, Berg CD, *et al.* Reduced lung-cancer mortality with low-dose computed tomographic screening. *N Engl J Med* 2011; 365: 395–409.

6. Field JK, Smith RA, Aberle DR, *et al.* International Association for the Study of Lung Cancer Computed Tomography Screening Workshop 2011 report. *J Thorac Oncol* 2012; 7: 10–19.
7. Field JK, Hansell DM, Duffy SW, *et al.* CT screening for lung cancer: countdown to implementation. *Lancet Oncol* 2013; 14: e591–e600.
8. Humphrey LL, Deffebach M, Pappas M, *et al.* Screening for lung cancer with low-dose computed tomography: a systematic review to update the US preventive services task force recommendation. *Ann Intern Med* 2013; 159: 411–420.
9. Centers for Medicare and Medicaid Services. Decision memo for screening for lung cancer with low dose computed tomography (LDCT) (CAG-00439N). www.cms.gov/medicare-coverage-database/details/nca-decision-memo.aspx?NCAId=274 Date last accessed: March 14, 2015. Date last updated: February 5, 2015.
10. Black WC, Gareen IF, Soneji SS, *et al.* Cost-effectiveness of CT screening in the National Lung Screening Trial. *N Engl J Med* 2014; 371: 1793–1802.
11. Tammemagi MC, Katki HA, Hocking WG, *et al.* Selection criteria for lung-cancer screening. *N Engl J Med* 2013; 368: 728–736.
12. Kovalchik SA, Tammemagi M, Berg CD, *et al.* Targeting of low-dose CT screening according to the risk of lung-cancer death. *N Engl J Med* 2013; 369: 245–254.
13. Goulart BH, Bensink ME, Mummy DG, *et al.* Lung cancer screening with low-dose computed tomography: costs, national expenditures, and cost-effectiveness. *J Natl Compr Canc Netw* 2012; 10: 267–275.
14. Whynes DK. Could CT screening for lung cancer ever be cost effective in the United Kingdom? *Cost Eff Resour Alloc* 2008; 6: 5.
15. Pastorino U, Bellomi M, Landoni C, *et al.* Early lung-cancer detection with spiral CT and positron emission tomography in heavy smokers: 2-year results. *Lancet* 2003; 362: 593–597.
16. Infante M, Lutman FR, Cavuto S, *et al.* Lung cancer screening with spiral CT: baseline results of the randomized DANTE trial. *Lung Cancer* 2008; 59: 355–363.
17. Blanchon T, Brechot JM, Grenier PA, *et al.* Baseline results of the Depiscan study: a French randomized pilot trial of lung cancer screening comparing low dose CT scan (LDCT) and chest X-ray (CXR). *Lung Cancer* 2007; 58: 50–58.
18. Lopes Pegna A, Picozzi G, Mascalchi M, *et al.* Design, recruitment and baseline results of the ITALUNG trial for lung cancer screening with low-dose CT. *Lung Cancer* 2009; 64: 34–40.
19. van Klaveren RJ, Oudkerk M, Prokop M, *et al.* Management of lung nodules detected by volume CT scanning. *N Engl J Med* 2009; 361: 2221–2229.
20. Pedersen J, Ashraf H, Dirksen A, *et al.* The Danish randomized lung cancer CT screening trial - overall design and results of the prevalence round. *J Thorac Oncol* 2009; 5: 608–614.
21. Becker N, Motsch E, Gross ML, *et al.* Randomized study on early detection of lung cancer with MSCT in Germany: study design and results of the first screening round. *J Cancer Res Clin Oncol* 2012; 138: 1475–1486.
22. Baldwin DR, Duffy SW, Wald NJ, *et al.* UK Lung Screen (UKLS) nodule management protocol: modelling of a single screen randomised controlled trial of low-dose CT screening for lung cancer. *Thorax* 2011; 66: 308–313.
23. Infante M, Cavuto S, Lutman F, *et al.* A randomized study of lung cancer screening with spiral computed tomography: three-year results from the DANTE trial. *Am J Respir Crit Care Med* 2009; 180: 445–453.
24. Pastorino U, Rossi M, Rosato V, *et al.* Annual or biennial CT screening *versus* observation in heavy smokers: 5-year results of the MILD trial. *Eur J Cancer Prev* 2012; 21: 308–315.
25. Field JK, van Klaveren R, Pedersen JH, *et al.* European randomized lung cancer screening trials: Post NLST. *J Surg Oncol* 2013; 108: 280–286.
26. Tammemagi MC, Church TR, Hocking WG, *et al.* Evaluation of the lung cancer risks at which to screen ever- and never-smokers: screening rules applied to the PLCO and NLST cohorts. *PLoS Med* 2014; 11: e1001764.
27. Cassidy A, Myles JP, van Tongeren M, *et al.* The LLP risk model: an individual risk prediction model for lung cancer. *Br J Cancer* 2008; 98: 270–276.
28. Raji OY, Duffy SW, Agbaje OF, *et al.* Predictive accuracy of the Liverpool Lung Project risk model for stratifying patients for computed tomography screening for lung cancer: a case–control and cohort validation study. *Ann Intern Med* 2012; 157: 242–250.
29. McRonald FE, Yadegarfar G, Baldwin DR, *et al.* The UK Lung Screen (UKLS): demographic profile of first 88,897 approaches provides recommendations for population screening. *Cancer Prev Res (Phila)* 2014; 7: 362–371.
30. Horeweg N, van der Aalst CM, Thunnissen E, *et al.* Characteristics of lung cancers detected by computer tomography screening in the randomized NELSON trial. *Am J Respir Crit Care Med* 2013; 187: 848–854.
31. Van't Westeinde SC, van Klaveren RJ. Screening and early detection of lung cancer. *Cancer J* 2011; 17: 3–10.
32. Heuvelmans MA, Oudkerk M, de Bock GH, *et al.* Optimisation of volume-doubling time cutoff for fast-growing lung nodules in CT lung cancer screening reduces false-positive referrals. *Eur Radiol* 2013; 23: 1836–1845.
33. Henschke CI, Yip R, Yankelevitz DF, *et al.* Definition of a positive test result in computed tomography screening for lung cancer: a cohort study. *Ann Intern Med* 2013; 158: 246–252.
34. Bach PB, Mirkin JN, Oliver TK, *et al.* Benefits and harms of CT screening for lung cancer: a systematic review. *JAMA* 2012; 307: 2418–2429.

35. American College of Radiology. Lung CT Screening Reporting and Data System (Lung-RADS). www.acr.org/quality-safety/resources/lungrads Date last accessed: April 27, 2015.
36. Pinsky PF, Gierada DS, Black W, *et al.* Performance of Lung-RADS in the National Lung Screening Trial: a retrospective assessment. *Ann Intern Med* 2015; 162: 485–491.
37. Horeweg N, van Rosmalen J, Heuvelmans MA, *et al.* Lung cancer probability in patients with CT-detected pulmonary nodules: a prespecified analysis of data from the NELSON trial of low-dose CT screening. *Lancet Oncol* 2014; 15: 1332–1341.
38. Nair A, Screaton NJ, Holemans JA, *et al.* Performance of trained radiographers in lung nodule detection: prospective comparison with experienced radiologists in lung cancer screening. *Insights Imaging* 2013; 4: S385–S386.
39. Duffy SW, Field JK, Allgood PC, *et al.* Translation of research results to simple estimates of the likely effect of a lung cancer screening programme in the United Kingdom. *Br J Cancer* 2014; 110: 1834–1840.
40. van der Aalst CM, van den Bergh KA, Willemsen MC, *et al.* Lung cancer screening and smoking abstinence: 2 year follow-up data from the Dutch–Belgian randomised controlled lung cancer screening trial. *Thorax* 2010; 65: 600–605.
41. Chen YF, Madan J, Welton N, *et al.* Effectiveness and cost-effectiveness of computer and other electronic aids for smoking cessation: a systematic review and network meta-analysis. *Health Technol Assess* 2012; 16: 1–205.
42. Hoogendoorn M, Feenstra TL, Hoogenveen RT, *et al.* Long-term effectiveness and cost-effectiveness of smoking cessation interventions in patients with COPD. *Thorax* 2010; 65: 711–718.
43. Tammemagi MC, Berg CD, Riley TL, *et al.* Impact of lung cancer screening results on smoking cessation. *J Natl Cancer Inst* 2014; 106: dju084.
44. Field JK. Perspective: the screening imperative. *Nature* 2014; 513: S7.

---

Disclosures: D.R. Baldwin has received grants from NIHR, during the conduct of the study; educational grants from Roche, Agfa and Irwin Mitchell, and a travel grant from OncImmune, outside the submitted work.

Chapter 3

# Tobacco control

Thierry Urban[1], Michel Underner[2], José Hureaux[1] and Xavier Quantin[3]

Tobacco control is the major contributor to the decline in adult tobacco use as a result of reduced initiation and increased cessation, and to subsequent declines in smoking-related mortality, particularly for lung cancer in men. The smoking prevalence has reached a plateau at 20–30% in developed countries and is on the rise in developing nations. The World Health Organization Framework Convention on Tobacco Control has been developed in response to the globalisation of the tobacco epidemic.

In lung cancer patients, smoking cessation and relapse prevention are opportunities to improve cancer survival rates, reduce the complications of treatment and improve quality of life. Data provide sufficient evidence to deliver advice to quit at diagnosis, particularly in the case of lung surgery. In advanced disease, both chemotherapy and radiation treatment are likely to produce fewer complications and less morbidity among nonsmokers than smokers. Supportive and cognitive behavioural therapies combined with pharmacological treatments are needed to provide the best chance to quit smoking.

The health consequences of smoking have been recently reported in the 2014 US surgeon general's report [1]. Active smoking is a major risk factor for lung cancer and ~30% of all cancer deaths are due to tobacco. Efforts by governments, nongovernmental organisations and the private sector, known as "tobacco control", are the principal contributors to the decline in adult tobacco use as a result of reduced initiation and increased cessation [2, 3], and to the subsequent declines in smoking-related mortality. Particular focus on smoking cessation is justified, since quitting smoking before the age of 40 years will reduce by ~90% the risk of death associated with continued smoking. The benefits of smoking cessation in patients with lung cancer should be considered, although lung cancer patients and oncologists are generally not familiar with these benefits.

## Tobacco smoke and lung cancer

### Active smoking

Jha *et al.* [4] reported the relationship between smoking history and mortality to provide estimates of the 21st century hazards of smoking and the benefits of smoking cessation in a

[1]Pulmonology Dept, Academic Hospital, Angers, France. [2]Pulmonology Dept, Academic Hospital, Poitiers, France. [3]Pulmonology Dept, Academic Hospital, Montpellier, France.

Correspondence: Thierry Urban, Département de Pneumologie, CHU ANGERS, 4, rue Larrey, 49000, Angers, France.
E-mail: thurban@chu-angers.fr

 Print ISBN: 978-1-84984-061-3. Online ISBN: 978-1-84984-062-0. Print ISSN: 2312-508X. Online ISSN: 2312-5098.

prospective cohort of 216917 adults. They showed that, for participants who were 25–79 years of age, the rate of death from any cause among current smokers was about three times that among never-smokers (hazard ratio (HR) for women: 3.0, 99% CI 2.7–3.3; HR for men: 2.8, 99% CI 2.4–3.1). Most of the excess mortality was due to neoplastic, vascular or respiratory diseases. Among current smokers, survival was shortened by 11 years for women and by 12 years for men, as compared with never-smokers. These data confirmed the results of four other reports [5–8].

Thun *et al.* [8] compared temporal trends in mortality across three time periods, using data from two historical cohort studies and five pooled contemporary cohort studies, among participants aged 55 years or older during follow-up. For female current smokers, as compared with female never-smokers, the relative risks of death from lung cancer were 2.73, 12.65 and 25.66 in the 1960s, 1980s and contemporary cohorts, respectively; the corresponding relative risks for male current smokers, as compared with male never-smokers, were 12.22, 23.81 and 24.97.

### Second-hand smoke

More than 10% of lung cancers occur in lifetime nonsmokers as a result of exposure to environmental smoke [9]. An analysis of 37 epidemiological studies showed that never-smokers who lived with a smoker were at a 26% increased risk of lung cancer when compared with those who did not live with a smoker [10]. A meta-analysis of 18 case–control studies found that, among never-smokers, the odds ratios comparing those ever exposed to second-hand smoke with those never exposed were 1.26 (95% CI 1.10–1.44) for ADC, 1.41 (95% CI 0.99–1.99) for SCC, and 3.09 (95% CI 1.62–5.89) for SCLC [11].

## Tobacco control

### Awareness of the need for tobacco control

Lung cancer was a rare disease prior to the 20th century. The tobacco industry then developed commercial cigarettes, facilitating inhalation of tobacco smoke into the lungs, with rapid nicotine delivery to the brain, making cigarette smoking very addictive. The adoption of cigarettes by tobacco users was followed by an increase in lung cancer deaths.

In 1954, two studies concluded that smokers increased their odds of dying from lung cancer [12] and the link between human smoking habits and death rates had been proven [13]. The World Health Organization (WHO) and government health agencies concluded that cigarettes were a major cause of lung cancer [14].

In a conspiracy to challenge scientific evidence, the tobacco industry claimed that these findings did not prove that cigarettes caused cancer. Cigarette companies became major television sponsors. Smoking was permitted nearly everywhere without restriction.

In 1964, the US surgeon general's report, recognising smoking as a cause of lung cancer, was a turning point in tobacco control [2]. Significant growth in the awareness of the harms of cigarette smoking led to a shift in public attitudes towards cigarette smoking and a persistent decline in cigarette consumption, and to increasing efforts to regulate the use, sale and advertising of tobacco products. In response, cigarette companies introduced cigarettes with filters and lower tar and lower nicotine, and many people switched to newer cigarettes. Data suggest that this switch made smoking even more dangerous, by allowing deeper inhalation of smoke into the airways [8].

### Tobacco control strategies

Subsequently, new tobacco control strategies were developed. These included higher prices for cigarettes by means of an increased excise tax, restrictions on smoking in public places, bans on tobacco advertising and promotion, public education about the hazards of smoking and the benefits of cessation, and easy access to cessation efforts. The public's perception of smoking shifted to towards the serious health risks and smoking became less acceptable as a social practice. Tobacco control was marked by significant reductions in tobacco use and was subsequently followed, in some countries, by a reduction in lung cancer incidence and mortality [1, 15]. Since then, and despite significant state-to-state variability, smoking prevalence has reached a plateau at 20–30% in developed countries. National surveys estimate that 70% of smokers in the USA say they want to quit and 50% have tried to quit at least once in the preceding year. Almost all (95%) of those who tried to quit on their own relapsed [16].

### WHO Framework Convention on Tobacco Control

The spread of the tobacco epidemic is facilitated by global marketing, trade liberalisation, direct foreign investment, transnational tobacco advertising, promotion and sponsorship. The international movement of contraband and counterfeit cigarettes or e-commerce have also contributed to the explosive increase in tobacco use [17].

The WHO Framework Convention on Tobacco Control is an international treaty adopted in May 2003 and brought into force in February 2005 [17]. It was developed in response to the globalisation of the tobacco epidemic and represents a milestone for the promotion of public health and for international health cooperation. Importantly, article 5.3 requires that "in setting and implementing their public health policies with respect to tobacco control, Parties shall act to protect these policies from commercial and other vested interests of the tobacco industry in accordance with national law". It comprises numerous tobacco control measures, including: price and tax measures as well as non-price measures to reduce the demand for tobacco; protection from exposure to tobacco smoke; regulation of the contents of tobacco products; regulation of tobacco product disclosures; regulation of the packaging and labelling of tobacco products; education, communication, training and public awareness; tobacco advertising, promotion and sponsorship; and demand reduction measures concerning tobacco dependence and cessation. Other measures concern the illicit trade in tobacco products, sales to and by minors, and provision of support for economically viable alternative activities.

Raising prices is an effective means of increasing smoking cessation. When the price of cigarettes increases by >10%, the rate of abstinence increases by 3% [18]. Smoking restrictions in public places, work places and households are another effective way of promoting abstinence and avoiding environmental exposure. Complete advertising bans on tobacco are another effective strategy, reducing smoking rates by 6% [18].

However, these public health measures are not enough for the 20–30% of adults who are addicted to nicotine and continue to smoke. Additional measures are needed to treat these patients' addictions [19]. Tobacco control should be particularly focused on children, known as the "replacement smokers".

### General pharmacotherapy

Behavioural interventions for tobacco and smoking cessation consist of individual counselling along with medications. This combination doubles abstinence rates compared with either type of intervention alone [20]. A Cochrane review of behavioural interventions for smoking cessation found a benefit from more intensive support (relative risk 1.16, 95% CI 1.09–1.24) for abstinence at the longest follow-up [21].

Nicotine replacement therapies (NRTs) are designed to suppress cravings for cigarettes and mitigate nicotine withdrawal symptoms by providing steady stimulation to the nicotinic receptors and preventing rapid fluctuations in the release of dopamine in the forebrain. NRT is safe, as it does not contain the thousands of non-nicotine products present in cigarettes [22] and increase the abstinence rate by twofold compared with placebo.

Varenicline is a nicotinic receptor agonist [23], attenuating the release of dopamine in the forebrain and preventing the binding of these receptors to nicotine.

## Tobacco control and lung cancer

### Prevalence of current smoking

The prevalence of smoking peaked around 1960 among US men and about two decades later among US women [16, 24]. The prevalence of current smokers was then more than halved between 1965 and 2010, from 42% to 19% [25, 26]. In the USA, a recent report estimated that 18% of adults are still smoking cigarettes and the prevalence of smoking changed little between 2004 and 2010 [27]. Data recently reported from 18 European countries, concerning individuals aged 15 years or older, found that 27.2% of participants were current smokers (30.6% of men and 24.1% of women) [28]. Nevertheless, smoking rates are on the rise in developing nations, particularly in East Asia and other parts of the Western Pacific region, where nearly two out of three adult males are smokers [18].

### Smoking cessation and survival

Peto *et al.* [29] showed that for men who stopped at 60, 50, 40 and 30 years of age the cumulative risks of lung cancer by age 75 years were 10%, 6%, 3% and 2%, respectively. In a cohort of 216917 adults between 1997 and 2004, Jha *et al.* [4] showed that adults who had quit smoking at 25–34, 35–44, 45–54 or 55–64 years of age gained about 10, 9, 6 and 4 years of life, respectively, as compared with those who continued to smoke. Nevertheless, smokers who had quit by about 39 years of age still had a 20% excess risk (HR 1.2), as compared with those who had never smoked. This hazard is substantial, although it is much smaller than the excess risk (HR 3.0) among those who continued to smoke [4]. These data were confirmed in a study of women [6].

The residual effects of smoking on lung cancer risk remain most notable in former smokers and a significant proportion of lung cancer is now diagnosed in former smokers [30]. In a study of 5628 lung cancer patients, 89% had a smoking history and 49% were former smokers [31]. Despite smoking cessation, the lung cancer risk persists, as shown in the Nurses Lung Health Study, in which the HR for lung cancer was 21.8 and 4.93 for current and former smokers, respectively, compared with nonsmokers [32].

## Smoking reduction

Pisinger *et al.* [33] identified 25 studies related to smoking reduction and concluded that "smoking reduction is associated with a 25% decline in biomarkers and incidence of lung cancer". Lee [34] identified three case–control studies and three cohort studies estimating change in lung cancer risk after reducing consumption and reported a lower lung cancer risk in reducers. Compared with non-reducers, the analysis showed a significantly lower risk (relative risk 0.81, 95% CI 0.74–0.88) for any reduction.

The limited number of studies providing relevant results, limited dose–response data, incomplete adjustment for baseline consumption, and the varying definitions of reduction used affects the establishment of a clear relationship.

## Tobacco control and lung cancer incidence

In Europe, the peak of lung cancer cases seems to have been reached in men, but not in women [35, 36]. Over the 1998–2007 period, a significant decline in lung cancer incidence rates was observed in 14 out of the 26 European countries among middle-aged men (35–64 years old) and in 15 countries among older men (65–74 years old) [36]. More marked declines were observed in older men. These analyses reveal that the gap between male and female lung cancer incidence is narrowing, particularly in Northern and Western Europe, with lung cancer rates in women aged 35–64 years old in 2006–2008 even higher than rates in men in Denmark, Iceland and Sweden. The lung cancer incidence for men aged 35–74 years old differed markedly between countries, with the highest rate in Belarus (161 cases per 100 000 in 2007) and the lowest rate in Sweden (40 cases per 100 000 in 2009), in the most recent period.

## Tobacco control and lung cancer mortality

The combined tobacco control efforts, since the 1964 US surgeon general's report until 2012, were associated with the avoidance of an estimated 8.0 million (credible range 7.4–8.3 million) premature smoking-attributable deaths [37]. The decrease in tobacco smoking averted approximately 146 000 lung cancer deaths among US men during 1991–2003 [38]. Moolgavkar *et al.* [39] estimated that 800 000 lung cancer deaths were avoided between 1975 and 2000. However, 70% of lung cancer deaths could have been prevented if cigarette companies had stopped marketing their products in 1964.

In Europe, Bray *et al.* [40], extracting data from the WHO mortality databank by age, sex and year of death (1970–2007) for 36 countries, concluded that lung cancer mortality in men has tended to decrease in many European countries during the past two decades, particularly in Northern and Western Europe. However, among women, mortality rates are still increasing in many countries, although in a few populations the rates are beginning to stabilise, notably in high-risk countries in Eastern Europe and Northern Europe. Men and women are in different phases of the smoking epidemic.

### Emerging areas

Through aggressive marketing in emerging markets, cigarette smoking continues to grow and constitutes a major threat to global public health [41]. Worldwide, about 30 million young adults begin smoking each year, and current patterns of behaviour suggest continued increases [42]. In 2008, the number of newly diagnosed lung cancers in developing countries exceeded that in developed countries by 22% [43]. The increase in smoking prevalence in Chinese males observed several decades ago led to a 27% increase in lung cancer mortality rates between 1990 and 2010 [44].

## Tobacco control in patients with lung cancer

### Biological rationale

Carcinogens in tobacco smoke act as genetic inducers, but may also act to promote progression of the cancer [45]. Nicotine induces polycyclic aromatic hydrocarbons (PAHs) in tobacco smoke, which are some of the major lung carcinogens [46, 47]. PAHs are inducers of hepatic enzymes, and many drugs are substrates for hepatic CYP1A2 and their metabolism can be induced in smokers. NRT does not contribute to these pharmacokinetic drug interactions. *In vitro*, nicotine can induce the proliferation of lung cancer cell lines, promote angiogenesis, and promote resistance to cisplatin-induced apoptosis [48, 49].

### Motivation for smoking cessation

Approximately 40% of patients with newly diagnosed lung cancer smoke [50], and the majority would like to stop smoking at this teachable moment [51]. Physicians should deliver clear advice to quit and a systematic referral to specialised tobacco treatment units, and education regarding the effect of smoking cessation, pharmacotherapy for withdrawal symptoms and likelihood of abstinence. In 201 smoking lung cancer patients, who were given targeted smoking cessation treatment, the abstinence rate after 6 months was 22% [51]. The recidivism rates remain high [52]. Other patients continue to smoke even after their diagnosis, demonstrating major tobacco dependence. In a recent study, of the 242 current smokers at diagnosis, 136 (56%) had quit 1 year after diagnosis [53].

### Tobacco smoking and survival in lung cancer patients

It is still unclear how smoking affects lung tumour progression, recurrence and metastasis, and whether smoking could be used as a predictor of lung cancer treatment outcome. In a study of 5229 patients with lung cancer, the median survival times among those who had never smoked, former smokers and current smokers were 1.4, 1.3 and 1.1 years, respectively ($p<0.01$). The relative risk per 10 years of smoking abstinence was 0.85, demonstrating a direct effect of smoking on survival [54].

The effect of smoking intensity on overall survival and the interactions between smoking and clinicopathological factors in lung cancer progression were investigated in four cohorts [55]. Patients who smoked more than 61 packs/year had an increased risk for lung cancer recurrence (HR 1.41, 95% CI 1.03–1.94; log-rank $p=0.032$) and shorter overall survival period (log-rank $p=0.033$). There were significant interactions between smoking and clinical stage ($p=0.02$), as well as patient age and tumour differentiation ($p=0.03$) in lung cancer progression. Heavy smoking at diagnosis could be an independent, significant prognostic factor.

An analysis of long-term outcomes in a cohort of 5185 patients with cancer from 13 different disease sites showed that current smoking at diagnosis in patients with lung cancer increases all-cause mortality and disease-specific mortality compared with never-smokers, former smokers and recent quitters (within 12 months of diagnosis) [56]. With a minimum of 12 years of follow-up, current smokers at the time of cancer diagnosis had a higher overall mortality risk compared with recent quitters (HR 1.17, 95% CI 1.03–1.32), former smokers (HR 1.29, 95% CI 1.17–1.42) and never-smokers (HR 1.38, 95% CI 1.23–1.54). Furthermore, current smokers had a higher disease-specific mortality risk than former smokers (HR 1.23, 95% CI 1.09–1.39) and never-smokers (HR 1.18, 95% CI 1.03–1.36).

Data from 4200 lung cancer patients, who participated in the National Comprehensive Cancer Network's NSCLC Database Project, were analysed including 618 never-smokers, 1483 current smokers, 380 smokers who had recently quit, and 1719 former smokers (who quit >12 months before diagnosis) [57]. Among patients with stage I–III disease, only never-smokers had better survival than current smokers (HR 0.47 (95% CI 0.26–0.85) *versus* 0.51 (95% CI, 0.38–0.68), respectively). Among patients with stage IV disease, the impact of smoking depended on age. Among younger patients (<55 years old), being a never-smoker and a former smoker for >12 months increased survival. Patients who were smoking at the time of diagnosis had worse survival compared with never-smokers. Among younger patients with stage IV disease, current smokers also had worse survival compared with former smokers who quit >12 months before diagnosis.

## Smoking cessation at diagnosis in lung cancer patients

A meta-analysis on patients with lung cancer suggested an advantage for abstaining from smoking in terms of survival, disease recurrence and risk for second primary cancer after adjusting for other risk factors, particularly cardiovascular risk factors [58]. In most of the studies included, most patients were diagnosed as having an early stage lung tumour. Continued smoking was associated with a significantly increased risk of all-cause mortality (HR 2.94, 95% CI 1.15–7.54) and recurrence (HR 1.86, 95% CI 1.01–3.41) in early stage NSCLC, and all-cause mortality (HR 1.86, 95% CI 1.33–2.59), development of a second primary tumour (HR 4.31, 95% CI 1.09–16.98) and recurrence (HR 1.26, 95% CI 1.06–1.50) in limited stage SCLC. Life table modelling on the basis of these data estimated 33% 5-year survival in 65 year-old patients with early stage NSCLC who continued to smoke compared with 70% in those who quit smoking [58]. The most important limitations of the study were the absence of data from randomised controlled trials, preventing any causal inferences, and the poor definition of smoking abstinence in many studies. In another review of phase III studies in patients with advanced lung cancer, ever-smoking had no conclusive relationship with outcome in patients with lung cancer [59].

Patients with lung cancer have an increased risk of developing a second lung tumour. In a study involving 569 patients who had undergone resection for stage I NSCLC and who were followed for a median of 5.9 years, the authors reported no cases of second lung cancer in 45 never-smokers, 2.72 second lung cancers per 100 patient-years in active smokers, and 1.77 per 100 patient-years in former smokers [60]. The HR for second lung cancer in active smokers *versus* former smokers was 1.9.

Data provide sufficient evidence to deliver advice to quit to early stage lung cancer patients. Such an intervention should be based on robust evidence that quitting smoking actually improves outcomes.

## Smoking cessation and lung cancer surgery

Nonsmokers are at decreased risk of postoperative complications compared with smokers [61–64]. Current smoking is considered as a risk factor for the development of postoperative complications following many types of surgery.

A systematic review and meta-analysis including nine studies compared postoperative complications in patients undergoing any type of surgery who stopped smoking within 8 weeks prior to surgery and those who continued to smoke [65]. One study found a beneficial effect of recent quitting compared with continuing smoking, and none identified any detrimental effects. In meta-analyses, quitting smoking within the 8 weeks before surgery was not associated with any increase or decrease in overall postoperative complications for all available studies (relative risk 0.78, 95% CI 0.57–1.07), for a group of three studies with high quality scores (relative risk 0.57, 95% CI 0.16–2.01), and for four studies specifically evaluating pulmonary complications (relative risk 1.18, 95% CI 0.95–1.46). Two other studies reported similar results [66, 67].

Conversely, in another systematic review and meta-analysis, the pooled data demonstrated a relative risk reduction of 41% (95% CI 15–59; $p<0.01$) for prevention of postoperative complications [68]. In this study, each week of cessation increased the magnitude of the effect by 19%. Trials of at least 4 weeks of smoking cessation had a significantly larger treatment effect than shorter trials ($p<0.04$). Analysis of 15 observational studies demonstrated important effects of smoking cessation on decreasing total complications (relative risk 0.76, 95% CI 0.69–0.84; $p<0.0001$), wound healing complications (relative risk 0.73, 95% CI 0.61–0.87; $p=0.0006$) and pulmonary complications (relative risk 0.81, 95% CI 0.70–0.93; $p<0.003$).

A Cochrane database review concluded that interventions that begin 4–8 weeks before surgery, including weekly counselling, and using NRT were most likely to have an impact on long-term smoking cessation and a beneficial effect on complication rates [66].

Most of the studies presented methodological limitations, different smoking classifications, different designs across the observational studies, and most had small sample sizes or heterogeneous reporting of outcomes. No firm conclusions can be drawn concerning the effect of preoperative smoking cessation on operative outcomes in patients undergoing surgery for lung cancer [67]. Patients should be advised to stop smoking at diagnosis. However, surgery in active smokers should not be postponed in order to allow smoking cessation, because of the lack of evidence that smoking cessation during the delay results in improved outcomes.

## Smoking cessation and advanced lung cancer patients

Both chemotherapy and radiation treatment are likely to produce fewer complications and less morbidity among nonsmokers than smokers [69]. Smoking could have detrimental effects on the efficacy of chemotherapy, including chemoresistance and altered chemotherapeutic levels [70, 71], and on the pharmacokinetics and toxicity profile of some drugs [72]. The EGFR inhibitor erlotinib is metabolised more actively in smokers as a result of cytochrome P450 induction and is therefore less effective, and twice the normal dose was suggested to produce the necessary circulating levels of the drug in smokers compared with never-smokers [73]. Exposure to nicotine might negatively impact on the apoptotic potential of cisplatin [48].

Some studies have suggested that lung cancer patients who smoke, compared with nonsmokers, have a greater risk of experiencing radiation pneumonitis [74], infection during radiotherapy [75], common side-effects of radiation such as oral mucositis, xerostomia, weight loss and fatigue [76], or a lower survival rate after radiation therapy [77]. A benefit of smoking cessation on radiochemotherapy was reported by a Canadian study of 215 patients with limited-stage SCLC. Patients with smoking cessation during therapy had an increased median survival time (18.0 *versus* 13.6 months) and 5-year survival rate (4% *versus* 8.9%; p=0.017) compared with current smokers [78].

### Smoking cessation and quality of life

Smoking cessation has been associated with improved quality of life, cognitive function, psychological well-being and self-esteem [79–82], and a majority of patients with cancer felt guilty when they kept on smoking. Lung cancer patients report decreased fatigue and shortness of breath, increased activity level, and improved performance status, appetite, sleep and mood after successful smoking cessation [83, 84]. These benefits may be of importance because patients with lung cancer have a greater symptom burden than patients with other cancers [85]. Quality of life was also decreased by smoking in patients with lung cancer, as well as in family members and caregivers of patients with lung cancer [86].

### Smoking cessation and lung cancer screening

Recent development in low-dose CT (LDCT) scanning is an opportunity to test the screening experience as a teachable moment for nicotine dependence intervention. Concomitant intervention for smoking cessation should be required in screened patients. The reported rates of new abstinence among smokers who underwent LDCT scans were noted to be higher than the predicted background rate in the general population in lung cancer screening trials, with abstinence rates during a 1-year follow-up period ranging from 14% to 16% [87, 88]. Positive LDCT scan results may motivate smoking cessation attempts, but questions have been raised about the impact of a negative LDCT scan on the reinforcement of smoking behaviour or the risk of relapse among recent quitters, because they think they have a clean bill of health. In a recent study, TAMMEMÄGI *et al.* [89] evaluated the impact of lung cancer screening results on smoking cessation among participants and showed that patients with normal screens had a sharply declining prevalence of smoking over time.

### Tobacco control pharmacotherapy in lung cancer patients

While many lung cancer patients may quit on their own or require minimal advice to quit, the treatment of tobacco use in other patients may require a more intensive and comprehensive approach. Supportive and cognitive behavioural therapies combined with pharmacological treatments are needed to provide the best chance to quit smoking [90]. A recent study found that, while they may ask about tobacco use and encourage patients to quit using tobacco, most oncologists do not discuss medications or provide cessation support [91]. The main limitations included patient resistance to treatment and inexperience in getting patients to quit. An alternative approach is to refer these patients to specialised units.

All of smoking cessation medication can be used readily, with a few exceptions (table 1). Varenicline can exacerbate chemotherapy-induced nausea [93], and oral NRTs may be irritating to a patient's oral mucosa [94]. There is evidence that varenicline is more effective in heavy smokers. Preclinical data have suggested that exposure to nicotine may decrease the effectiveness of radiotherapy and/or chemotherapy *in vitro* and *in vivo* [95]. However, NRT is not associated with any increase in the incidence of cancer, even in long-term follow-up [96]. At the present time, NRT should still be considered to be a proven cessation aid that eliminates the other diverse chemicals present in tobacco smoke.

The recent increase in use of smokeless tobacco and e-cigarettes, particularly among young adults, could modulate these results in future. E-cigarettes are non-tobacco-containing nicotine delivery devices that have experienced a rapid increase in use and are now marketed by the major US tobacco companies. If e-cigarettes are used instead of tobacco cigarettes, the adverse health effects are likely to be considerably less than those of cigarettes in terms of the risk of lung cancer. However, the use of e-cigarettes in combination with tobacco cigarettes may offset some of the potential benefits in young patients. Moreover smoking cessation rate remain to be evaluated with e-cigarettes [97].

## Conclusion

Tobacco control is the principal contributor to the decline in smoking-related morbidity and mortality. In patients with lung cancer, the current data provide sufficient evidence to deliver advice to quit tobacco, even if more evidence are needed that quitting smoking actually improves outcomes. In 2013, the American Society of Clinical Oncology published an important policy statement on tobacco: "providing oncology providers with the evidence-based and practical information they need to successfully integrate tobacco cessation activities into their practices" [98].

Table 1. Pharmacological interventions for smoking cessation

| | Placebo | Single NRT | Bupropion | Nicotine patch | Nicotine gum | Other NRT# | Combination NRT |
|---|---|---|---|---|---|---|---|
| **NRT** | 1.84 (1.71–1.99) | | | | | | |
| **Bupropion** | 1.82 (1.60–2.06) | 0.99 (0.86–1.13) | | | | | |
| **Varenicline** | 2.88 (2.40–3.47) | 1.57 (1.29–1.91) | 1.59 (1.29–1.96) | 1.51 (1.22–1.87) | 1.72 (1.38–2.13) | 1.42 (1.12–1.79) | 1.06 (0.75–1.48) |

Data are presented as OR (95% credible interval). NRT: nicotine replacement therapy. #: including inhalers, sprays, tablets and lozenges. Data from Cahill *et al.* [92].

## References


1. US Department of Health and Human Services. The Health Consequences of of Smoking—50 Years of Progress. A Report of the Surgeon General. Rockville, US Department of Health and Human Services, 2014.
2. US Department of Health, Education and Welfare. Smoking and Health: Report of the Advisory Committee to the Surgeon General of the Public Health Service. (Public Health Service Publication No. 1103). Washington, Public Health Service, 1964.
3. Cokkinides V, Bandi P, McMahon C, *et al.* Tobacco control in the United States – recent progress and opportunities. *CA Cancer J Clin* 2009; 59: 352–365.
4. Jha P, Ramasundarahettige C, Landsman V, *et al.* 21st-century hazards of smoking and benefits of cessation in the United States. *N Engl J Med* 2013; 368: 341–350.
5. Doll R, Peto R, Boreham J, *et al.* Mortality in relation to smoking: 50 years' observations on male British doctors. *BMJ* 2004; 328: 1519–1533.
6. Pirie K, Peto R, Reeves GK, *et al.* The 21st century hazards of smoking and benefits of stopping: a prospective study of one million women in the UK. *Lancet* 2013; 381: 133–134.
7. Sakata R, McGale P, Grant EJ, *et al.* The effect of smoking on mortality and life expectancy in Japan. *BMJ* 2012; 345: e7093.
8. Thun MJ, Carter BD, Feskanich D, *et al.* 50-year trends in smoking-related mortality in the United States. *N Engl J Med* 2013; 368: 351–364.
9. US Department of Health and Human Services. The health consequences of involuntary exposure to tobacco smoke: a report of the Surgeon General. Atlanta, US Department of Health and Human Services, Centers for Disease Control and Prevention, 2006.
10. Hackshaw AK, Law MR, Wald NJ. The accumulated evidence on lung cancer and environmental tobacco smoke. *BMJ* 1997; 315: 980–988.
11. Kim CH, Lee YC, Hung RJ, *et al.* Exposure to secondhand tobacco smoke and lung cancer by histological type: a pooled analysis of the International Lung Cancer Consortium (ILCCO). *Int J Cancer* 2014; 135: 1918–1930.
12. Doll R, Hill AB. The mortality of doctors in relation to their smoking habits. *BMJ* 1954; 1: 1451–1455.
13. Hammond EC, Horn D. The relationship between human smoking habits and death rates: a follow-up study of 187,766 men. *JAMA* 1954; 155: 1316–1328.
14. Proctor RN. The history of the discovery of the cigarette lung cancer link: evidentiary traditions, corporate denial, global toll. *Tob Control* 2012; 21: 87–91.
15. Jha P, Chaloupka FJ. Curbing the epidemic – governments and the economics of tobacco control. Washington, World Bank, 1999.
16. Centers for Disease Control and Prevention (CDC). Quitting smoking among adults – United States, 2001–2010. *MMWR Morb Mortal Wkly Rep* 2011; 60: 1513–1519.
17. World Health Organization. WHO Framework Convention on Tobacco Control. Geneva, World Health Organization, 2003.
18. World Health Organization. WHO Report on the Global Tobacco Epidemic 2009: Implementing Smoke-free Environments. Geneva, World Health Organization, 2009.
19. Hughes JR, Keely J, Naud S. Shape of the relapse curve and long-term abstinence among untreated smokers. *Addiction* 2004; 99: 29–38.
20. Fiore MC, Jaén CR, Baker TB, *et al.* Clinical Practice Guideline. Treating Tobacco Use and Dependence: 2008 Update. Rockville, US Department of Health and Human Services, Public Health Service, 2008.
21. Stead LF, Lancaster T. Behavioural interventions as adjuncts to pharmacotherapy for smoking cessation. *Cochrane Database Syst Rev* 2012; 12: CD009670.
22. Tran K, Asakawa K, Cimon K, *et al.* Pharmacologic-based Strategies for Smoking Cessation: Clinical and Cost-Effectiveness Analyses. (Technology report no 130.) Ottawa, Canadian Agency for Drugs and Technologies in Health, 2010.
23. Hays JT, Ebbert JO. Varenicline for tobacco dependence. *N Engl J Med* 2008; 359: 2018–2024.
24. Forey B, Hamling J, Hamling J, *et al.* International smoking statistics 2006-2012. Sutton, P N Lee Statistics & Computing Ltd, 2012. http://pnlee.co.uk/Downloads/ISS/ISS-Methods_121004.pdf
25. National Center for Health Statistics. Health, United States, 2010: with Special Feature on Death and Dying. Hyattsville, US Department of Health and Human Services, 2011.
26. Warner KE, Sexton D, Gillespie DB, *et al.* The impact of tobacco control on adult per capita cigarette consumption in the United States. *Am J Public Health* 2014; 104: 83–89.
27. Agaku IT, King BA, Dube SR *et al.* Current cigarette smoking among adults - United States, 2005 2012. *MMWR Morb Mortal Wkly Rep* 2014; 63: 29–34.
28. Gallusa S, Lugoa A, La Vecchiaa C, *et al.* Pricing Policies And Control of Tobacco in Europe (PPACTE) project: cross-national comparison of smoking prevalence in 18 European countries. *Eur J Canc Prev* 2014; 23: 177–185.

29. Peto R, Darby S, Deo H, *et al.* Smoking, smoking cessation, and lung cancer in the UK since 1950: combination of national statistics with two case control studies. *BMJ* 2000; 321: 323–329.
30. Mong C, Garon EB, Fuller C, *et al.* High prevalence of lung cancer in a surgical cohort of lung cancer patients a decade after smoking cessation. *J Cardiothorac Surg* 2011; 6: 19.
31. Yang P, Allen MS, Aubry MC, *et al.* Clinical features of 5,628 primary lung cancer patients: experience at Mayo Clinic from 1997 to 2003. *Chest* 2005; 128: 452–462.
32. Kenfield S, Stampfer MJ, Rosner BA, *et al.* Smoking and smoking cessation in relation to mortality in women. *JAMA* 2008; 299: 2037–2047.
33. Pisinger C, Godtfredsen NS. Is there a health benefit of reduced tobacco consumption? A systematic review. *Nicotine Tob Res* 2007; 9: 631–646.
34. Lee PN. The effect of reducing the number of cigarettes smoked on risk of lung cancer, COPD, cardiovascular disease and $FEV_1$ – a review. *Regul Toxicol Pharmacol* 2013; 67: 372–381.
35. Malvezzi M, Bosetti C, Rosso T, *et al.* Lung cancer mortality in European men: trends and predictions. *Lung Cancer* 2013; 80: 138–145.
36. Lortet-Tieulent J, Renteria E, Sharp L, *et al.* Convergence of decreasing male and increasing female incidence rates in major tobacco-related cancers in Europe in 1988-2010. *Eur J Canc* 2013 [In press DOI: 10.1016/j.ejca.2013.10.014].
37. Holford TR, Meza R, Warner KE, *et al.* Tobacco control and the reduction in smoking-related premature deaths in the United States, 1964–2012. *JAMA* 2014; 311: 164–171.
38. Thun MJ, Jemal A. How much of the decrease in cancer death rates in the United States is attributable to reductions in tobacco smoking? *Tob Control* 2006; 15: 345–347.
39. Moolgavkar SH, Holford TR, Levy DT, *et al.* Impact of reduced tobacco smoking on lung cancer mortality in the United States during 1975–2000. *J Natl Cancer Inst* 2012; 104: 541–548.
40. Bray FI, Weiderpass E. Lung cancer mortality trends in 36 European countries: secular trends and birth cohort patterns by sex and region 1970-2007. *Int J Cancer* 2010; 126: 1454–1466.
41. Bartecchi CE, MacKenzie TD, Schrier RW. The global tobacco epidemic. *Sci Am* 1995; 272: 44–51.
42. Giovino GA, Mirza SA, Samet JM, *et al.* Tobacco use in 3 billion individuals from 16 countries: an analysis of nationally representative cross-sectional household surveys. *Lancet* 2012; 380: 668–679.
43. Jemal A, Bray F, Center MM, *et al.* Global cancer statistics. *CA Cancer J Clin* 2011; 61: 69–90.
44. Yang G, Wang Y, Zeng Y, *et al.* Rapid health transition in China, 1990–2010: findings from the Global Burden of Disease Study 2010. *Lancet* 2013; 381: 1987–2015.
45. Hecht SS. Tobacco smoke carcinogens and lung cancer. *J Natl Cancer Inst* 1999; 91: 1194–1210.
46. Hoffmann D, Hoffmann I. The changing cigarette, 1950–1995. *J Toxicol Environ Health* 1997; 50: 307–364.
47. Zevin S, Benowitz NL. Drug interactions with tobacco smoking: an update. *Clin Pharmacokinet* 1999; 36: 425–438.
48. Xu J, Huang H, Pan C, *et al.* Nicotine inhibits apoptosis induced by cisplatin in human oral cancer cells. *Int J Oral Maxillofac Surg* 2007; 36: 739–744.
49. Dasgupta P, Rizwani W, Pillai S, *et al.* Nicotine induces cell proliferation, invasion and epithelialmesenchymal transition in a variety of human cancer cell lines. *Int J Cancer* 2009; 124: 36–45.
50. Park ER, Japuntich SJ, Rigotti NA, *et al.* A snapshot of smokers after lung and colorectal cancer diagnosis. *Cancer* 2012; 118: 3153–3164.
51. Sanderson Cox L, Patten CA, Ebbert JO, *et al.* Tobacco use outcomes among patients with lung cancer treated for nicotine dependence. *J Clin Oncol* 2002; 20: 3461–3469.
52. Walker MS, Vidrine DJ, Gritz ER, *et al.* Smoking relapse during the first year after treatment for early-stage non-small-cell lung cancer. *Cancer Epidemiol Biomarkers Prev* 2006; 15: 2370–2377.
53. Eng L, Su J, Qiu X, *et al.* Second-hand smoke as a predictor of smoking cessation among lung cancer survivors. *J Clin Oncol* 2014; 32: 564–570.
54. Ebbert JO, Yang P, Vachon CM, *et al.* Lung cancer risk reduction after smoking cessation: observations from a prospective cohort of women. *J Clin Oncol* 2003; 21: 921–926.
55. Guo NL, Tosun K, Horn K. Impact and interactions between smoking and traditional prognostic factors in lung cancer progression. *Lung Cancer* 2009; 66: 386–392.
56. Warren GW, Kasza KA, Reid M, *et al.* Smoking at diagnosis and survival in cancer patients. *Int J Cancer* 2013; 132: 401–410.
57. Ferketich AK, Niland JC, Mamet R, *et al.* Smoking status and survival in the national comprehensive cancer network non-small cell lung cancer cohort. *Cancer* 2013; 119: 847–853.
58. Parsons A, Daley A, Begh R, *et al.* Influence of smoking cessation after diagnosis of early stage lung cancer on prognosis: systematic review of observational studies with meta-analysis. *BMJ* 2010; 340: b5569.
59. Mitchell P, Mok T, Barraclough H, *et al.* Smoking history as a predictive factor of treatment response in advanced non-small-cell lung cancer: a systematic review. *Clin Lung Cancer* 2012; 13: 239–251.
60. Rice D, Kim HW, Sabichi A, *et al.* The risk of second primary tumors after resection of stage I nonsmall cell lung cancer. *Ann Thorac Surg* 2003; 76: 1001–1007.

61. Møller A, Villebro N, Pedersen T, *et al.* Effect of preoperative smoking intervention on postoperative complications: a randomised clinical trial. *Lancet* 2002; 359: 114–117.
62. Barrera R, Shi W, Amar D, *et al.* Smoking and timing of cessation: impact on pulmonary complications after thoracotomy. *Chest* 2005; 127: 1977–1983.
63. Yildizeli B, Fadel E, Mussot S, *et al.* Morbidity, mortality, and long-term survival after sleeve lobectomy for non-small cell lung cancer. *Eur J Cardiothorac Surg* 2007; 31: 95–102.
64. Suzuki M, Otsuji M, Baba M, *et al.* Bronchopleural fistula after lung cancer surgery: multivariate analysis of risk factors. *J Cardiovasc Surg* 2002; 43: 263–267.
65. Myers K, Hajek P, Hinds C, *et al.* Stopping smoking shortly before surgery and postoperative complications: a systematic review and meta-analysis. *Arch Intern Med* 2011; 171: 983–989.
66. Thomsen T, Villebro N, Møller AM. Interventions for preoperative smoking cessation. *Cochrane Database Syst Rev* 2010; 7: CD002294.
67. Schmidt-Hansen M, Page R, Hasler E. The effect of preoperative smoking cessation or preoperative pulmonary rehabilitation on outcomes after lung cancer surgery: a systematic review. *Clin Lung Cancer* 2013; 14: 96–102.
68. Mills E, Eyawo O, Lockhart I, *et al.* Smoking cessation reduces postoperative complications: a systematic review and meta-analysis. *Am J Med* 2011; 124: 144–154.
69. Cooley ME, Wang Q, Johnson BE, *et al.* Factors associated with smoking abstinence among smokers and recent-quitters with lung and head and neck cancer. *Lung Cancer* 2012; 76: 144–149.
70. Duarte RL, Luiz RR, Paschoal ME. The cigarette burden (measured by the number of pack-years smoked) negatively impacts the response rate to platinum-based chemotherapy in lung cancer patients. *Lung Cancer* 2008; 61: 244–254.
71. Mohan A, Singh P, Kumar S, *et al.* Effect of change in symptoms, respiratory status, nutritional profile and quality of life on response to treatment for advanced non-small cell lung cancer. *Asian Pac J Cancer Prev* 2008; 9: 557–562.
72. van der Bol JM, Mathijssen RHJ, Loos WJ, *et al.* Cigarette smoking and irinotecan treatment: pharmacokinetic interaction and effects on neutropenia. *J Clin Oncol* 2007; 25: 2719–2726.
73. Shepherd FA, Rodrigues Pereira J, Ciuleanu T, *et al.* Erlotinib in previously treated non-small cell lung cancer. *N Engl J Med* 2005; 353: 123–132.
74. Monson J, Stark P, Reilly J. Clinical radiation pneumonitis and radiographic changes after thoracic radiation therapy for lung carcinoma. *Cancer* 1998; 82: 842–850.
75. Sarihan S, Ercan I, Saran A, *et al.* Evaluation of infections in non-small cell lung cancer patients treated with radiotherapy. *Cancer Detect Prev* 2005; 29: 181–188.
76. Gritz E, Lam CY, Vidrine DJ, *et al.* Cancer prevention: tobacco dependence and its treatment. *In*: DeVita VT Lawrence TS Rosenberg SA DePinho RA Weinberg RA, eds. Cancer: Principles and Practice of Oncology. Volume 2. 8th Edn. Philadelphia, Lippincott Williams and Williams, 2008; pp. 593–608.
77. Fox JL, Rosenzweig KE, Ostroff JS. The effect of smoking status on survival following radiation therapy for non-small cell lung cancer. *Lung Cancer* 2004; 44: 287–293.
78. Videtic GM, Stitt LW, Dar AR, *et al.* Continued cigarette smoking by patients receiving concurrent chemoradiotherapy for limited-stage small-cell lung cancer is associated with decreased survival. *J Clin Oncol* 2003; 21: 1544–1549.
79. Balduyck B, Sardari Nia P, Cogen A, *et al.* The effect of smoking cessation on quality of life after lung cancer surgery. *Eur J Cardiothorac Surg* 2011; 40: 1432–1437.
80. Chen J, Qi Y, Wampfler JA, *et al.* Effect of cigarette smoking on quality of life in small cell lung cancer patients. *Eur J Cancer* 2012; 48: 1593–1601.
81. Myrdal G, Valtysdottir S, Lambe M, *et al.* Quality of life following lung cancer surgery. *Thorax* 2003; 58: 194–197.
82. Sarna L, Padilla G, Holmes C, *et al.* Quality of life of long-term survivors of non-small-cell lung cancer. *J Clin Oncol* 2002; 20: 2920–2929.
83. Garces YI, Yang P, Parkinson J, *et al.* The relationship between cigarette smoking and quality of life after lung cancer diagnosis. *Chest* 2004; 126: 1733–1741.
84. Baser S, Shannon V, Eapen G, *et al.* Smoking cessation after diagnosis of lung cancer is associated with a beneficial effect on performance status. *Chest* 2006; 130: 1784–1790.
85. Cooley ME. Symptoms in adults with lung cancer. A systematic research review. *J Pain Symptom Manage* 2000; 19: 137–153.
86. Weaver KE, Rowland JH, Augustson E, *et al.* Smoking concordance in lung and colorectal cancer patient-caregiver dyads and quality of life. *Cancer Epidemiol Biomarkers Prev* 2011; 20: 239–248.
87. Cox LS, Clark MM, Jett JR, *et al.* Change in smoking status after spiral chest computed tomography scan screening. *Cancer* 2003; 98: 2495–2501.
88. Styn MA, Land SR, Perkins KA, *et al.* Smoking behavior 1 year after computed tomography screening for lung cancer: effect of physician referral for abnormal CT findings. *Cancer Epidemiol Biomarkers Prev* 2009; 18: 3484–3489.

89. Tammemägi MC, Berg CD, Riley TL, *et al.* Impact of lung cancer screening results on smoking cessation. *J Natl Cancer Inst* 2014; 106: dju084.
90. Nayan S, Gupta MK, Sommer DD. Evaluating smoking cessation interventions and cessation rates in cancer patients: a systematic review and meta-analysis. *ISRN Oncol* 2011; 2011: 849023.
91. Warren GW, Marshall JR, Cummings KM, *et al.* Practice patterns and perceptions of thoracic oncology providers on tobacco use and cessation in cancer patients. *J Thorac Oncol* 2013; 8: 543–548.
92. Cahill K, Stevens S, Perera R, *et al.* Pharmacological interventions for smoking cessation: an overview and network meta-analysis. *Cochrane Database Syst Rev* 2013; 5: CD009329.
93. Jiménez-Ruiz C, Berlin I, Hering T. Varenicline: a novel pharmacotherapy for smoking cessation. *Drugs* 2009; 69: 1319–1338.
94. Wallström M, Sand L, Nilsson F, *et al.* The long-term effect of nicotine on the oral mucosa. *Addiction* 1999; 94: 417–423.
95. Warren GW, Romano MA, Kudrimoti MR, *et al.* Nicotinic modulation of therapeutic response *in vitro* and *in vivo*. *Int J Cancer* 2012; 131: 2519–2527.
96. Murray RP, Connett JE, Zapawa LM. Does nicotine replacement therapy cause cancer? Evidence from the Lung Health Study. *Nicotine Tob Res* 2009; 11: 1076–1182.
97. McRobbie H, Bullen C, Hartmann-Boyce J, *et al.* Electronic cigarettes for smoking cessation and reduction. *Cochrane Database Syst Rev* 2014; 12: CD010216.
98. Hanna N, Mulshine J, Wollins DS, *et al.* Tobacco cessation and control a decade later: American Society of Clinical Oncology Policy Statement Update. *J Clin Oncol* 2013; 31: 3147–3157.

Disclosures: None declared.

Chapter 4

# The association with COPD

Juan P. de-Torres and Javier J. Zulueta

Epidemiological and case–control studies have shown that COPD is an independent risk factor for lung cancer. The presence of airway obstruction and/or emphysema increases the risk of having lung cancer by two to three fold. Recent research has highlighted several potential common pathways that may explain this deadly association. These include chronic retention of airborne carcinogens, the presence of chronic inflammation, and common genetic and epigenetic risk factors.

Smoking prevention and smoking cessation are the most important measures for primary prevention of both COPD and lung cancer. Recent data suggest that lung cancer screening in patients with COPD, especially those with mild-to-moderate disease, could potentially decrease lung cancer mortality, one of the most common causes of death.

The association between COPD and lung cancer means that the clinical management of these patients requires a multidisciplinary team that includes a respiratory medicine physician. The pulmonologist's role ranges from determining preoperative risk to handling the consequences of oncologic treatments, such as COPD exacerbations.

COPD and lung cancer are amongst the top five causes of death, and both diseases have seen their death tolls increase in the last few decades [1]. In addition to sharing the main aetiological factor, *i.e.* tobacco smoking, it has been suggested that each disease has specific biopathogenic pathways that confer a synergistic relationship between them with bidirectional implications [2]. Most of this information is speculative and should be confirmed in specifically designed studies.

Lung cancer patients have a worse outcome if they also have COPD [3]. However, individuals with COPD have an increased risk of developing lung cancer, independent of smoking history, age and sex [4]. Several authors have suggested that radiological emphysema is one of the strongest markers of lung cancer risk and might be an important criterion in the selection of high-risk individuals who may benefit most from lung cancer screening programmes [5, 6].

Lung cancer screening and emphysema as selection criteria for screening are areas of the field with novel information and the most promising results.

Pulmonary Dept, Clínica Universidad de Navarra, Pamplona, Spain.

Correspondence: Juan P. de-Torres, Pulmonary Dept, Clínica Universidad de Navarra, Pamplona, 31200, Spain. E-mail: jpdetorres@unav.es

 Print ISBN: 978-1-84984-061-3. Online ISBN: 978-1-84984-062-0. Print ISSN: 2312-508X. Online ISSN: 2312-5098.

## Evidence of the association between COPD and lung cancer

As well as being amongst the most important causes of death worldwide [1], both lung cancer and COPD are amongst the top four causes of years of life lost, years living with a disability and disability-adjusted life years [1]. Despite the enormous impact on the lives of patients and their relatives, as well as on healthcare systems, COPD is greatly underdiagnosed and undertreated globally [7, 8]. Lung cancer has a dismal prognosis because it is usually diagnosed at an advanced, incurable stage [9]. However, the recent publication of the results of the National Lung Screening Trial (NLST) [10] and of numerous guidelines [11–15], which favourably recommend lung cancer screening with low-dose CT (LDCT) in high-risk individuals, has completely changed the future of this disease. The link between lung cancer and COPD has been suggested by several epidemiological, pharmacological and observational studies. These are summarised in table 1.

Between 1985 and 2005, several studies observed that impaired lung function, as measured by $FEV_1$, was associated with an increased risk of lung cancer [4, 16–21]. The findings of these studies are summarised below.

Skillrud *et al.* [4] were the first to postulate the idea of an independent relationship between COPD and lung cancer. For 10 years, they followed 113 smokers with COPD and $FEV_1$% >70%, and 113 controls without COPD with the same age, sex and pack-years history. They found that lung cancer incidence was four times higher in COPD patients than in controls.

Tockman *et al.* [16] examined lung cancer development in a sample of patients with moderate-to-severe obstruction who were included in the Intermittent Positive Pressure Breathing Trial, and a sample of patients with no-to-moderate obstruction from the Johns

Table 1. Studies supporting the association between COPD, emphysema and lung cancer

| First author [ref.] | Patients n | Effect of COPD/emphysema on lung cancer risk | Lung cancer |
|---|---|---|---|
| **Skillrud [4]** | 226 | Increased incidence of lung cancer in patients with COPD | Incidence |
| **de Torres [5]** | 1166 | Increased incidence of lung cancer in individuals with emphysema | Incidence |
| **Wilson [6]** | 3638 | Increased incidence of lung cancer in individuals with emphysema | Incidence |
| **Tockman [16]** | 4395 | Increased mortality with decreased $FEV_1$ % | Mortality |
| **Kuller [17]** | 361 662 | Increased mortality with decreased $FEV_1$ % | Mortality |
| **Wasswa-Kintu [18]** | Meta-analysis | Increased mortality with decreased $FEV_1$ % | Diagnosis |
| **Anthonisen [19]** | 5887 | 33% of mild COPD patients died from lung cancer | Mortality |
| **de Torres [20]** | 2507 | 23.7% of COPD patients died from lung cancer | Mortality |
| **Mannino [21]** | 5402 | Increased mortality with decreased $FEV_1$ % | Incidence |
| **Smith [22]** | Meta-analysis | Visually determined emphysema was shown to better assess lung cancer risk than the software evaluated | Incidence/mortality |

Hopkins Lung Project. They found that in smokers, the presence of COPD was more of an indicator of subsequent development of lung cancer than age or the level of smoking.

Kuller *et al.* [17] studied men participating in the Multiple Risk Factor Intervention Trial, evaluating the relationship between baseline $FEV_1$ and lung cancer mortality among smokers between the third and 10th year of follow-up. $FEV_1$ was a powerful predictor of lung cancer death, with increased mortality rates (3.02 deaths per 1000 person-years) among those in the lowest $FEV_1$ quintile, as compared to 0.43 deaths per 1000 person-years among those in the highest quintile (better lung function), even after adjusting for smoking dose, duration of smoking, or age at onset of smoking.

Wasswa-Kintu *et al.* [18] performed a systematic review and meta-analysis of the studies published in PubMed and EMBASE from January 1966 to January 2005. They found that the risk of lung cancer increased with decreasing $FEV_1$. When compared with the highest $FEV_1$ quintile (>100% predicted), the lowest $FEV_1$ quintile (approximately <70% pred) was associated with a 2.23-fold increase in the risk of lung cancer in men (95% CI 1.73–2.86) and a 3.97-fold increase in women (95% CI 1.93–8.25). Even relatively small decrements of $FEV_1$ (~90% pred) increased the risk of lung cancer by 30% in men (95% CI 1.05–1.62) and 2.64 fold in women (95% CI 1.30–5.31) [18]. More recently, several pharmacological studies (TORCH (Towards a Revolution in COPD Health) and UPLIFT (Understanding Potential Long-term Impacts on Function with Tiotropium)) have suggested that lung cancer is amongst the most common causes of death in COPD patients, reporting lung cancer mortality in 15–25% of the patients [23, 24]. Another hallmark study was the Lung Health Study (LHS) [19], a randomised clinical trial of smoking cessation in 5887 smokers 35–60 years of age with evidence of mild to moderate airway obstruction followed for about 14.5 years. The LHS found that 32–33% of the participants died of lung cancer. Finally, the BODE (body mass index (BMI), airflow obstruction, dyspnoea, exercise capacity) study, which had a 5-year mean follow-up, showed that 24% of the 2507 patients died of lung cancer [20].

Mannino *et al.* [21] analysed data from the First National Health and Nutrition Examination Survey (NHANES), which has up to 22 years of follow-up, and found that the presence of moderate or severe obstruction was associated with a higher risk of incident lung cancer (hazard ratio 2.8; 95% CI 1.8–4.4) [21]. In the above-mentioned BODE study, de Torres *et al.* [20] observed an inverse relationship between the degree of airway obstruction and lung cancer death. In comparison with patients at Global Initiative for Chronic Obstructive Lung Disease (GOLD) stages III and IV, those at GOLD stages I and II had a 2–3-fold greater risk of dying from lung cancer [20]. This surprising finding challenges the notion that the risk of lung cancer increases as lung function worsens; specifically designed studies are required to confirm these findings.

To consider this from a different angle, spirometrically documented airway obstruction is present at the time of lung cancer diagnosis in up to 73% of men and 52% of women. In a matched controlled community-based study, the prevalence of COPD in individuals with and without lung cancer was 50% and 8%, respectively [25].

## The importance of emphysema

The use of detailed imaging techniques, such as CT, in large lung cancer screening studies conducted in the last 20 years has led to important advances in the understanding of emphysema and its potential role in the association between COPD and lung cancer. DE TORRES *et al.* [5] and WILSON *et al.* [6] conducted similar studies in the setting of lung cancer screening trials, and came to very similar conclusions: the presence of emphysema on a baseline LDCT increases the risk of lung cancer 2–3 fold, independent of tobacco history, age, sex, airway obstruction and body mass index [5, 6]. These findings have subsequently been confirmed by other studies [26]. Interestingly, in a meta-analysis in which all of the studies reported the association between emphysema and lung cancer, it was found that this association holds true only when emphysema is determined qualitatively by a radiologist [22]. In studies in which quantitative determinations were performed with image analysis software, the association between emphysema and lung cancer was not significant [26, 27]. The reasons for this paradox are yet to be explained.

### Histological types of lung cancer in patients with COPD

Traditionally, the most frequent histological type of lung cancer in patients with COPD is NSCLC, present in up to 80–85% of the cases, with ADC incidence tending to surpass that of SCC in both sexes [28].

In a case–control study of 86 lung cancer patients and 54 controls, PAPI *et al.* [29] showed that airflow obstruction is a risk factor for SCC. In the aforementioned study by DE TORRES *et al.* [20], SCC was the most frequent histological type in GOLD stages II and III, although ADC was the most common in GOLD stage I.

## Mechanistic links between COPD and lung cancer

There are certain hallmark pathogenic pathways in COPD and emphysema (increased apoptosis, matrix degradation and repair, activation of the immune response) that are essentially opposed to those associated with lung cancer (decreased apoptosis, DNA damage/repair, genome instability, clonal expansion, invasion angiogenesis). However, it has been hypothesised that several basic mechanisms link both diseases. Table 2 summarises the proposed mechanisms to explain this association.

All of these suggested mechanisms are merely speculative and based on research that was not performed in COPD patients with lung cancer. Ongoing investigations are trying to confirm these hypotheses in appropriately designed animal and human studies.

### Chronic retention of airborne carcinogens

COPD is characterised by two different pathological processes: parenchymal destruction, namely emphysema; and small airway obstruction, represented by chronic bronchitis [8]. These phenotypes have in common the presence of chronic nonreversible airway obstruction that causes air retention and suppression of the clearance of secretions. Several investigators have postulated that this scenario causes chronic exposure to carcinogens and repetitive stimulation of bronchoalveolar stem cells, a potential initial step in lung carcinogenesis [30]. This is a speculative hypothesis that is not supported by objective data.

Table 2. Summary of the mechanisms proposed to explain the association between COPD and lung cancer

| |
|---|
| **Chronic inflammation** |
| "Useless" cycles of tissue injury and repair |
| Unstable DNA-replicative activity susceptible to mutagenic hits from inflammatory mediators |
| Shift from M1 to M2 polarised macrophages in COPD airways that may weaken anti-tumoural surveillance |
| STAT3 and NF-κβ activation |
| In emphysema, neutrophil elastase and MMP-12 that could promote tumour loci and growth |
| **Retention of airborne carcinogens** |
| Chronic exposure to carcinogens |
| Repetitive stimulation of BASC |
| **Genetic factors: candidate genes** |
| *CHRNA3/5* |
| *HHIP* |
| *TERT* |
| **Epigenetics factors** |
| DNA hypermethylation |
| HDACs |
| HATs |
| Micro RNA |

STAT3: signal transducer and activator of transcription 3; NF-κβ: nuclear factor-κβ; MMP-12: matrix metallopeptidase-12; BASC: bronchoalveolar stem cell; *CHRNA3/5*: acetyl cholinergic nicotinic receptor subunits α3 and α5; *HHIP*: hedgehog interacting protein; *TERT*: telomerase reverse transcriptase; HDAC: histone deacetylase; HAT: histone acetylase.

## Chronic inflammation

Chronic low grade inflammation is present in ~25–30% of patients with COPD [31] and data from epidemiological studies suggest that its presence predicts the development of the most frequent comorbidities of the disease [32]. The association between inflammation and cancer development is well known: persistent tissue inflammation can trigger malignant transformation and promote tumour progression [33]. Indeed, in the setting of chronic inflammation, the abundance of "useless" cycles of tissue injury and repair is key in the progression to malignant degeneration [33].

Cellular damage can activate two events: the induction of cell death, which recruits more inflammatory cells; and the loss of tissue integrity, which triggers a regenerative response with the recruitment of quiescent tissue stem cells into the cell cycle [34]. In this tissue repair phase, there is a highly unstable DNA-replicative activity susceptible to mutagenic hits from inflammatory mediators and/or environmental carcinogens (cigarette smoke). A small percentage of cells will escape the pro-apoptotic safety switches and will accumulate sufficient genetic and epigenetic changes to progress towards the path of dysplasia, *in situ* carcinoma and invasive cancer [35]. In normal circumstances, there is an active "immune surveillance" operating against the emergence of malignant cell clones. The recruitment of innate inflammatory cells can result in the suppression of this protection [36]. These are myeloid-derived suppressor cells (MDSCs), a heterogeneous population of immature leukocytes that includes monocytes/macrophages and neutrophils. In humans, there is an unclear line separating MDSCs from tumour-associated macrophages, which are present in injured tissue and which execute a molecular programme that suppresses cellular immunity while supporting tissue repair [37].

A recent report revealed the potential role of Langerhans' cells (antigen-presenting cells distributed in the bronchial epithelium), which metabolise polycyclic aromatic hydrocarbons to carcinogenic intermediates [38]. As a recent report showed that Langerhans' cells are increased in the small airways of COPD patients [39], one could speculate that these cells may enhance the carcinogenic effect of tobacco smoke.

Several reports have linked inflammation and oncogenesis by suggesting that the intracellular protein STAT3 (signal transducer and activator of transcription 3) has an essential role. The activation of this transcription factor occurs downstream of pathways associated with interleukin (IL)-6, EGF and VEGF, which are involved in inflammation, epithelial repair and angiogenesis, respectively [40]. On its own, STAT3 activity controls most of the classic and emerging hallmarks of carcinogenesis, promoting inflammation and the avoidance of immune destruction [41].

Another possible association of inflammation and carcinogenesis in COPD patients is *via* the activation of nuclear factor (NF)-κβ after smoke exposure in the airways and in the lung parenchyma [42]. Nuclear translocation of NF-κβ could be indirectly oncogenic through pro-inflammatory mediators, and directly oncogenic by activating anti-apoptotic proteins [43].

The potential role of neutrophil elastase and matrix metallopeptidase (MMP)-12 has also been suggested in patients with emphysema. Neutrophil elastase can degrade insulin receptor substrate (IRS)1, increasing the interaction between Pl3K and platelet-derived growth factor receptor, resulting in increased proliferation of tumour cells [44, 45]. MMP-12 can sustain chronic inflammation and tissue remodelling years after smoking cessation, but most importantly, this process could lead to pulmonary foci of ADC in an IL-6/STAT3-dependent manner [46]).

## Genetic and epigenetic factors

Genome-wide association studies have demonstrated common chromosomal loci and candidate genes that might be implicated in the shared genetic susceptibility for COPD and lung cancer [47]. One of these loci is 15q25, which encodes for *CHRNA3/5* (acetyl cholinergic nicotinic receptor subunits α3 and α5) [48]. In addition to its neurotropic properties, which are associated with nicotine addiction, it also affects bronchial epithelial cells. Nicotinic receptor activation in normal airway epithelial cells boosts a response towards malignant degeneration by increasing the proliferation rate, inhibiting apoptosis and inducing inflammation [49]. The loci 4q31, which encodes *HHIP* (hedgehog interacting protein), is a transmembrane protein of an ancient intercellular communication pathway involved in organ development and stem cell biology [50]. Hedgehog signalling in the lung is involved in bronchial tree embryogenesis [51] and participates in the repeated cycles of injury and repair that lead to an increased risk of malignant degeneration in the presence of mutagenic factors. The hedgehog pathway's effects on the epithelial mesenchymal transition (EMT) mean it provides a potential common pathogenic background through the expression of mesenchymal proteins, loss of epithelial integrity and increase cell motility [52]. Among the candidate genes, hTERT (human telomerase reverse transcriptase) has been identified in the 5p15.33 region [53]. Both COPD and lung cancer have been associated with signs of early senescence, including reduced telomerase activity and shorter telomere length [54, 55]. Telomere signals have been shown to decrease significantly even in squamous metaplasia, indicating that telomere shortening could be an early genetic marker of bronchial carcinogenesis [56].

Epigenetics define many types of phenotype or gene expression alterations that are not encoded in the DNA sequence. DNA hypermethylation at promoter regions is a typical epigenetic mechanism that affects gene transcription involved in oncogenesis, particularly in lung cancer. Hypermethylation has been described in COPD and has been associated with quicker lung function decline. It has also been described in association with progression from cell hyperplasia, to squamous metaplasia and carcinoma *in situ* [57]. The second major epigenetic mechanism occurs through histone acetyltransferase (HAT) and histone deacetylaces (HDACs), which affect the degree of chromatin winding around histone complexes, thus controlling the access of RNA polymerases and transcription factors to gene promoter regions. Decreased levels of HDAC activity have been described with increasing severity of COPD [58]. Oxidative stress and chronic inflammation, both of which are increased in COPD patients, are associated with deactivation of HDACs while simultaneously stimulating HAT. Some HDACs (such as HDAC-3) deacetylate NF-κβ, resulting in the termination of pro-inflammatory gene transcription [59]. Conversely, NF-κβ acetylation promotes prolonged NF-κβ activity, a phenomenon reported in cancer, providing further evidence of the epigenetic link between inflammation and oncogenesis [43].

Lastly, non-coding RNA, called microRNAs (miRNAs), can selectively repress the translation of many biologically related genes at once [60]. These short single strands of RNA specifically bind to sequences at the 3-unstranslated end of mRNA strands, and either block protein translation or lead to degradation of target mRNA, miRNA hybrid. A recent study showed that miRNAs are significantly downregulated in COPD patients [61]. The fact that some miRNAs work as tumour suppressor agents and that their levels predict prognosis in lung cancer [62], adds support to a potential role in carcinogenesis in COPD patients.

## Clinical consequences of the COPD–lung cancer association

The links between COPD and lung cancer may have important implications in the clinical management of both disease, particularly in the realms of prevention and treatment.

### Primary prevention

There is no doubt that foremost in the battle against COPD and lung cancer is smoking prevention and smoking cessation. Smoking cessation should be offered to all smokers as early as possible as available data indicate that the age of quitting is key in determining future risk [63].

## Secondary prevention

This strategy mainly focuses on reducing the risk of developing lung cancer in patients already diagnosed with COPD. It includes pharmacological treatments and nonpharmacological interventions.

### *Pharmacological treatment*

Several studies suggest the potential beneficial effects of statins on inflammatory cytokine production, neutrophil influx, matrix degradation and EMT [64]. Conflicting data have been published that explore the possible preventive effects of these agents in lung cancer. An observational study from Denmark has shown that statin use commenced before cancer diagnosis was associated with reduced cancer-related mortality [65]. In contrast, a large meta-analysis that included 175 000 statin-using individuals from 27 randomised trials, failed to demonstrate a reduction in the incidence of cancer mortality, including lung cancer [66].

Preliminary studies generated enthusiasm about the use of inhaled corticosteroids for the reduction of lung cancer mortality in COPD patients [67]. However, large prospective trials have failed to demonstrate such a benefit [23].

Cyclooxygenase (COX) signalling was considered another potential target of chemoprevention due to its potential role in carcinogenesis through the production of prostaglandin (PG)$E_2$, a promoter of resistance to apoptosis, increased dysplasia and enhanced invasion [68]. A recent phase IIb trial of the $PGE_2$ inhibitor celecoxib in a high-risk population of smokers, demonstrated a reduction of proliferating antigens in the bronchial epithelium, a surrogate marker for lung cancer risk [69]. Unfortunately, celecoxib's high cardiovascular risk profile limits its use, especially in patients with COPD who already have a high risk for cardiovascular events. Another way to interact with the COX pathway is to enhance the production of $PGI_2$, a counterpart to $PGE_2$, which is usually underexpressed in cancer. Furthermore, oral prostacyclin (iloprost) was recently tested in smokers with endobronchial dysplasia with promising results [70].

Epigenetic pathways have also been investigated as potential targets for chemoprevention. By activating HDAC2, theophylline indirectly suppresses NF-κβ, thus restoring sensitivity to corticosteroids in COPD patients. In experimental studies with mice, this strategy reduces carcinogen-induced cancers [71]. Studies in humans are underway.

### *Nonpharmacological measures: lung cancer screening*

Lung cancer screening may be most effective in individuals with COPD, particularly in patients who also have emphysema [5, 6]. In a preliminary study, de Torres *et al.* [72] analysed the effect of lung cancer screening, comparing two cohorts of COPD patients matched for lung function, sex, age, smoking and demographics. One cohort underwent screening and the other did not. In comparison with the cohort in which screening was not performed, where 100% of the cancers were diagnosed in advanced stages, 80% of lung cancer cases in the screening cohort were diagnosed at stage I or II. Interestingly, the number of screenings that needed to be performed to diagnose one lung cancer case in the screening cohort was only 34.

Patients with COPD seem to be good candidates for lung cancer screening. With this in mind, de Torres *et al.* [73] recently proposed the COPD Lung Cancer Screening Score (COPD-LUCSS), a 0–10-point score (predictor variables included: >60 years of age, >60 pack-years, BMI <25 and emphysema presence on the CT) that helped identify those who were at high risk (7–10 points) and were potentially the best candidates for screening. Although COPD-LUCSS is derived from a USA-based screening population and validated in a Spanish screening cohort of COPD patients, it should also be validated in different COPD populations. An ongoing study in Japan is investigating the potential role of screening COPD in the primary care setting [74].

## Treatment implications

### *COPD patients*

The diagnosis of lung cancer in a COPD patient is usually associated with a dismal prognosis due to the fact that most are diagnosed at advanced incurable stages (III–IV). In view of the high incidence of lung cancer in COPD patients, lung cancer screening may turn out to be the most effective intervention known to date for the reduction of mortality. However, several issues regarding curative treatment of lung cancer in COPD patients will have to be considered. To begin with, the risk of perioperative complications is higher in COPD patients [75]. Preoperative evaluations will therefore need to be thorough. The role of limited resection as compared to lobectomy, the current gold standard, has been evaluated in a randomised controlled study [76]. This might be very important for COPD patients with lung function limitations. Several reports have shown that surgical removal of lung cancer may result in improved lung function in individuals with emphysema because of lung volume reduction [77]. As more patients with COPD are diagnosed with lung cancer at earlier stages, these surgical issues will have to be considered more frequently. In patients with nonsurgical, early stage lung cancer due to limited lung function, other therapeutic options, such as stereotactic modulated radiation therapy, could be considered [78].

### *Lung cancer patients*

The prevalence of COPD in individuals diagnosed with lung cancer is also high [79]. Oncologists and thoracic surgeons should keep it in mind that COPD requires continuous treatment. Furthermore, complications derived from oncological treatments can significantly affect the natural history of COPD, particularly by promoting exacerbations of the disease. As we foresee increasingly early stage lung cancer diagnoses in patients with COPD, multidisciplinary teams that include respiratory medicine specialists are mandatory in the management of patients with both conditions.

## References


1. Murray CJ, Lopez AD. Measuring the global burden of disease. *N Engl J Med* 2013; 369: 448–457.
2. Vermaelen K, Brusselle G. Exposing a deadly alliance: novel insights into the biological links between COPD and lung cancer. *Pulm Pharmacol Ther* 2013; 26: 544–554.
3. Young RP, Hopkins RJ, Christmas T, *et al.* COPD prevalence is increased in lung cancer, independent of age, sex and smoking history. *Eur Respir J* 2009; 34: 380–386.
4. Skillrud DM, Offord KP, Miller RD. Higher risk of lung cancer in chronic obstructive pulmonary disease. A prospective, matched, controlled study. *Ann Intern Med* 1986; 105: 503–507.
5. de Torres JP, Bastarrika G, Wisnivesky JP, *et al.* Assessing the relationship between lung cancer risk and emphysema detected on low-dose CT of the chest. *Chest* 2007; 132: 1932–1938.
6. Wilson DO, Weissfeld JL, Balkan A, *et al.* Association of radiographic emphysema and airflow obstruction with lung cancer. *Am J Respir Crit Care Med* 2008; 178: 738–744.
7. Soriano JB, Lamprecht B. Chronic obstructive pulmonary disease: a worldwide problem. *Med Clin North Am* 2012; 96: 671–680.
8. Vestbo J, Hurd SS, Agustí AG, *et al.* Global strategy for the diagnosis, management, and prevention of chronic obstructive pulmonary disease: GOLD executive summary. *Am J Respir Crit Care Med* 2013; 187: 347–365.

9. Pirozynski M. 100 years of lung cancer. *Respir Med* 2006; 100: 2073–2084.
10. Aberle D, Adams A, Berg C, *et al.* Reduced lung-cancer mortality with low-dose computed tomographic screening. *N Engl J Med* 2011; 365: 395–409.
11. American Lung Association. Providing guidance on lung cancer screening to patients and physicians. April 23, 2012. http://www.lung.org/lung-disease/lung-cancer/lung-cancer-screening-guidelines/lung-cancer-screening.pdf. Date last accessed: October 17, 2013.
12. Detterbeck FC, Mazzone PJ, Naidich DP, *et al.* Screening for lung cancer: diagnosis and management of lung cancer, 3rd ed: American College of Chest Physicians evidence-based clinical practice guidelines. *Chest* 2013; 143: e78S–e92S.
13. Jaklitsch MT, Jacobson FL, Austin JHM, *et al.* The American Association for Thoracic Surgery guidelines for lung cancer screening using low-dose computed tomography scans for lung cancer survivors and other high-risk groups. *J Thorac Cardiovasc Surg* 2012; 144: 33–38.
14. Wender R, Fontham ETH, Barrera E, *et al.* American Cancer Society lung cancer screening guidelines. *CA Cancer J Clin* 2013; 63: 107–117.
15. Moyer VA, U.S. Preventive Services Task Force. Screening for lung cancer: US Preventive Services Task Force recommendation statement. *Ann Intern Med* 2014; 160: 330–338.
16. Tockman MS, Anthonisen NR, Wright EC, *et al.* Airway obstruction and the risk for lung cancer. *Ann Intern Med* 1987; 106: 512–518.
17. Kuller LH, Ockene J, Meilahn E, *et al.* Relation of forced expiratory volume in one second (FEV1) to lung cancer mortality in the Multiple Risk Factor Intervention Trial (MRFIT). *Am J Epidemiol* 1990; 132: 265–274.
18. Wasswa-Kintu S, Gan WQ, Man SF, *et al.* Relationship between reduced forced expiratory volume in one second and the risk of lung cancer: a systematic review and meta-analysis. *Thorax* 2005; 60: 570–575.
19. Anthonisen NR1, Skeans MA, Wise RA, *et al.* The effects of a smoking cessation intervention on 14.5-year mortality: a randomized clinical trial. *Ann Intern Med* 2005; 142: 233–239.
20. de Torres JP, Marín JM, Casanova C, *et al.* Lung cancer in patients with chronic obstructive pulmonary disease-incidence and predicting factors. *Am J Respir Crit Care Med* 2011; 184: 913–919.
21. Mannino DM, Aguayo SM, Petty TL, *et al.* Low lung function and incident lung cancer in the United States: data from the First National Health and Nutrition Examination Survey follow-up. *Arch Intern Med* 2003; 163: 1475–1480.
22. Smith BM, Pinto L, Ezer N, *et al.* Emphysema detected on computed tomography and risk of lung cancer: a systematic review and meta-analysis. *Lung Cancer* 2012; 77: 58–63.
23. Calverley PM, Anderson JA, Celli B, *et al.* Salmeterol and fluticasone propionate and survival in chronic obstructive pulmonary disease. *N Engl J Med* 2007; 356: 775–789.
24. Tashkin DP, Celli B, Senn S, *et al.* A 4-year trial of tiotropium in chronic obstructive pulmonary disease. *N Engl J Med* 2008; 359: 1543–1554.
25. Loganathan RS1, Stover DE, Shi W, *et al.* Prevalence of COPD in women compared to men around the time of diagnosis of primary lung cancer. *Chest* 2006; 129: 1305–1312.
26. Zueluta JJ, Wisnivesky JP, Henschke C. *et al*, Emphysema socres predict death from COPD and lung cancer. *Chest* 2012; 141: 1216–1223.
27. Sverzellati N, Randi G, Calabro E, *et al.* Relationshp between lung cancer and pulmonary emphysema. *Insights into Imagingm* 2011; 2: S135–S324.
28. Gabrielson E. Worldwide trends in lung cancer pathology. *Respirology* 2006; 11: 533–538.
29. Papi A, Casoni G, Caramori G, *et al.* COPD increases the risk of squamous histological subtype in smokers who develop non-small cell lung carcinoma. *Thorax* 2004; 59: 679–681.
30. Houghton AM, Mouded M, Shapiro SD. Common origins of lung cancer and COPD. *Nat Med* 2008; 14: 1023–1024.
31. Agustí A, Edwards LD, Rennard SI, *et al.* Persistent systemic inflammation is associated with poor clinical outcomes in COPD: a novel phenotype. *PLoS One* 2012; 7: e37483.
32. Miller J, Edwards LD, Agustí A, *et al.* Comorbidity, systemic inflammation and outcomes in the ECLIPSE cohort. *Respir Med* 2013; 107: 1376–1384.
33. Vakkila J, Lotze MT. Inflammation and necrosis promote tumour growth. *Nat Rev Immunol* 2004; 4: 641–648.
34. Ferguson LR, Laing WA. Chronic inflammation, mutation and human disease. *Mutat Res* 2010; 690: 1–2.
35. Dixon K1, Kopras E. Genetic alterations and DNA repair in human carcinogenesis. *Semin Cancer Biol* 2004; 14: 441–448.
36. Ben-Baruch A. Inflammation-associated immune suppression in cancer: the roles played by cytokines, chemokines and additional mediators. *Semin Cancer Biol* 2006; 16: 38–52.
37. Gabrilovich DI, Ostrand-Rosenberg S, Bronte V. Coordinated regulation of myeloid cells by tumours. *Nat Rev Immunol* 2012; 12: 253–268.
38. Modi BG1, Neustadter J, Binda E, *et al.* Langerhans cells facilitate epithelial DNA damage and squamous cell carcinoma. *Science* 2012; 335: 104–108.
39. Van Pottelberge GR, Bracke KR, Demedts IK, *et al.* Selective accumulation of langerhans-type dendritic cells in small airways of patients with COPD. *Respir Res* 2010; 11: 35.

40. Li Y, Du H, Qin Y, *et al.* Activation of the signal transducers and activators of the transcription 3 pathway in alveolar epithelial cells induces inflammation and adenocarcinomas in mouse lung. *Cancer Res* 2007; 67: 8494–8503.
41. Hanahan D, Weinberg RA. Hallmarks of cancer: the next generation. *Cell* 2011; 144: 646–674.
42. Di Stefano A, Caramori G, Oates T, *et al.* Increased expression of nuclear factor-kappaB in bronchial biopsies from smokers and patients with COPD. *Eur Respir J* 2002; 20: 556–563.
43. Lee H, Herrmann A, Deng JH, *et al.* Persistently activated Stat3 maintains constitutive NF-kappaB activity in tumors. *Cancer Cell* 2009; 15: 283–293.
44. Bracke K1, Cataldo D, Maes T, *et al.* Matrix metalloproteinase-12 and cathepsin D expression in pulmonary macrophages and dendritic cells of cigarette smoke-exposed mice. *Int Arch Allergy Immunol* 2005; 138: 169–179.
45. Molet S1, Belleguic C, Lena H, *et al.* Increase in macrophage elastase (MMP-12) in lungs from patients with chronic obstructive pulmonary disease. *Inflamm Res* 2005; 54: 31–36.
46. Houghton AM, Quintero PA, Perkins DL, *et al.* Elastin fragments drive disease progression in a murine model of emphysema. *J Clin Invest* 2006; 116: 753–759.
47. Young RP, Hopkins RJ, Gamble GD, *et al.* Genetic evidence linking lung cancer and COPD: a new perspective. *Appl Clin Genet* 2011; 4: 99–111.
48. Young RP, Hopkins RJ, Hay BA, *et al.* Lung cancer gene associated with COPD: triple whammy or possible confounding effect? *Eur Respir J* 2008; 32: 1158–1164.
49. West KA, Brognard J, Clark AS, *et al.* Rapid Akt activation by nicotine and a tobacco carcinogen modulates the phenotype of normal human airway epithelial cells. *J Clin Invest* 2003; 111: 81–90.
50. Van Durme YM, Eijgelsheim M, Joos GF, *et al.* Hedgehog-interacting protein is a COPD susceptibility gene: the Rotterdam Study. *Eur Respir J* 2010; 36: 89–95.
51. Chuang PT, Kawcak T, McMahon AP. Feedback control of mammalian Hedgehog signaling by the Hedgehog-binding protein, Hip1, modulates Fgf signaling during branching morphogenesis of the lung. *Genes Dev* 2003; 17: 342–347.
52. Sohal SS, Reid D, Soltani A, *et al.* Evaluation of epithelial mesenchymal transition in patients with chronic obstructive pulmonary disease. *Respir Res* 2011; 12: 130.
53. Wauters E, Smeets D, Coolen J, J. *et al.* The TERT-CLPTM1L locus for lung cancer predisposes to bronchial obstruction and emphysema. *EurRespir J* 2011; 38: 924–931.
54. Albrecht E, Sillanpää E, Karrasch S, *et al.* Telomere length in circulating leukocytes is associated with lung function and disease. *Eur Respir J* 2014; 43: 983–992.
55. Seow WJ, Cawthon RM, Purdue MP, *et al.* Telomere length in white blood cell DNA and lung cancer: a pooled analysis of three prospective cohorts. *Cancer Res* 2014; 74: 4090–4098.
56. Kumaki F, Kawai T, Hiroi S, *et al.* Telomerase activity and expression of human telomerase RNA component and human telomerase reverse transcriptase in lung carcinomas. *Human Pathol* 2001; 32: 188–195.
57. Sundar IK, Mullapudi N, Yao H, *et al.* Lung cancer and its association with chronic obstructive pulmonary disease: update on nexus of epigenetics. *Curr Opin Pulm Med* 2011; 17: 279–285.
58. Ito K, Ito M, Elliott WM, *et al.* Decreased histone deacetylase activity in chronic obstructive pulmonary disease. *N Engl J Med* 2005; 352: 1967–1976.
59. Chen L, Fischle W, Verdin E, *et al.* Duration of nuclear NF-kappaB action regulated by reversible acetylation. *Science* 2001; 293: 1653–1657.
60. Belinsky SA, Nikula KJ, Palmisano WA, *et al.* Aberrant methylation of p16(INK4a) is an early event in lung cancer and a potential biomarker for early diagnosis. *PNAS* 1998; 95: 11891–11896.
61. Pottelberge GR, Mestdagh P, Bracke KR, *et al.* MicroRNA expression in induced sputum of smokers and patients with chronic obstructive pulmonary disease. *Am J Respir Crit Care Med* 2011; 183: 898–906.
62. Takamizawa J, Konishi H, Yanagisawa K, *et al.* Reduced expression of the let-7 microRNAs in human lung cancers in association with shortened postoperative survival. *Cancer Res* 2004; 64: 3753–3756.
63. Peto R1, Darby S, Deo H, *et al.* Smoking, smoking cessation, and lung cancer in the UK since 1950: combination of national statistics with two case-control studies. *BMJ* 2000; 321: 323–329.
64. Young RP, Hopkins R, Eaton TE. Pharmacological actions of statins: potential utility in COPD. *Eur Respir Rev* 2009; 18: 222–232.
65. Nielsen SF, Nordestgaard BG, Bojesen SE. Statin Use and reduced cancer-related mortality. *NEJM* 2012; 367: 1792–1802.
66. Emberson JR, Kearney PM, Blackwell L. *et al.* Lack of effect of lowering LDL cholesterol on cancer: meta-analysis of individual data from 175,000 people in 27 randomised trials of statin therapy. *PloS One* 2012; 7: e29849.
67. Parimon T, Chien JW, Bryson CL, *et al.* Inhaled corticosteroids and risk of lung cancer among patients with chronic obstructive pulmonary disease. *Am J Respir Crit Care Med* 2007; 175: 712–719.
68. Greenhough A, Smartt HJ, Moore AE, *et al.* The COX-2/PGE2 pathway: key roles in the hallmarks of cancer and adaptation to the tumour microenvironment. *Carcinogenesis* 2009; 30: 377–386.
69. Mao JT, Roth MD, Fishbein MC, *et al.* Lung cancer chemoprevention with celecoxib in former smokers. *Cancer Prev Res (Phila)* 2011; 4: 984–993.

70. Keith RL, Blatchford PJ, Kittelson J, *et al.* Oral iloprost improves endobronchial dysplasia in former smokers. *Cancer Prev Res (Phila)* 2011; 4: 793–802.
71. Adcock IM, Chung KF, Caramori G, *et al.* Kinase inhibitors and airway inflammation. *Eur J Pharmacol* 2006; 533: 118–132.
72. de Torres JP, Casanova C, Marín JM, *et al.* Exploring the impact of screening with low-dose CT on lung cancer mortality in mild to moderate COPD patients: a pilot study. *Respir Med* 2013; 107: 702–707.
73. de Torres JP, Wilson DO, Sanchez-Salcedo P, *et al.* Lung cancer in patients with chronic obstructive pulmonary disease: development and validation of the COPD Lung Cancer Screening Score. *Am J Respir Crit Care Med* 2015; 191: 285–291.
74. Sekine Y, Fujisawa T, Suzuki K, *et al.* Detection of chronic obstructive pulmonary disease in community-based annual lung cancer screening: Chiba Chronic Obstructive Pulmonary Disease Lung Cancer Screening Study Group. *Respirology* 2014; 19: 98–104.
75. Raviv S, Hawkins KA, DeCamp MM Jr, *et al.* Lung cancer in chronic obstructive pulmonary disease: enhancing surgical options and outcomes. *Am J Respir Crit Care Med* 2011; 183: 1138–1146.
76. Smith CB, Kale M, Mhango G, *et al.* Comparative outcomes of elderly stage I lung cancer patients treated with segmentectomy *via* video-assisted thoracoscopic surgery *versus* open resection. *J Thorac Oncol* 2014; 9: 383–389.
77. Choong CK, Mahesh B, Patterson GA, *et al.* Concomitant lung cancer resection and lung volume reduction surgery. *Thorac Surg Clin* 2009; 19: 209–216.
78. Kimura T, Nishibuchi I, Murakami Y, *et al.* Functional image-guided radiotherapy planning in respiratory-gated intensity-modulated radiotherapy for lung cancer patients with chronic obstructive pulmonary disease. *Int J Radiat Oncol Biol Phys* 2012; 82: e663–e670.
79. Maldonado F, Bartholmai BJ, Swensen SJ, *et al.* Are airflow obstruction and radiographic emphysema risk factors for lung cancer? A nested case-control study using quantitative emphysema analysis. *Chest* 2010; 138: 1295–1302.

---

Support statement: This work was supported in part by a grant (RD12/0036/0062) from Red Temática de Investigación Cooperativa en Cáncer (RTICC), Instituto de Salud Carlos III (ISCIII), the Spanish Ministry of Economy and Competitiveness, and the European Regional Development Fund (ERDF) "Una manera de hacer Europa", Spanish Ministry of Health FIS Projects: PI04/2404, PI07/0792, PI10/01652, PI11/01626.

Disclosures: None declared.

Chapter 5

# Idiopathic pulmonary fibrosis

Carlos Robalo Cordeiro, Tiago M. Alfaro, Sara Freitas and Jessica Cemlyn-Jones

Idiopathic pulmonary fibrosis seems to be increasingly likely as an independent risk factor for lung cancer, although its precise frequency is uncertain. Studies focussing on the cellular and molecular pathways have shown that the main findings concern changes in cell proliferation, genetics, oncogenic pathways, cell communication and tissue invasion. Cigarette smoking is the most significant risk factor. In this subset of patients, there seems to be a predominance of SCC, although tumours tend to be peripheral. Prognosis is poor and treatment is challenging if we are to assure that patients receive the best treatment for each condition.

There seems to be an increased risk of lung cancer present in several interstitial lung diseases (ILD), with a more evident link in idiopathic pulmonary fibrosis (IPF), systemic sclerosis and some forms of pneumoconioses, such as asbestosis.

IPF is a rare but increasingly recognised ILD, of unknown aetiology, with a highly variable natural history, from an insidious onset to a rapid clinical and functional decline. Major risk factors are associated with male sex, smoking habit and age, which are in line with some of the leading risk factors for lung cancer. The low IPF prevalence rates, which are inconsistent within the literature, do not preclude the need for more careful screening for the disease given the poor prognosis (median survival 2–5 years) and the lack of a curative therapy.

The association of IPF and lung cancer poses some interesting questions regarding pathogenic similarities, difficulties in diagnosis and the absence of therapeutic measures to prevent the more severe prognosis that characterises this association.

This is the context for this chapter, which will focus on the association between IPF and lung cancer, both from a cellular and molecular perspective as well as on a clinical level.

## Cellular and molecular changes

A number of studies have found significant associations between lung cancer and pulmonary fibrosis at a cellular and molecular level. Some results suggest that pulmonary fibrosis may be a preneoplastic lesion, which increases the risk of lung cancer, whereas others indicate that there are similarities between them, suggesting a common pathogenesis.

Centre of Pneumology, Coimbra University Hospital, Coimbra, Portugal

Correspondence: Carlos Robalo Cordeiro, Centre of Pneumology, Coimbra University Hospital, 3000 Coimbra, Portugal. E-mail: carlos.crobalo@gmail.com

 Print ISBN: 978-1-84984-061-3. Online ISBN: 978-1-84984-062-0. Print ISSN: 2312-508X. Online ISSN: 2312-5098.

The main findings concern changes in cell proliferation, genetics, oncogenic pathways, cell communication and tissue invasion (fig. 1).

### Cell proliferation and apoptosis

Cancer is usually defined as uncontrolled cellular proliferation and invasion. Pulmonary fibrosis is also characterised by increased cellular proliferation. Lung fibroblasts from IPF patients display enhanced proliferation in serum-free cultures [1]. These cells show sustained growth *via* the autocrine production of TGF-β and a decrease in both production and sensitivity of the anti-fibrotic prostaglandin $E_2$ [2, 3]. Tumour necrosis factor-α receptor 1 is a mediator of cell death and inhibits cell growth in fibroblasts. Fibroblasts from patients with pulmonary fibrosis were found to show a decrease in the expression of this receptor, leading to enhanced proliferation and decreased collagen degradation [2].

IPF is also associated with significant changes in cellular apoptosis. Apoptosis, a form of programmed cell death, is essential for the maintenance of normal tissue homeostasis, by eliminating damaged cells. It is also an important component of the resolution phase of tissue response to injury, removing previously recruited inflammatory cells and mesenchymal cells [4]. In IPF lungs, an increase in apoptosis in type II alveolar epithelial cells coexists with resistance to apoptosis by myofibroblasts. This has led previous authors to coin the term "apoptosis paradox" [4]. Korfei *et al.* [5] have shown that 70–80% of type II alveolar epithelial cells (AECs) in IPF lungs display signs of apoptosis. AECs show an increase in pro-apoptotic proteins and a decrease in anti-apoptotic proteins [6]. Furthermore, the increase in apoptosis is seen both in areas overlapping myofibroblasts as well as normal alveoli [7]. This increase in type II AEC apoptosis is thus considered to be an important factor in the overall pathophysiology of IPF [8]. The evidence of the myofibroblast resistance to apoptosis is weaker. However, histological studies from IPF lungs usually show a lack of apoptosis in fibroblasts [6, 9, 10]. The reasons for this decrease

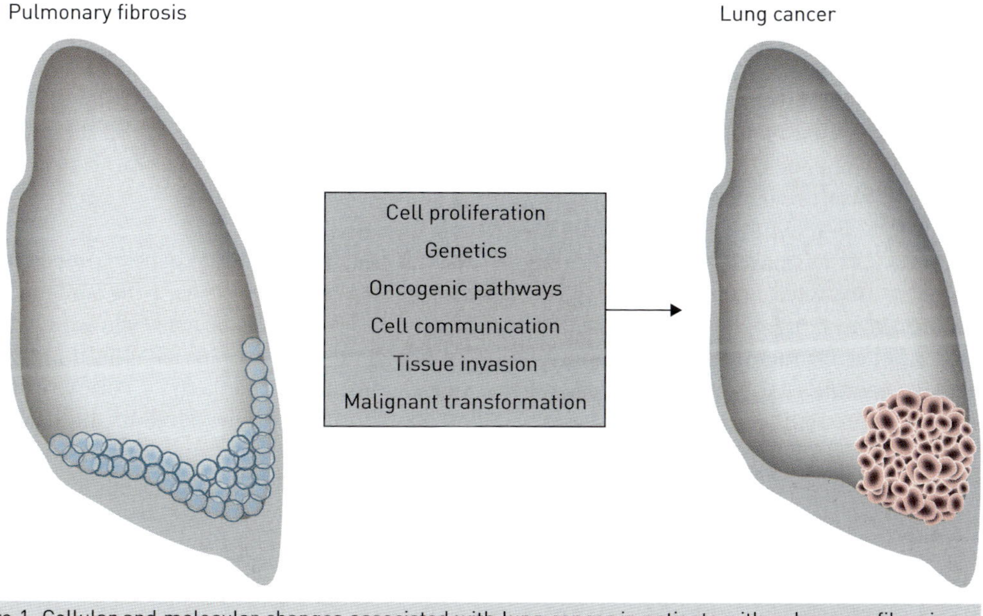


Figure 1. Cellular and molecular changes associated with lung cancer in patients with pulmonary fibrosis.

in apoptosis include changes in the concentration of mediators that activate or prevent apoptosis [11], changes in the expression on surface receptors involved in apoptosis [12], and changes in the interactions with the extracellular matrix [13].

## Genetic changes

Cytogenetic changes are a key factor in the development and progression of several types of cancer, including lung cancer. Some of the most frequently changed genes are the tumour suppressors involved in the control of normal cell proliferation and apoptosis, such as p53, KRAS (Kirsten rat sarcoma viral oncogene homologue) and FHIT [14]. These genes have also been shown to be altered in pulmonary fibrosis, especially in the honeycombing areas [15–17]. Microsatellite instability and loss of heterozygosity, typically seen in lung cancer, have also been shown in a proportion of IPF patients [18].

Smoking has been associated with an increased risk for both IPF and lung cancer. The genetic changes that are caused by smoking include the dysregulation of ageing-related genes and reduction of telomere length in the small airway epithelium [19]. Importantly, both IPF and lung cancer have been associated with changes in telomere length. Telomeres are repetitive DNA sequences located at the ends of linear chromosomes with an important role in maintaining chromosome stability and preventing fusion events between chromosomes. Ageing is associated with progressive telomere shortening, leading to cell senescence [20]. Changes in telomerase, the enzyme that ensures telomere integrity, have been associated with familial forms of IPF, and a significant proportion of non-familial IPF patients have decreased telomere length [21]. In lung cancer, although the results are not definitive, there are several reports of an association between telomere length and telomerase expression and both the risk and prognosis of the disease. Antitelomerase drugs are regarded as a possible therapeutic target for lung cancer [20, 22].

Epigenetics are changes in gene expression and chromatin organisation that are independent of the DNA sequence and that can be inherited in a stable manner over cell divisions. This includes changes in patterns of histone acetylation and methylation, usually as a result of environmental exposure to smoking, diet and ageing. The methylation of tumour suppressor genes and hypomethylation of oncogenes have important roles in carcinogenesis [23]. In IPF, a reduced pattern of methylation of the gene Thy-1 has been shown and is associated with a transformation of fibroblasts into myofibroblasts within the fibroblastic foci [24]. The mechanism for the increased resistance to apoptosis of the IPF fibroblast also seems to be related to epigenetic changes [25, 26].

MicroRNAs are small, non-protein coding RNAs that negatively regulate gene expression. Lung cancer is associated with changes in the expression of several microRNAs, with some acting as oncogenes and others as tumour suppressors [27]. In IPF, several studies have shown alterations in a number of microRNAs, including miR-21, miR-200 and let-7d [28, 29]. In an array study of 470 microRNAs from IPF lungs, ~10% were significantly changed in comparison with control lungs [30]. Finally, free circulating DNA was found in higher levels in both IPF [31] and lung cancer patients [32], and is being studied as a potential biomarker for both diseases.

## Oncogenic signalling pathways

Aberrant expression of developmentally active signalling pathways is a recognised component of the pathogenesis of cancer [33]. Two of these pathways, wnt (wingless-type protein)/β-Catenin and PI3K (phosphatidylinositol-4,5-bisphosphate 3-kinase)/AKT, are also altered in IPF. wnt is part of a highly conserved family of secreted glycoproteins with a range of actions. Its major (canonical) pathway is transferred to the nucleus *via* β-catenin and has been linked to increased carcinogenesis through genetic regulation. A detailed description of the wnt/β-catenin pathway is outside the scope of this chapter and can be found elsewhere [34]. An increase in nuclear β-catenin in IPF lungs has been reported by CHILOSI *et al.* [35], indicating activation of the pathway. Another study found more evidence of wnt pathway activation, showing increased phosphorylation of Lrp6 (low density lipoprotein receptor-related protein 6) and Gsk-3β (glycogen synthase kinase 3β) (both part of the canonical wnt/β-catenin pathway), as well as increased expression of the wnt target genes cyclin D1, matrix metalloproteinase-7 and fibronectin 1 [36]. The pro-fibrotic cytokine TGF-β may activate the wnt pathway through the phosphorylation of ERK 1/2 (extracellular signal-regulated kinase 1/2) causing inhibition of GSK-3 phosphorylation. The fibroblast proliferation effects of TGF-β are dependent on the activation of the PI3K pathway, indicating another common characteristic between cancer and IPF, and a new possible therapeutic target in this disease [37]. A recent study of IPF patients by STELLA *et al.* [38] found expression of the lung cancer-associated molecular pathways P-mTOR (phospho-mammalian target of rapamycin), P-met (phospho-MET) and P-ERM (phospho-ezrin/radixin/moesin) in fibroblastic foci. Two of these patients, both former smokers, had EGFR mutations. The authors concluded that these are possible therapeutic targets for the prevention of disease progression.

### Cell communication

Gap junctions are pathways for intercellular communication and have a key role in tissue homeostasis, regulation of mitosis, differentiation and apoptosis. They are membrane channels formed by aggregates of proteins named connexins [39]. The most important connexin in human lung fibroblasts is connexin 43 (CX43) [40]. As with many other types of cancer, lung cancer is characterised by a deficiency in the presence and action of gap junction intercellular communication; this deficiency is believed to be involved in carcinogenesis [41]. A reduction in the expression of CX43 has been found in primary lung fibroblasts from IPF patients, as well as human lung carcinoma cell lines [40, 42]. Possible causes of the decrease in CX43 expression in IPF lung fibroblasts are oxidative stress, activation of protein kinase C [43] or induction of the epithelial–mesenchymal transition (EMT), which is associated with a decrease in CX43 expression [44, 45]. This may constitute a new therapeutic target, as the transfection of human lung carcinoma cell lines with CX43 cDNA has been shown to lead to decreased cell growth [46].

### Tissue invasion

Lung cancer is a complex tissue composed of carcinoma cells, stromal cells and extracellular matrix (ECM). The fibroblasts that are found in association with a tumour have been termed "cancer-associated fibroblasts" (CAF) [47]. A number of studies have shown that CAFs have a role in tumour initiation, tumour-stimulatory inflammation, growth, angiogenesis, metabolism, metastatic process, drug response and immune surveillance [48]. The origin of CAFs may include recruitment from resident fibroblasts of the surrounding tissue, recruitment from bone marrow-derived mesenchymal stem cells or transition from epithelial cells [49]. The main mediator for the differentiation of local cells to CAF is TGF-β. TGF-β has opposing paradoxical effects, acting as a tumour suppressant in premalignant conditions and promoting tumour growth, invasion, angiogenesis and metastasis formation in advanced tumours. CAFs that are exposed to TGF-β produce inflammatory mediators and MMP which facilitate protein invasion. These cells also produce more TGF-β, which acts in an autocrine way, leading to further CAF activation, and in a paracrine fashion, enhancing the malignant behaviour of neoplastic cells [50, 51].

Fibroblasts are the key modulators of pulmonary fibrosis. In IPF, fibroblasts cluster in areas of previously normal tissue and evolve into myofibroblasts, creating structures called fibroblastic foci (FF). These foci are the origin of excessive deposition of ECM, leading to the progressive destruction of tissue architecture, which is typical of IPF [52]. A three-dimensional study of IPF lungs has shown that FF are not independent structures. They are part of an interconnected reticulum (the fibroblast reticulum) that infiltrates the pulmonary parenchyma much like a neoplasm [53].

One other common factor in the pathogenesis of pulmonary fibrosis and cancer is EMT. EMT is the process by which epithelial cells acquire a fibroblast-like phenotype. There are robust data on the relevance of EMT in the pathogenesis of cancer, including in malignant transformation, formation of cancer stem cells, invasion and metastatic capacity [54]. The data on the importance of EMT in pulmonary fibrosis is weaker [55]. Chilosi *et al.* [56] found the expression of the migratory markers laminin, fascin and heat shock protein-27 in the epithelial cells to be above that of the fibroblastic foci of IPF patients, forming a "sandwich pattern". These markers are important for cancer invasion [57–59]. The mechanisms of EMT have been studied in fibrosis and cancer, and seem to be similar, also underlining a shared mechanism [55].

## Epidemiology

Several studies have identified the association between IPF and lung cancer; the earliest report occurred in 1957, in a study performed by Spain [60]. However, within the literature there are different perspectives on this association, with highly variable prevalence rates (from 4.8% to 48%) [61–65], but they all lead to the conclusion that IPF patients are at a higher risk of developing lung cancer than the general population (prevalence rates of 2.0–6.4%) [61–65]. The lowest prevalence rate of 4.8% was reported by Wells and Mannino [61] in a large US autopsy study. At the other end of the spectrum, Matsushita *et al.* [62] performed a 200-patient autopsy study and reported a prevalence rate of 48%. These contradictory results may be explained by the different methodology and diagnostic criteria used, which could lead to misclassification. More recent studies have established that IPF is an independent risk factor for lung cancer [64–66], with increasing cumulative incidence over time after diagnosis [67, 68].

Combined pulmonary fibrosis and emphysema (CPFE), a more recently described syndrome that combines features of both, is thought to be related to higher rates of lung cancer than either IPF or emphysema alone. However, only a few studies have focussed on this topic and it remains controversial. One of the most recent studies did establish that CPFE patients are definitely at higher risk than emphysema patients, but no significant difference was found between the CPFE and IPF groups [69].

### Risk factors

Cigarette smoking is probably the most important risk factor for the development of lung cancer in IPF patients and for each of the diseases on its own. The studies by Matsushita *et al.* [62] and HUBBARD *et al.* [65] confirmed the relationship between smoking burden and the risk of lung cancer in IPF patients, and concluded that there is a direct association between the smoking index and lung cancer risk. However, HUBBARD *et al.* [65] also demonstrated that IPF is a risk factor independent of smoking status.

Male sex and age seem to be important risk factors for both IPF and lung cancer. AUBRY *et al.* [63] found a male:female ratio of 7:1 in IPF patients with lung cancer. In contrast, LEE *et al.* [70] did not find such a significant difference and in this study, sex was not considered to be an independent risk factor, after multivariate analysis. In the work of OZAWA *et al.* [67], age was confirmed as an independent risk factor for the development of lung cancer in IPF patients, after using a Cox proportional hazards regression model.

Other malignancies and exposure to metal dusts or asbestos have also been described as independent risk factors in some reports [67, 71].

The same risk factors seem to be implied in CPFE patients with lung cancer, but further and larger studies are needed to fully characterise this population [72].

## Clinical features

### Symptoms

IPF is characterised by progressive exertional dyspnoea and dry cough of insidious onset and daytime worsening [73]. Given the high frequency of comorbidities, including lung cancer, it is recommended that aggravated dyspnoea or cough, fever, haemoptysis or finger clubbing should prompt lung cancer screening. Finger clubbing seems to be much more prevalent in IPF with lung cancer (95%) than IPF alone (63%) [74].

### CT findings

IPF diagnosis relies heavily on a usual interstitial pneumonia (UIP) pattern, which is present on a high-resolution CT (HRCT) scan. Typical features include a subpleural reticular pattern located predominantly in the lower lobes, with septal thickening and honeycombing with or without traction bronchiectasis in advanced disease. Ground-glass opacities are rare and usually only present in early stages of the disease [73]. The diagnosis of lung cancer in these patients poses some difficulties, especially in the initial stages, when lung cancer may present as a solid nodule or ground-glass opacity, with a stellate or band-like shape that intermingles with fibrotic alterations; this can lead to a delay in diagnosis (fig. 2) [75].

Anatomical locations of lung cancer lesions show a predominance of peripheral and basal sites within IPF-related areas [74–76]. In the study by MATSUSHITA *et al.* [62], surgical specimens from IPF patients showed that the majority of lung cancer cases arose in the border between the honeycombing areas and non-fibrotic areas. However, the studies by PARK *et al.* [64] and KREUTER *et al.* [77] had dissonant outcomes, with an almost even distribution of lesions in upper and lower lobes, though sustaining the more peripheral location for most lesions, with poor correlation with fibrotic areas. MIZUSHIMA and KOBAYASHI [78] reported the peripheral location of the lung cancer lesions to be as high as 91%, but figures between 55% and 90% are common [76, 77, 79].

Although lung cancer is a frequent comorbidity of IPF, routine imaging screening, such as HRCT or low-dose CT, is not currently recommended [73].

### Histology

ADC was first associated with IPF, supporting the "scar carcinoma" concept [80, 81]. However, subsequent studies came to the conclusion that there is a predominance of SCC in IPF patients, with ADC as the second most common lung cancer, except when considering female sex alone [62, 63, 77, 79]. Typically, SCC is centrally located, but in this subset of patients, it is predominantly peripheral.

There are also important but variable figures for small cell carcinoma, which range from 12% to 30% [62, 63, 77, 79].

CPFE patients seem to share the same histological distribution, with a slightly higher predominance of SCC. The majority of the cancer lesions are also located in fibrotic areas rather than in emphysematous spaces [69, 72, 82].

Some studies have reported synchronous lung tumours as a form of presentation of lung cancer in IPF patients [78, 83]. The most common synchronous multiple lung cancer combinations found in a large Japanese study were SCC plus small cell carcinoma, and ADC plus small cell carcinoma [78]. However, this predominance of small cell carcinomas was not seen in other studies. Rohwedder and Weatherbee [83] concluded that SCC–SCLC, SCC–SCC and SCC–ADC are the most common combinations of lung cancer seen in IPF patients. Whether it is single or multiple lung cancer that impacts on the survival of these patients is unknown.

## Treatment options

Active treatment of both IPF and lung cancer poses some questions that have not yet been answered consistently. One treatment approach is to offer patients the best therapy

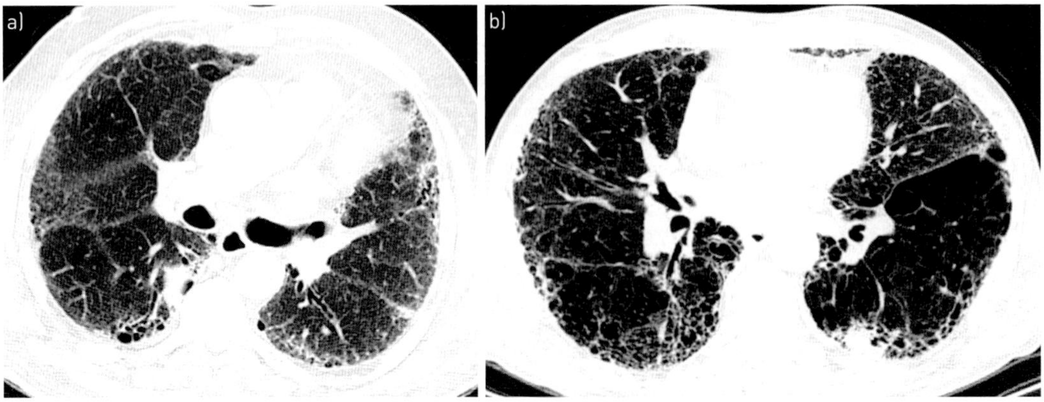


Figure 2. CT scans in two patients with lung cancer and pulmonary fibrosis. a) A nodule is seen in the posterior segment of the right lower lobe. b) A nodule is seen in the posterior segment of the left lower lobe.

for each of the conditions, depending on the patient's physiological status and the stage of the disease.

IPF is a progressive disease with an extremely poor prognosis and without curative treatment. Current guidelines address the stabilisation of the disease and the improvement of quality of life according to the condition of the patient. Mild-to-moderate disease has two new therapeutic agents that have recently been approved for the treatment of IPF: nintedanib and pirfenidone [84]. Both compounds have been shown to decrease functional decline, which is consistent with a slowing of disease progression [85, 86]. Corticosteroids, other immunosupressants and *N*-acetylcysteine have shown conflicting results and are now reserved for only a small number of patients [73].

Lung cancer should be addressed in the same way as for the general population. Where appropriate, surgery, chemotherapy and radiotherapy should be used according to the condition of the patient and the staging of the disease; the possibility of multimodal treatment should be considered.

However, an increasing amount of evidence relates lung cancer treatment options to significant morbidity and mortality in IPF patients that is much higher than in the general population, whether or not surgery or conventional chemotherapy are considered [77]. Larger, prospectively conducted studies are needed to clarify the best treatment available. CPFE patients undergo the same therapeutic orientation as IPF alone [82].

## Surgery

Surgical resection of lung cancer in patients with IPF is the best option for early stage disease, with a potentially curative role. However, surgery in IPF patients is associated with significant postoperative morbidity and mortality, causing adverse events such as acute exacerbation of IPF (AEIPF), pneumonia, bronchopleural fistulas and persistent air leaks [87, 88].

AEIPF is the most frequent adverse event, with an incidence of $\leqslant$20% and a mortality rate of >50%. It is defined as: 1) a previous or concurrent diagnosis of IPF; 2) unexplained worsening or development of dyspnoea within 30 days; 3) HRCT with new bilateral ground-glass abnormality and/or consolidation superimposed on a background reticular or honeycomb pattern consistent with a UIP pattern; 4) worsening hypoxaemia from a known baseline arterial blood gas; 5) no evidence of pulmonary infection *via* endotracheal aspiration or bronchoalveolar lavage; 6) exclusion of alternative causes, including left heart failure, pulmonary embolism and identifiable causes of acute lung injury [89].

Some studies have tried to focus on preoperative parameters that could help predict postoperative complications. Clinical findings, lung function and HRCT features have been evaluated for that purpose, with contradictory results. In a study by Suzuki *et al.* [90], only the extent of fibrosis was significantly correlated with the onset of AEIPF. Other studies, however, recognised that some function parameters were associated with a higher risk of AEIPF. The most consistent parameters were a lower $D_{LCO}$, a lower vital capacity (VC) and a higher composite physiological index (CPI) [88, 91, 92]:

$$CPI = 91.0 - (0.65 \times D_{LCO}\ \%\ \text{predicted}) - (0.53 \times FVC\ \%\ \text{predicted}) + (0.34 \times FEV_1\ \%\ \text{predicted})$$

Concerning procedure-specific morbidity and mortality, pneumonectomy (33% *versus* 5%) and lobectomy (12% *versus* 3%) had a much higher risk of mortality in IPF patients compared with the control group [91]. The incidence of postoperative complications associated with VATS is low but cannot prevent AEIPF events [93]. In a study by Goto *et al.* [94], IPF was identified as a risk factor for postoperative mortality, regardless of the extent of disease or functional impairment. Iwata *et al.* [95] recently described a statistically significant decrease in AEIPF events in patients due to undergo lung surgery who were previously treated with pirfenidone for 2–5 weeks, in comparison with control subjects. However, the study was retrospective and performed in a small population; a wider, prospective study is therefore required to consistently confirm these promising results.

### Chemotherapy

Few studies published to date report on chemotherapy in IPF patients with lung cancer. Current recommendations use the same therapeutic approaches as for the general population; however, larger and prospective studies are needed as most of the existing reports only enrol small groups of patients [96–98]. Cytotoxic combination chemotherapy with platinum (cisplatin or carboplatin) is the standard first-line treatment for NSCLC, and platinum plus etoposide is the standard for SCLC.

The occurrence of AEIPF in relation to chemotherapy is highly variable, ranging 0–23% [77, 99]. Other complications associated with chemotherapy are pneumonia, respiratory or cardiovascular failure and cytopenia.

Nintedanib is a recently approved treatment for both IPF [86] and NSCLC of ADC tumour histology, as a second-line option [100]. As yet, no studies have been published that focus on the use of this drug for the concomitant treatment of IPF and lung cancer of ADC type but it is likely that this will be assessed in the near future.

### Radiotherapy

Although widely used in lung cancer treatment, radiotherapy does not seem to be a suitable therapeutic option in this subset of patients, given the risk of radiation pneumonitis, which would add to fibrotic worsening. Infection is also a possible complication that could significantly affect the outcome of these patients [77]. Few articles mention this form of treatment in IPF–lung cancer patients and larger studies are needed to truly understand the potential role of this technique in treating these patients.

## Prognosis

Generally, IPF and lung cancer are diseases with a poor prognosis. When combined, the outcome is even worse, with reduced overall survival and lower relapse-free survival or PFS compared with lung cancer alone, regardless of age, sex, histological type and disease staging [70, 76, 101]. Lee *et al.* [70] performed a cox regression hazard ratio analysis to identify variables that affect survival in IPF patients; lung cancer was the most significant independent predictor of survival.

IPF–lung cancer patients have increased rates of mortality due to respiratory failure. As seen in the study by TOMASSETTI *et al.* [101], 43% of deaths were due to respiratory failure, 13% to lung cancer progression and 17% to lung cancer treatment-related complications.

The same findings apply to the CPFE subgroup [82].

## Conclusions and perspectives

A significant amount of knowledge concerning the association between pulmonary fibrosis and cancer has been gathered. Clinical studies have shown an increased risk of lung cancer in fibrosis patients, and molecular and cellular studies have shown similarities and common pathogenic pathways in these disorders.

Many vital questions and challenges are, however, still unanswered. An early diagnosis is usually required for improved treatment outcomes in both pulmonary fibrosis and cancer. The identification of high-risk patients and biomarkers for the development of cancer in IPF patients would allow these improvements. Possible candidates include peripheral blood microRNAs and free DNA.

Another important target for future studies is the identification of the best treatment strategies for these patients. This includes improving current strategies and identifying new therapeutic targets. Some of these targets are presented in table 1.

There has been increasing awareness of IPF in the general and respiratory scientific community. This suggests that the near future will also bring important developments in this area. Meanwhile, clinicians will have to rely on the diagnostic and treatment strategies that are available for both diseases, together with good clinical sense when treating these complex patients.

Table 1. A noncomprehensive list of therapeutic targets in lung cancer and pulmonary fibrosis

| |
|---|
| **Proliferation and apoptosis** |
| TGF-β inhibition [102] |
| Use of mitogens [103, 104] |
| **Genetic changes** |
| Reduction of methylation of a microRNA gene [105] |
| Use of miR-29 [106] |
| **Signalling** |
| Inhibition of wnt/β-catenin signalling [107] |
| **Cell communication** |
| Normalisation of CX43 expression [108] |
| **Tissue invasion** |
| Inhibition of hyaluronan synthase 2 [109] |

wnt: wingless-type protein; CX43: connexin 43.

## References


1. Raghu G, Chen YY, Rusch V, *et al.* Differential proliferation of fibroblasts cultured from normal and fibrotic human lungs. *Am Rev Respir Dis* 1988; 138: 703–708.
2. Vancheri C, Sortino MA, Tomaselli V, *et al.* Different expression of TNF-alpha receptors and prostaglandin E(2) production in normal and fibrotic lung fibroblasts: potential implications for the evolution of the inflammatory process. *Am J Respir Cell Mol Biol* 2000; 22: 628–634.
3. McAnulty RJ, Hernandez-Rodriguez NA, Mutsaers SE, *et al.* Indomethacin suppresses the anti-proliferative effects of transforming growth factor-beta isoforms on fibroblast cell cultures. *Biochem J* 1997; 321: 639–643.
4. Thannickal VJ, Horowitz JC. Evolving concepts of apoptosis in idiopathic pulmonary fibrosis. *Proc Am Thorac Soc* 2006; 3: 350–356.
5. Korfei M, Ruppert C, Mahavadi P, *et al.* Epithelial endoplasmic reticulum stress and apoptosis in sporadic idiopathic pulmonary fibrosis. *Am J Respir Crit Care Med* 2008; 178: 838–846.
6. Plataki M, Koutsopoulos AV, Darivianaki K, *et al.* Expression of apoptotic and antiapoptotic markers in epithelial cells in idiopathic pulmonary fibrosis. *Chest* 2005; 127: 266–274.
7. Barbas-Filho JV, Ferreira MA, Sesso A, *et al.* Evidence of type II pneumocyte apoptosis in the pathogenesis of idiopathic pulmonary fibrosis (IFP)/usual interstitial pneumonia (UIP). *J Clin Pathol* 2001; 54: 132–138.
8. Gunther A, Korfei M, Mahavadi P, *et al.* Unravelling the progressive pathophysiology of idiopathic pulmonary fibrosis. *Eur Respir Rev* 2012; 21: 152–160.
9. Uhal BD, Joshi I, Hughes WF, *et al.* Alveolar epithelial cell death adjacent to underlying myofibroblasts in advanced fibrotic human lung. *Am J Physiol* 1998; 275: L1192–L1199.
10. Yoshida K, Kuwano K, Hagimoto N, *et al.* MAP kinase activation and apoptosis in lung tissues from patients with idiopathic pulmonary fibrosis. *J Pathol* 2002; 198: 388–396.
11. Tanaka T, Yoshimi M, Maeyama T, *et al.* Resistance to Fas-mediated apoptosis in human lung fibroblast. *Eur Respir J* 2002; 20: 359–368.
12. Buhling F, Wille A, Rocken C, *et al.* Altered expression of membrane-bound and soluble CD95/Fas contributes to the resistance of fibrotic lung fibroblasts to FasL induced apoptosis. *Respir Res* 2005; 6: 37.
13. Kobayashi T, Liu X, Kim HJ, *et al.* TGF-beta1 and serum both stimulate contraction but differentially affect apoptosis in 3D collagen gels. *Respir Res* 2005; 6: 141.
14. Rom WN, Hay JG, Lee TC, *et al.* Molecular and genetic aspects of lung cancer. *Am J Respir Crit Care Med* 2000; 161: 1355–1367.
15. Maeshima AM, Maeshima A, Kawashima O, *et al.* K-ras gene point mutation in neogenetic lesions of subpleural fibrotic lesions: either an early genetic event in lung cancer development or a non-specific genetic change during the inflammatory reparative process. *Pathol Int* 1999; 49: 411–418.
16. Hojo S, Fujita J, Yamadori I, *et al.* Heterogeneous point mutations of the p53 gene in pulmonary fibrosis. *Eur Respir J* 1998; 12: 1404–1408.
17. Uematsu K, Yoshimura A, Gemma A, *et al.* Aberrations in the fragile histidine triad (FHIT) gene in idiopathic pulmonary fibrosis. *Cancer Res* 2001; 61: 8527–8533.
18. Demopoulos K, Arvanitis DA, Vassilakis DA, *et al.* MYCL1, FHIT, SPARC, p16(INK4) and TP53 genes associated to lung cancer in idiopathic pulmonary fibrosis. *J Cell Mol Med* 2002; 6: 215–222.
19. Walters MS, De BP, Salit J, *et al.* Smoking accelerates aging of the small airway epithelium. *Respir Res* 2014; 15: 94.
20. Gansner JM, Rosas IO. Telomeres in lung disease. *Transl Res* 2013; 162: 343–352.
21. Cronkhite JT, Xing C, Raghu G, *et al.* Telomere shortening in familial and sporadic pulmonary fibrosis. *Am J Respir Crit Care Med* 2008; 178: 729–737.
22. Fernandez-Garcia I, Ortiz-de-Solorzano C, Montuenga LM. Telomeres and telomerase in lung cancer. *J Thorac Oncol* 2008; 3: 1085–1088.
23. Herceg Z, Vaissiere T. Epigenetic mechanisms and cancer: an interface between the environment and the genome. *Epigenetics* 2011; 6: 804–819.
24. Sanders YY, Pardo A, Selman M, *et al.* Thy-1 promoter hypermethylation: a novel epigenetic pathogenic mechanism in pulmonary fibrosis. *Am J Respir Cell Mol Biol* 2008; 39: 610–618.
25. Huang SK, Scruggs AM, Donaghy J, *et al.* Histone modifications are responsible for decreased Fas expression and apoptosis resistance in fibrotic lung fibroblasts. *Cell Death Dis* 2013; 4: e621.
26. Cisneros J, Hagood J, Checa M, *et al.* Hypermethylation-mediated silencing of p14(ARF) in fibroblasts from idiopathic pulmonary fibrosis. *Am J Physiol Lung Cell Mol Physiol* 2012; 303: L295–L303.
27. Lin PY, Yu SL, Yang PC. MicroRNA in lung cancer. *Br J Cancer* 2010; 103: 1144–1148.
28. Pandit KV, Milosevic J, Kaminski N. MicroRNAs in idiopathic pulmonary fibrosis. *Transl Res* 2011; 157: 191–199.
29. Yang S, Banerjee S, de Freitas A, *et al.* Participation of miR-200 in pulmonary fibrosis. *Am J Pathol* 2012; 180: 484–493.

30. Pandit KV, Corcoran D, Yousef H, *et al.* Inhibition and role of let-7d in idiopathic pulmonary fibrosis. *Am J Respir Crit Care Med* 2010; 182: 220–229.
31. Casoni GL, Ulivi P, Mercatali L, *et al.* Increased levels of free circulating DNA in patients with idiopathic pulmonary fibrosis. *Int J Biol Markers* 2010; 25: 229–235.
32. Zhang R, Shao F, Wu X, *et al.* Value of quantitative analysis of circulating cell free DNA as a screening tool for lung cancer: a meta-analysis. *Lung Cancer* 2010; 69: 225–231.
33. Mazieres J, He B, You L, *et al.* Wnt signaling in lung cancer. *Cancer Lett* 2005; 222: 1–10.
34. Clevers H, Nusse R. Wnt/beta-catenin signaling and disease. *Cell* 2012; 149: 1192–1205.
35. Chilosi M, Poletti V, Zamo A, *et al.* Aberrant Wnt/beta-catenin pathway activation in idiopathic pulmonary fibrosis. *Am J Pathol* 2003; 162: 1495–1502.
36. Konigshoff M, Balsara N, Pfaff EM, *et al.* Functional Wnt signaling is increased in idiopathic pulmonary fibrosis. *PLoS One* 2008; 3: e2142.
37. Conte E, Fruciano M, Fagone E, *et al.* Inhibition of PI3K prevents the proliferation and differentiation of human lung fibroblasts into myofibroblasts: the role of class I P110 isoforms. *PLoS One* 2011; 6: e24663.
38. Stella GM, Inghilleri S, Pignochino Y, *et al.* Activation of oncogenic pathways in idiopathic pulmonary fibrosis. *Transl Oncol* 2014; 7: 650–655.
39. Naus CC, Laird DW. Implications and challenges of connexin connections to cancer. *Nat Rev Cancer* 2010; 10: 435–441.
40. Trovato-Salinaro A, Trovato-Salinaro E, Failla M, *et al.* Altered intercellular communication in lung fibroblast cultures from patients with idiopathic pulmonary fibrosis. *Respir Res* 2006; 7: 122.
41. King TJ, Bertram JS. Connexins as targets for cancer chemoprevention and chemotherapy. *Biochim Biophys Acta* 2005; 1719: 146–160.
42. Cesen-Cummings K, Fernstrom MJ, Malkinson AM, *et al.* Frequent reduction of gap junctional intercellular communication and connexin43 expression in human and mouse lung carcinoma cells. *Carcinogenesis* 1998; 19: 61–67.
43. Lin D, Takemoto DJ. Oxidative activation of protein kinase Cgamma through the C1 domain. Effects on gap junctions. *J Biol Chem* 2005; 280: 13682–13693.
44. de Boer TP, van Veen TA, Bierhuizen MF, *et al.* Connexin43 repression following epithelium-to-mesenchyme transition in embryonal carcinoma cells requires Snail1 transcription factor. *Differentiation* 2007; 75: 208–218.
45. Johnson LN, Koval M. Cross-talk between pulmonary injury, oxidant stress, and gap junctional communication. *Antioxid Redox Signal* 2009; 11: 355–367.
46. Zhang ZQ, Zhang W, Wang NQ, *et al.* Suppression of tumorigenicity of human lung carcinoma cells after transfection with connexin43. *Carcinogenesis* 1998; 19: 1889–1894.
47. Kalluri R, Zeisberg M. Fibroblasts in cancer. *Nat Rev Cancer* 2006; 6: 392–401.
48. Bhowmick NA, Neilson EG, Moses HL. Stromal fibroblasts in cancer initiation and progression. *Nature* 2004; 432: 332–337.
49. Madar S, Goldstein I, Rotter V. 'Cancer associated fibroblasts' – more than meets the eye. *Trends Mol Med* 2013; 19: 447–453.
50. Calon A, Tauriello DV, Batlle E. TGF-beta in CAF-mediated tumor growth and metastasis. *Semin Cancer Biol* 2014; 25: 15–22.
51. Valcz G, Sipos F, Tulassay Z, *et al.* Importance of carcinoma-associated fibroblast-derived proteins in clinical oncology. *J Clin Pathol* 2014; 67: 1026–1031.
52. King TE Jr, Pardo A, Selman M. Idiopathic pulmonary fibrosis. *Lancet* 2011; 378: 1949–1961.
53. Cool CD, Groshong SD, Rai PR, *et al.* Fibroblast foci are not discrete sites of lung injury or repair: the fibroblast reticulum. *Am J Respir Crit Care Med* 2006; 174: 654–658.
54. Thiery JP. Epithelial-mesenchymal transitions in tumour progression. *Nat Rev Cancer* 2002; 2: 442–454.
55. Bartis D, Mise N, Mahida RY, *et al.* Epithelial-mesenchymal transition in lung development and disease: does it exist and is it important? *Thorax* 2014; 69: 760–765.
56. Chilosi M, Zamo A, Doglioni C, *et al.* Migratory marker expression in fibroblast foci of idiopathic pulmonary fibrosis. *Respir Res* 2006; 7: 95.
57. Masuda R, Kijima H, Imamura N, *et al.* Laminin-5gamma2 chain expression is associated with tumor cell invasiveness and prognosis of lung squamous cell carcinoma. *Biomed Res* 2012; 33: 309–317.
58. Li A, Dawson JC, Forero-Vargas M, *et al.* The actin-bundling protein fascin stabilizes actin in invadopodia and potentiates protrusive invasion. *Curr Biol* 2010; 20: 339–345.
59. Pavan S, Musiani D, Torchiaro E, *et al.* HSP27 is required for invasion and metastasis triggered by hepatocyte growth factor. *Int J Cancer* 2014; 134: 1289–1299.
60. Spain DM. The association of terminal bronchiolar carcinoma with chronic interstitial inflammation and fibrosis of the lungs. *Am Rev Tuberc* 1957; 76: 559–566.
61. Wells C, Mannino DM. Pulmonary fibrosis and lung cancer in the United States: analysis of the multiple cause of death mortality data, 1979 through 1991. *South Med J* 1996; 89: 505–510.

62. Matsushita H, Tanaka S, Saiki Y, *et al.* Lung cancer associated with usual interstitial pneumonia. *Pathol Int* 1995; 45: 925–932.
63. Aubry MC, Myers JL, Douglas WW, *et al.* Primary pulmonary carcinoma in patients with idiopathic pulmonary fibrosis. *Mayo Clin Proc* 2002; 77: 763–770.
64. Park J, Kim DS, Shim TS, *et al.* Lung cancer in patients with idiopathic pulmonary fibrosis. *Eur Respir J* 2001; 17: 1216–1219.
65. Hubbard R, Venn A, Lewis S, *et al.* Lung cancer and cryptogenic fibrosing alveolitis. A population-based cohort study. *Am J Respir Crit Care Med* 2000; 161: 5–8.
66. Le Jeune I, Gribbin J, West J, *et al.* The incidence of cancer in patients with idiopathic pulmonary fibrosis and sarcoidosis in the UK. *Respir Med* 2007; 101: 2534–2540.
67. Ozawa Y, Suda T, Naito T, *et al.* Cumulative incidence of and predictive factors for lung cancer in IPF. *Respirology* 2009; 14: 723–728.
68. Dalleywater W, Powell H, Jones G, *et al.* P277 The incidence of lung cancer in people with idiopathic pulmonary fibrosis and connective tissue disease associated pulmonary fibrosis in the UK: a population based study. *Thorax* 2014; 69: A195.
69. Kwak N, Park CM, Lee J, *et al.* Lung cancer risk among patients with combined pulmonary fibrosis and emphysema. *Respir Med* 2014; 108: 524–530.
70. Lee KJ, Chung MP, Kim YW, *et al.* Prevalence, risk factors and survival of lung cancer in the idiopathic pulmonary fibrosis. *Thorac Cancer* 2012; 3: 150–155.
71. Ma Y, Seneviratne CK, Koss M. Idiopathic pulmonary fibrosis and malignancy. *Curr Opin Pulm Med* 2001; 7: 278–282.
72. Girard N, Marchand-Adam S, Naccache JM, *et al.* Lung cancer in combined pulmonary fibrosis and emphysema: a series of 47 Western patients. *J Thorac Oncol* 2014; 9: 1162–1170.
73. Raghu G, Collard HR, Egan JJ, *et al.* An official ATS/ERS/JRS/ALAT statement: idiopathic pulmonary fibrosis: evidence-based guidelines for diagnosis and management. *Am J Respir Crit Care Med* 2011; 183: 788–824.
74. Bouros D, Hatzakis K, Labrakis H, *et al.* Association of malignancy with diseases causing interstitial pulmonary changes. *Chest* 2002; 121: 1278–1289.
75. Yoshida R, Arakawa H, Kaji Y. Lung cancer in chronic interstitial pneumonia: early manifestation from serial CT observations. *AJR Am J Roentgenol* 2012; 199: 85–90.
76. Lee T, Park JY, Lee HY, *et al.* Lung cancer in patients with idiopathic pulmonary fibrosis: clinical characteristics and impact on survival. *Respir Med* 2014; 108: 1549–1555.
77. Kreuter M, Ehlers-Tenenbaum S, Schaaf M, *et al.* Treatment and outcome of lung cancer in idiopathic interstitial pneumonias. *Sarcoidosis Vasc Diffuse Lung Dis* 2015; 31: 266–274.
78. Mizushima Y, Kobayashi M. Clinical characteristics of synchronous multiple lung cancer associated with idiopathic pulmonary fibrosis. A review of Japanese cases. *Chest* 1995; 108: 1272–1277.
79. Nagai A, Chiyotani A, Nakadate T, *et al.* Lung cancer in patients with idiopathic pulmonary fibrosis. *Tohoku J Exp Med* 1992; 167: 231–237.
80. Kawai T, Yakumaru K, Suzuki M, *et al.* Diffuse interstitial pulmonary fibrosis and lung cancer. *Acta Pathol Jpn* 1987; 37: 11–19.
81. Fraire AE, Greenberg SD. Carcinoma and diffuse interstitial fibrosis of lung. *Cancer* 1973; 31: 1078–1086.
82. Minegishi Y, Kokuho N, Miura Y, *et al.* Clinical features, anti-cancer treatments and outcomes of lung cancer patients with combined pulmonary fibrosis and emphysema. *Lung Cancer* 2014; 85: 258–263.
83. Rohwedder JJ, Weatherbee L. Multiple primary bronchogenic carcinoma with a review of the literature. *Am Rev Respir Dis* 1974; 109: 435–445.
84. National Clinical Guideline C. National Institute for Health and Clinical Excellence: Guidance. Diagnosis and Management of Suspected Idiopathic Pulmonary Fibrosis: Idiopathic Pulmonary Fibrosis. London, Royal College of Physicians (UK) National Clinical Guideline Centre, 2013.
85. King TE Jr, Bradford WZ, Castro-Bernardini S, *et al.* A phase 3 trial of pirfenidone in patients with idiopathic pulmonary fibrosis. *N Engl J Med* 2014; 370: 2083–2092.
86. Richeldi L, du Bois RM, Raghu G, *et al.* Efficacy and safety of nintedanib in idiopathic pulmonary fibrosis. *N Engl J Med* 2014; 370: 2071–2082.
87. Kawasaki H, Nagai K, Yoshida J, *et al.* Postoperative morbidity, mortality, and survival in lung cancer associated with idiopathic pulmonary fibrosis. *J Surg Oncol* 2002; 81: 33–37.
88. Kushibe K, Kawaguchi T, Takahama M, *et al.* Operative indications for lung cancer with idiopathic pulmonary fibrosis. *Thorac Cardiovasc Surg* 2007; 55: 505–508.
89. Hyzy R, Huang S, Myers J, *et al.* Acute exacerbation of idiopathic pulmonary fibrosis. *Chest* 2007; 132: 1652–1658.
90. Suzuki H, Sekine Y, Yoshida S, *et al.* Risk of acute exacerbation of interstitial pneumonia after pulmonary resection for lung cancer in patients with idiopathic pulmonary fibrosis based on preoperative high-resolution computed tomography. *Surg Today* 2011; 41: 914–921.

91. Kumar P, Goldstraw P, Yamada K, *et al.* Pulmonary fibrosis and lung cancer: risk and benefit analysis of pulmonary resection. *J Thorac Cardiovasc Surg* 2003; 125: 1321–1327.
92. Shintani Y, Ohta M, Iwasaki T, *et al.* Predictive factors for postoperative acute exacerbation of interstitial pneumonia combined with lung cancer. *Gen Thorac Cardiovasc Surg* 2010; 58: 182–185.
93. Watanabe A, Kawaharada N, Higami T. Postoperative acute exacerbation of IPF after lung resection for primary lung cancer. *Pulm Med* 2011; 2011: 960316.
94. Goto T, Maeshima A, Oyamada Y, *et al.* Idiopathic pulmonary fibrosis as a prognostic factor in non-small cell lung cancer. *Int J Clin Oncol* 2014; 19: 266–273.
95. Iwata T, Yoshida S, Nagato K, *et al.* Experience with perioperative pirfenidone for lung cancer surgery in patients with idiopathic pulmonary fibrosis. *Surg Today* 2014 [In press DOI: 10.1007/s00595-014-1071-5].
96. Minegishi Y, Sudoh J, Kuribayasi H, *et al.* The safety and efficacy of weekly paclitaxel in combination with carboplatin for advanced non-small cell lung cancer with idiopathic interstitial pneumonias. *Lung Cancer* 2011; 71: 70–74.
97. Watanabe N, Taniguchi H, Kondoh Y, *et al.* Chemotherapy for extensive-stage small-cell lung cancer with idiopathic pulmonary fibrosis. *Int J Clin Oncol* 2014; 19: 260–265.
98. Watanabe N, Taniguchi H, Kondoh Y, *et al.* Efficacy of chemotherapy for advanced non-small cell lung cancer with idiopathic pulmonary fibrosis. *Respiration* 2013; 85: 326–331.
99. Minegishi Y, Takenaka K, Mizutani H, *et al.* Exacerbation of idiopathic interstitial pneumonias associated with lung cancer therapy. *Intern Med* 2009; 48: 665–672.
100. Reck M, Kaiser R, Mellemgaard A, *et al.* Docetaxel plus nintedanib *versus* docetaxel plus placebo in patients with previously treated non-small-cell lung cancer (LUME-Lung 1): a phase 3, double-blind, randomised controlled trial. *Lancet Oncol* 2014; 15: 143–155.
101. Tomassetti S, Gurioli C, Ryu JH, *et al.* The impact of lung cancer on survival of idiopathic pulmonary fibrosis. *Chest* 2015; 147: 157–164.
102. Iyer SN, Gurujeyalakshmi G, Giri SN. Effects of pirfenidone on transforming growth factor-beta gene expression at the transcriptional level in bleomycin hamster model of lung fibrosis. *J Pharmacol Exp Ther* 1999; 291: 367–373.
103. Deterding RR, Havill AM, Yano T, *et al.* Prevention of bleomycin-induced lung injury in rats by keratinocyte growth factor. *Proc Assoc Am Physicians* 1997; 109: 254–268.
104. Dohi M, Hasegawa T, Yamamoto K, *et al.* Hepatocyte growth factor attenuates collagen accumulation in a murine model of pulmonary fibrosis. *Am J Respir Crit Care Med* 2000; 162: 2302–2307.
105. Dakhlallah D, Batte K, Wang Y, *et al.* Epigenetic regulation of miR-17~92 contributes to the pathogenesis of pulmonary fibrosis. *Am J Respir Crit Care Med* 2013; 187: 397–405.
106. Xiao J, Meng XM, Huang XR, *et al.* miR-29 inhibits bleomycin-induced pulmonary fibrosis in mice. *Mol Ther* 2012; 20: 1251–1260.
107. Kim TH, Kim SH, Seo JY, *et al.* Blockade of the wnt/beta-catenin pathway attenuates bleomycin-induced pulmonary fibrosis. *Tohoku J Exp Med* 2011; 223: 45–54.
108. Koval M, Billaud M, Straub AC, *et al.* Spontaneous lung dysfunction and fibrosis in mice lacking connexin 40 and endothelial cell connexin 43. *Am J Pathol* 2011; 178: 2536–2546.
109. Li Y, Jiang D, Liang J, *et al.* Severe lung fibrosis requires an invasive fibroblast phenotype regulated by hyaluronan and CD44. *J Exp Med* 2011; 208: 1459–1471.

---

Disclosures: C.R. Cordeiro reports receiving personal fees from InterMune during the conduct of the study. T.M. Alfaro reports receiving travel support for the 2014 European Respiratory Society Congress from InterMune. S. Freitas reports receiving travel support from InterMune during the conduct of the study.

Chapter 6

# Histological diagnosis: recent developments

Gavin M. Laing, Andrea D. Chapman, Louise M. Smart and Keith M. Kerr

Contemporary management of patients with lung cancer requires a comprehensive diagnosis embracing anatomical, morphological and molecular features of the tumours. Accurate, consistent histological diagnosis also provides invaluable epidemiological information and contributes to our understanding of the pathogenesis of the disease. The World Health Organization (WHO) histological classification is fundamental, combined with TNM staging, to proper diagnosis of surgically resected cases and has recently been revised. Most patients, however, have only small biopsy or cytology specimens for diagnosis, where the WHO classification cannot be applied in full, and where IHC has become a key factor in refining the likely diagnosis. The increasing diversity of treatments offered to patients with all types of lung cancer and the recognition of therapeutically important biological differences between tumour subtypes has placed accurate pathological diagnosis in the spotlight. Subtyping of NSCLC and appropriate pathological assessment are required to follow current guidelines for the triage of cases for molecular pathology testing.

The histological diagnosis of lung cancer is important to determine the most appropriate management for the patient but it may also be extremely challenging [1]. Initial diagnosis is usually performed using small biopsy samples or cytological specimens. For most patients, this will be the only pathological sample available for diagnosis, as the majority of patients with lung cancer present with metastatic disease. In this context, confirmation of malignancy is clearly an important first step, followed by the classification of the disease, considering whether the cancer is primary to the lung or metastatic. The histological subclassification of the tumour then determines the subsequent investigation and treatment. In a minority of cases, the disease is diagnosed at an early stage and the patient is fit for radical resection of the tumour with curative intent. Resection rates for lung cancer vary enormously, depending on the case mix of the reporting centre, but in the UK, for example, resection rates are generally <15% [2, 3], and ranged from 5.6% to 12.3% in one survey of English health regions [4]. In this latter context, the histological diagnosis is in part confirmatory, assuming a preoperative diagnosis was obtained, but allows a complete, definitive diagnosis and classification of the tumour as well as pathological staging. This information helps prognostic assessment and informs any consideration of adjuvant therapy.

Dept of Pathology, Aberdeen University Medical School, Aberdeen Royal Infirmary, Aberdeen, UK.

Correspondence: Keith M. Kerr, Dept of Pathology, Aberdeen University Medical School, Aberdeen Royal Infirmary, Aberdeen, AB25 2ZD, UK. E-mail: k.kerr@abdn.ac.uk

 Print ISBN: 978-1-84984-061-3. Online ISBN: 978-1-84984-062-0. Print ISSN: 2312-508X. Online ISSN: 2312-5098.

Histological diagnosis also provides valuable epidemiological data on lung cancer; how the disease may vary according to geography, race, sex and aetiology. Accurate and consistent classification also underpins research into the pathogenesis of numerous forms of lung cancer.

The histological diagnosis of lung cancer can be challenging for a number of reasons. There is a wide range of tumour types, some, like ADC, demonstrating remarkable histological diversity [5]. Several of the common types of primary lung cancer have shared morphological features with carcinomas of other organs that may metastasise to the lung. Lung cancer is not infrequently diagnosed in a sample from an extrathoracic metastatic site where the differential diagnosis could be very broad. Because of difficulty in accessing intrathoracic tumours, and the frequent comorbidities suffered by many lung cancer patients, the samples obtained for diagnosis can be extremely small, posing significant limitations on the diagnostic process.

The first part of this chapter describes how to handle surgical resection specimens then gives a brief synopsis of the forthcoming revision of the World Health Organisation (WHO) classification of lung cancer, which is used for diagnosis of surgically resected tumours [6]. The second part of this chapter considers the issues in diagnosing and classifying lung cancer in small biopsy and cytology specimens, as well as brief reference to molecular testing, which is an integral part of contemporary lung cancer diagnosis, but which is discussed in detail elsewhere in this *Monograph*.

## Diagnosis of lung cancer in surgically resected cases

### Specimen preparation

Specimen preparation and examination are pivotal in facilitating the most complete and accurate diagnosis of surgically resected lung tumours. The types of specimen under consideration are lobectomy and pneumonectomy specimens, and sublobar resections including segmentectomy and wedge resections; essentially any specimen removed with the intent to completely resect the whole primary tumour.

Such specimens may be received in the pathology laboratory unfixed. If the ischaemia time is short, fresh tissue may be taken for tissue banking/research, assuming appropriate arrangements are in place (facilities, ethics, *etc.*). Intraoperative frozen section diagnosis may be requested on a bronchial or other resection margin, mediastinal lymph nodes, other lesions suspicious of tumour spread, or on the main lesion itself if preoperative confirmation of malignancy was not obtained. In general, however, intraoperative frozen section diagnosis should only be requested when a diagnosis is required to determine the progress and nature of the surgery subsequently undertaken. Further details of this process are beyond the scope of this chapter.

Resected tumour specimens require fixation, to preserve tissue and histological detail. This is best achieved by rapid transport of specimens from the operating theatre to the pathology laboratory, where they can be inflated with fixative (usually 10% neutral-buffered formalin (NBF)) either perbronchially or by parenchymal injection. Logistics may require samples to be placed in fixative in the operating theatre before transportation. Tumours fix less well if specimens are simply immersed in fixative and stiffening of the tissues restricts subsequent inflation. Inflation is useful to allow better anatomical assessment of the tumour, lymph nodes, airways and surrounding pulmonary parenchyma. Even if inflation with fixative is performed, transection of large tumours may be beneficial to allow access of fixative to the centre of the tumour mass.

Careful sectioning and examination of the tumour and the surrounding lung allow the best assessment of tumour character, size, extent and spread, all of which are important in the final diagnosis. Any associated pathological changes in the surrounding lung may be important for subsequent patient management.

## The WHO classification of lung tumours

The current WHO classification of lung tumours was published in 2004 [6] and is the standard used by most pathologists. This classification has been revised and is due for publication in Spring 2015. The classification presents the range of recognised tumour subtypes and their definitions, as well as descriptions of the criteria to be used, and other associated information regarding clinical features, imaging, macroscopic features, tumour behaviour, prognosis and molecular data. Differential diagnosis is briefly discussed. Primarily this classification is designed for whole-tumour specimens where the pathologist has the opportunity to sample the entire tumour to get an overall impression of the histopathological features. The 2004 classification does not adequately address the particular challenges of tumour diagnosis and subtyping of small biopsy and cytology samples. This problem was considered when the Pathology Committee of the International Association for the Study of Lung Cancer (IASLC), in conjunction with other representatives of the IASLC, the American Thoracic Society (ATS) and the European Respiratory Society (ERS) proposed a new multidisciplinary classification of pulmonary ADC [7, 8].

There follows below a brief synopsis of the lung cancer categories and their histological features, as will be presented in the forthcoming 2015 publication (table 1). Tumours other than the most common malignant epithelial malignancies are not discussed.

These are the main primary tumour categories in the 2004 and forthcoming 2015 WHO lung cancer classification. They are presented in the order they appear in each publication. More detail is provided in the text.

### *Adenocarcinoma*

The classification of ADCs follows the recommendations published by the IASLC/ATS/ERS panel [7]. Many of the issues driving the change in classification are reviewed elsewhere [5]

Table 1. The World Health Organization (WHO) classification of lung cancer: main lung tumour categories

| 2004 WHO classification | 2015 WHO classification |
|---|---|
| SCC | ADC |
| SCLC | SCC |
| ADC | Neuroendocrine tumours |
| Large cell lung carcinoma | Large cell lung carcinoma |
| Adenosquamous carcinoma | Adenosquamous carcinoma |
| Sarcomatoid carcinoma | Sarcomatoid carcinomas |
| Carcinoid tumour | Other and unclassified carcinomas |
| Salivary gland tumours | Salivary gland tumours |

and the clinical significance of these changes has been described [9, 10]. ADCs are still regarded as malignant epithelial tumours that show evidence of "glandular" differentiation. Most of these tumours arise in the peripheral parenchymal part of the lung, and may originate from pre-invasive, dysplastic lesions called atypical adenomatous hyperplasia, recognised as an ADC precursor lesion arising in the so-called terminal respiratory unit where thyroid transcription factor (TTF)1 expression is expected. However, not all ADCs arise from this epithelial compartment, probably in part explaining why only 80–85% of lung ADCs express this marker [11, 12].

The evidence for glandular differentiation is usually the identification of particular histological patterns. This normally requires a significant area of tumour to be observed to allow recognition of one or more of the lepidic, acinar, papillary, micropapillary or solid patterns of tumour. The vast majority of resected ADCs comprise more than one pattern and in the 2004 WHO classification, all of these cases would have been placed in the "mixed adenocarcinoma" category, most of the remaining categories being redundant. The new classification recommends that resected lung ADCs are reported according to their predominant histological pattern (*e.g.* ADC or predominantly micropapillary) and suggests that pathologists also describe all of the patterns of disease present, to the nearest 5% by area of tumour. The predominant pattern has been related to postoperative prognosis. Lepidic-predominant carcinomas have a relatively good postoperative course; solid and micropapillary predominant cases are aggressive and do relatively badly [13, 14]. Some studies consider acinar- and papillary-predominant cases a prognostically intermediate group but others have found papillary-predominant tumours to be more aggressive [15].

One of the most significant changes in the new classification is the discontinuation of the term "bronchioloalveolar carcinoma" (BAC). Historically used for any tumour spreading around alveolar walls in the lung, the definition of BAC was changed in the 1999 WHO classification [16] but confusion and old usage persisted. Although intended to classify a localised, noninvasive ADC [17], BAC continued to be used to describe all manner of ADCs, including advanced metastatic cases. "Lepidic adenocarcinoma" is the currently accepted descriptive term for ADC when it is growing around alveolar walls without destroying them. Readers may be interested in the origins of this terminology [18]. When this is the only pattern present, usually in the context of a localised lesion <2 cm in diameter, the lesion is diagnosed as ADC *in situ* (AIS). If the lesion is predominantly lepidic-pattern ADC but some invasion is present and the focus measures <5 mm, a diagnosis of minimally invasive ADC (MIA) is given. Both AIS and MIA appear to have no metastatic risk [7, 19, 20].

Another significant change is in the definition of solid-pattern ADC. The definition of a sheet-like NSCLC lacking glands or papillae but showing more than five mucin vacuoles in each of two or more high-power fields remains in place. However, a solid-pattern ADC is now also alternatively defined as an undifferentiated NSCLC, which expresses pneumocyte markers (TTF1 or napsin A) on IHC staining. This has also impacted upon the diagnosis of large cell carcinoma (see later).

Other changes in the ADC category include the reclassification of tumours formerly called "mucinous BAC" as invasive mucinous ADCs and the removal of a number of ADC variants.

Some of the new changes in ADC classification will change our epidemiological statistics of this disease in the future (so-called classification shift). The categories of AIS and MIA are now clearly defined in the new classification and identify cases with 100% 5-year survival. These cases would previously have been diagnosed as ADC, either "well-differentiated" ADC or BAC. Furthermore, the introduction of IHC into the definition of ADC will add to this category morphologically undifferentiated tumours with a generally poorer postoperative survival. In coming years, we may well read reports of falling postoperative survival times for resected ADCs due to these classification shifts. Classifying resected invasive ADCs by predominant pattern may also provide powerful prognostic data but the clinical utility of this is less clear.

### *Squamous cell carcinomas*

The diagnosis of resected SCC is generally less complicated than for ADC. This tumour is defined as a malignant epithelial tumour (carcinoma) showing morphological evidence of squamous differentiation (keratin production or intercellular bridges). Tumours are mostly centrally located, arising from large bronchi and many probably derive from precursor lesions of the bronchial epithelium (squamous dysplasia and SCC *in situ*). *In situ* bronchial disease is often present in adjacent airways but is not required to confirm primary disease. Increasingly, differential diagnosis of primary SCC of the lung is complicated by a history of SCC of head and neck. Where tobacco is aetiologically linked to both tumours, there are no mainstream methods to reliably distinguish the two. If the head and neck SCC is related to human papilloma virus (HPV) infection, it often has basaloid morphology and both these factors may help discriminate, although HPV expression in primary lung SCC has been reported [21–24]. This has, however, been a controversial area and some assert that a false-positive HPV test can arise due to technical problems [25]. It is worth noting that there appears to be an increasing prevalence or recognition of peripherally located primary SCCs of the lung [26]. As with most issues of differential diagnosis, these questions are often resolved by clinicopathological correlation.

The papillary, small cell and clear cell variants of SCC have been eliminated from the classification but basaloid carcinoma, which was a variant of large cell carcinoma in the 2004 WHO classification, has been retained as a variant of SCC. Whilst this tumour has similarities to SCC both morphologically and immunohistochemically, it also has differences in molecular profile [27] and has been recognised as an aggressive variant [28,29]. Other studies have suggested, however, that it is no more aggressive than poorly differentiated SCC [30], both of which appear to show relatively modest interobserver agreement regarding diagnosis [31].

Following from the acceptance of IHC in defining some resected undifferentiated NSCLCs as ADC, an undifferentiated tumour that abundantly expresses p63, p40 or cytokeratin 5/6 (squamous-associated markers) may be reclassified as nonkeratinising SCC.

### *Large cell carcinoma*

Probably the biggest change in the proposed 2015 WHO lung cancer classification concerns the large cell carcinoma category. The definition of an undifferentiated NSCLC lacking features of SCC or ADC also now excludes cases with IHC evidence of SCC or ADC markers. All variants of large cell carcinoma have been removed or moved to other categories (basaloid carcinoma to SCC, LCNEC to neuroendocrine carcinomas (see later) and lymphoepithelioma-like carcinoma (LELC) to "other carcinomas") whilst clear cell carcinoma and large cell carcinoma with rhabdoid phenotype have been deleted.

Morphologically undifferentiated large cell carcinomas are now reclassified as either solid ADC or non-keratinising SCC if the appropriate IHC is positive. If the IHC is not predictive, is negative or is unavailable, the diagnosis of large cell carcinoma is still valid but remains a diagnosis only to be made on surgically resected cases. Our own experience suggests about 30% of former large cell carcinomas would remain so after IHC was carried out. This change was made, given the importance of detecting targetable mutations in advanced lung cancer, because one important study of mutation profiling in lung cancer showed that the large cell carcinomas shared mutation profiles with other cancer types, mostly ADC [32]. However, current recommendations for molecular testing of lung cancer would not have excluded large cell carcinomas from testing and the prevalence of currently targetable mutations in large cell carcinomas is extremely low [33–35].

### *Sarcomatoid carcinomas*

The criteria for diagnosing these rare tumours in resection specimens have not changed. At least 10% of the tumour must show pleomorphic, spindle cell or giant cell carcinoma, and emphasis is given to calling these "pleomorphic carcinoma", as a collective term for all cases other than the exceptionally rare carcinosarcoma and pulmonary blastoma. Pleomorphic carcinomas are universally aggressive neoplasms that are typically chemotherapy resistant [36]; they usually have SCC or ADC components, but may exist in pure form as pleomorphic, spindle cell or giant cell carcinoma. Although the pleomorphic components of a tumour may express IHC markers associated with SCC or ADC, there is no proposal to reclassify these tumours on that basis. Classification of these tumours remains morphological.

### *Neuroendocrine tumours*

In the 2004 classification, the four main neuroendocrine tumours were dispersed into three different categories. From 2015, SCLC, LCNEC and the carcinoid tumours (typical and atypical) are in the same category. Pre-invasive, precursor lesions for SCLC and LCNEC are essentially unknown; a rare disease called diffuse idiopathic pulmonary neuroendocrine cell hyperplasia is associated with the development of often multiple, peripheral, spindle cell type carcinoid tumours. Diagnostic criteria for these neuroendocrine tumours remain the same.

SCLC is a highly malignant neuroendocrine carcinoma comprising mostly relatively small tumour cells with little cytoplasm, leading to characteristic "moulding" of featureless or finely granular nuclei, at least in certain sample types (fig. 1). Neuroendocrine features demonstrated by IHC are usual, not universal, and generally not required for diagnosis, although in practice, pathologists increasingly support a diagnosis of SCLC by IHC testing. An interesting new development is the finding of SCLC in repeat biopsy samples of around 2–14% of patients relapsing after treatment of an *EGFR*-mutated ADC by an EGFR-TKI [37]. The mechanism of this transformation is not known but may be due to emergence of pre-existing minor resistant clones of SCLC in the TKI-naïve tumour.

LCNECs are usually morphologically quite different from SCLC; cells are larger with abundant eosinophilic cytoplasm, vesicular nuclei and prominent nuclei. Organoid architecture (trabeculae, glands and rosettes) is usual and may mimic ADC. LCNEC is usually only confidently diagnosed in the resection specimen. It is rarely possible to make a confident diagnosis on small biopsy or cytology samples. Diagnosis requires demonstration of neuroendocine differentiation, which in practice usually means that two out of three immunostains (usually chromogranin, synaptophysin and CD56) should be positive. It is worth noting, especially given morphological similarities to ADC, that 50–60% of LCNECs

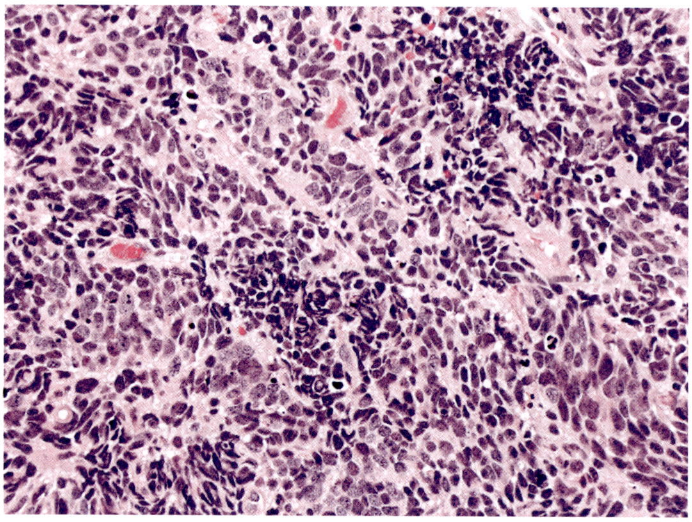

Figure 1. Endobronchial biopsy showing SCLC. The smearing artefact, indistinct nuclei, lack of cytoplasm, nuclear moulding, and abundance of both mitoses and apoptosis are characteristic features.

express TTF1. Genomic data based on mutational and gene expression profiles [32, 38] show significant overlap in findings between SCLC and LCNEC.

Carcinoid tumours are invasive malignant lesions that show a range of usually easily recognisable histological appearances. Insular, trabecular or glandular architecture is common, spindle cell morphology is less so and more often found in peripherally located lesions rather than in the archetypal, endobronchial polypoid tumour. Whilst typical carcinoid tumours show regional nodal spread in about 10% of cases and distant metastases are very rare, atypical carcinoid tumours are more aggressive, akin to SCC, with a tendency for bone and brain metastases. Atypical carcinoid is a very rare tumour and is distinguished from TC by the presence of tumour necrosis and/or the identification of more than two mitoses per 2 $mm^2$ of tumour. Generally this distinction can only be made in resected cases, although very occasionally, mitoses or necrosis may appear in a large biopsy sample. Genetically, carcinoid tumours are completely different from SCLC and LCNEC [38, 39] and will not transform into their highly malignant counterparts.

### *Other types of lung carcinoma*

Definitive diagnosis of adenosquamous carcinoma is reserved for resection specimens since each component should account for at least 10% of the whole tumour, usually in discrete zones. With the introduction of IHC into the definition of SCC and ADC comes the ability to diagnose adenosquamous carcinoma if, using appropriate markers on a resected undifferentiated tumour, there are discrete, respective immunopositive zones meeting the 10% rule. Salivary-type tumours are rare, occur mostly in the trachea or large bronchi, morphologically resemble their counterparts in the salivary glands and show variable low-to-moderate degrees of malignant behaviour. The "other carcinomas" category includes LELC, a largely Epstein–Barr virus-associated tumour, and a new entity, so-called NUT carcinoma, which is defined by the presence of *NUTM1* gene rearrangement, and leads to a pulmonary or mediastinal tumour, often resembling basaloid SCC, with occasional, "abrupt" keratin pearls, and which is IHC-positive for NUT protein [40].

## Diagnosis of lung cancer in "small" samples

As mentioned earlier, this is a much more frequent issue for pathologists than diagnosing resected primary lung cancer. Most patients with lung cancer will have a histological and/or cytological diagnosis of their tumour (~73% in the Scottish Lung Cancer Audit [41]), but relatively few of these will go on to have their tumour resected. Until relatively recently, the diagnosis of lung cancer in patients with advanced disease and no prospect of potentially curative surgical resection was relatively straightforward: the patients either had SCLC or they did not. If they did not have SCLC, even if they were given a pathological diagnosis of SCC, ADC or some other subtype, they were considered a single category, NSCLC, as the treatment for all these tumours was the same. In recent years, there has been relatively little change in the chemotherapy given for advanced SCLC. However, patients with SCC are now given different platinum doublet chemotherapy, unlike those with nonsquamous NSCLC [42].

The discovery of therapeutically targetable molecular changes in ADCs has made histological subtyping important for case triage for molecular testing [43–46], a subject discussed elsewhere in this *Monograph*. All cases of ADC or probable ADC (by predictive IHC), cases where ADC is a component of the tumour (adenosquamous, sarcomatoid with ADC, *etc.*), cases where ADC cannot be excluded, and all cases regarded as NSCLC not otherwise specified (NOS) after all possible examination of that case is completed should be routinely tested. *Bona fide* SCCs should be considered for testing if there is a never-smoking or long-time ex-smoking history [46]. Current guidelines regard *EGFR* mutation and *ALK* fusion gene testing to be routine.

Antiangiogenic agents like bevacizumab carry a risk of fatal haemorrhage in patients with SCC, leading to this agent being licensed for use only in nonsquamous NSCLC [47].

### Sample preparation

The standard procedure is to fix all small biopsy samples in 10% NBF as soon as they are removed from the patient. There are numerous other fixatives available, which may favour the conduct of particular diagnostic techniques, but 10% NBF is a safe solution for almost all diagnostic procedures that may be required. Fixation time of 6–48 h is recommended; long enough to preserve the material but not long enough to compromise DNA or antigenic integrity. Pathologists should be aware of the additional fixation and other chemical processing that may occur in modern automated tissue processors. If ultra-rapid processing is employed in order to meet demands for an extremely quick diagnostic turnaround time, pathologists and those making these demands should be aware that IHC and other techniques may be compromised by too short a fixation time.

Cytological techniques are frequently used in a very wide range of samples and there are dangers in making generalised comments about "cytology" in lung cancer diagnosis. The standard initial approach is to stain cellular material that is aspirated, brushed or washed from tumour-bearing tissue and spread on glass slides. This allows very rapid morphological assessment and often, definitive diagnosis. So called rapid on-site evaluation is widely practiced as a way of assessing diagnostic cytology material at the time of sampling for adequate yield of tumour cells [48]. This will also facilitate appropriate subsequent sample handling. Some samples may be suspended in liquid then deposited on slides (referred to as liquid-based cytology (LBC) preparation) [49]. The increasing dependence of cytological diagnosis on IHC, however, with the additional need for molecular testing in many cases, has placed greater emphasis on preparing material to facilitate these tests. The simplest routine way to do this is to prepare a cell pellet and create an artificial, paraffin wax-embedded cell block, which can then be handled and sectioned like a biopsy sample. The Cellient technique (Hologic, Bedford, MA, USA) may facilitate this process [50]. Cytology smears may also be used as a DNA source for molecular pathology and LBC samples allow IHC to be performed [49] but the cell block technique is convenient and allows limited material to be used in a range of tests [51].

## Diagnostic yield of sampling techniques in lung cancer cases

This issue has been extensively reviewed elsewhere [52, 53]. In brief, and despite a wide range of published figures for individual techniques, probably reflecting various biases, a number of basic conclusions may be drawn about the diagnostic yield, in terms of a diagnosis of "malignancy", in patients who have lung cancer. Of course, these figures are also a reflection of the skill of the operator acquiring the samples and of the pathologist reporting the case, factors which are frequently forgotten when published data are considered. Techniques that do not directly visualise or target the lesion generally do worse (sputum, endobronchial approaches in peripheral lesions invisible to the bronchoscopist) than those where the lesion is directly visualised, either at endoscopy or under radiological guidance. Inevitably, when a peripheral lung lesion is smaller, diagnostic yields for transthoracic, guided approaches fall from around 90% to around 60–70% [52, 54].

While normal practice is to obtain tumour tissue from the most easily accessible site, with the smallest risk to the patient, other considerations are now also important. As well as securing a tissue diagnosis of lung cancer, staging information is important and bronchoscopy is often combined with EBUS or EUS lymph node aspiration [55]. Distant metastatic sites are frequently biopsied and pleural or pericardial effusion fluid can be an excellent source of tumour tissue (fig. 2). Until such time as we understand any clinically significant differences in biomarker expression or other pathological features between primary tumour and metastatic sites, tumour from anywhere has equal diagnostic value. The important goal is to obtain enough tumour tissue to allow a full pathological diagnosis including morphological assessment, IHC and molecular studies.

## Limitations of diagnosis in small samples

Intuitively, an accurate and complete pathological diagnosis of lung cancer will be difficult, if not impossible, if the sample contains only a few tumour cells. In bronchial biopsy samples containing NSCLC, average tumour content is only around 20–25%, and between 33% and 50% of tissue fragments taken contain no tumour at all [56]. In some cases, it may be possible to confirm malignancy but little more, whilst in some we can distinguish SCLC from a NSCLC but, using standard morphology, no more. In limited material, definitive features of SCC (keratin and intercellular bridges) may be lacking and for ADC, where diagnosis is more reliant on large areas of tumour to show specific tumour patterns and architecture, accurate small sample diagnosis by morphology alone is even harder [57]. Recognition of these limitations led to the perfectly reasonable recommendation that where the evidence for a specific NSCLC subtype was lacking, a diagnosis of NSCLC-NOS should

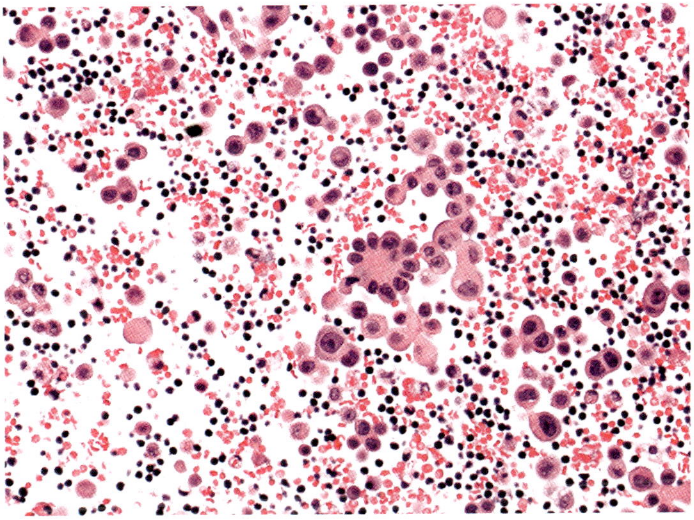

Figure 2. Cytology cell block of pleural effusion fluid showing clear papillary structures of ADC. There are also abundant small lymphocytes in the background. This case would be suitable for molecular testing.

be given [58, 59]. The need for specific subtyping of NSCLC to determine treatment has rendered the NSCLC-NOS diagnosis problematic.

### Resolving the NSCLC-NOS issue

IHC may be used to predict the likely NSCLC subtype when a small sample shows indeterminate morphology. IHC may be used on biopsy as well as suitably prepared cytology specimens [8, 60] and has a predictive accuracy of 80–85% in unselected cases, where predicted cell type is compared with that made on a subsequent surgical resection [61–64]. As a minimum, p63 or p40 to predict SCC (fig. 3) and TTF1 to predict ADC is recommended [7, 8] but cytokeratin 5/6 is also validated for SCC [61]. A mucin stain is also useful in identifying ADCs, especially when TTF1 IHC is negative or not available.

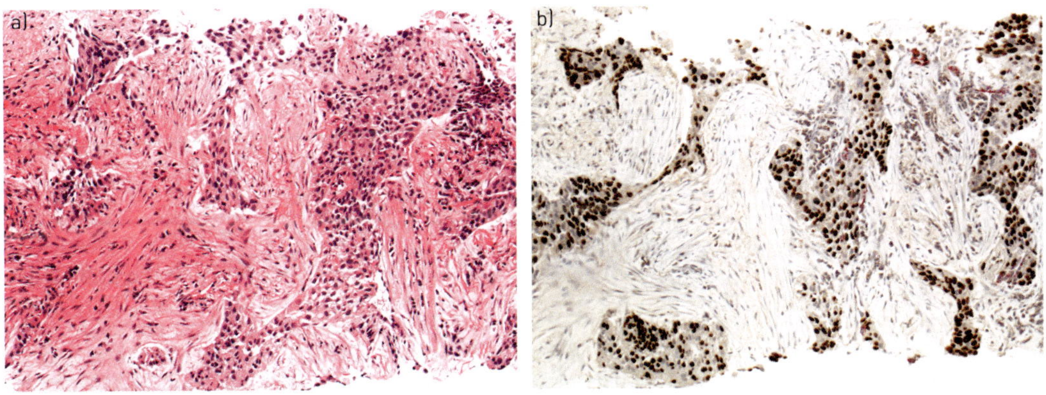


Figure 3. In this lung core biopsy, there is a) undifferentiated carcinoma, which would be called NSCLC not otherwise specified on morphological grounds, but as b) p63 IHC is diffusely positive, the correct diagnosis is NSCLC, probably SCC (table 2). Such a case would not be routinely submitted for molecular testing.

Extensive panels of IHC tests should be avoided, as they may exhaust the tissue and prevent subsequent molecular testing. A full clinical history accompanying the sample will help prevent overinvestigation by pathologists. Predictive IHC can reduce morphological NSCLC-NOS rates of around 40% in cytology samples and around 25% in biopsy samples to 6% [61]. IHC markers will not resolve every case and pathologists should not use large numbers of unvalidated, nonspecific markers to try to eliminate NSCLC-NOS. This is neither feasible nor reasonable, as a proportion of lung cancers are undifferentiated, both morphologically and with respect to IHC markers associated with differentiated cell types. Recommendations state that the reported NSCLC-NOS rates should be under 10% of cases [8]. Positive TTF1 staining is associated with *EGFR* mutation and *ALK* fusion genes in pulmonary ADCs [65, 66].

## Diagnostic categories for small samples

Recognising that this IHC approach to diagnosis is not, and cannot be, absolutely accurate in every case, it is recommended that diagnoses predicted by IHC are couched in terms of "probable" or "favoured" diagnoses. It is appropriate clinically to treat a favoured diagnosis in the same way as a definite diagnosis. The 10% rule that is applied to the definition of several tumour types in the resection setting (adenosquamous carcinoma and pleomorphic/sarcomatoid carcinoma), the need to assess mitoses in 2 $mm^2$ or more to distinguish typical from atypical carcinoid tumour and the fact that large cell carcinoma is still a diagnosis of exclusion mean that none of these specific diagnoses can be definitively made on small biopsies or on cytology. A mixture of squamous and glandular features, or sarcomatoid morphology, may be described but definitive diagnosis cannot be made. Occasionally, there will be good enough architecture to diagnose a salivary-type carcinoma. Potential small sample diagnoses are listed in table 2.

If there are pleomorphic/sarcomatoid features present in the tumour, this should be mentioned. If there are features of SCC and ADC, both should be described but a definitive diagnosis of adenosquamous carcinoma cannot be made.

Table 2. Diagnostic categories for small sample diagnosis

SCC
NSCLC, probably SCC[#]
ADC
NSCLC, probably ADC[#]
NSCLC, not otherwise specified[¶]
SCLC
High-grade neuroendocrine carcinoma[+]
Carcinoid tumour, not otherwise specified[§]

#: diagnosis predicted by IHC. ¶: IHC is not predictive, not available or cannot be carried out. +: some high-grade, undifferentiated carcinomas have morphological features that the pathologist may recognise as "neuroendocrine" but the appearances are not typical of SCLC; IHC will confirm neuroendocrine differentiation. This is a useful term to use in such cases. The pathologist may, however, indicate if they favour SCLC or a LCNEC. Occasionally there may be enough architecture to suggest a diagnosis of LCNEC is likely. §: carcinoid tumour is usually easy to diagnose and although IHC is not required, it is often used to support the diagnosis; there are no reliable approaches to distinguish typical from atypical carcinoid in small biopsy or cytology samples in most instances.

## Differential diagnosis

The importance of a good history accompanying the small diagnostic sample in a patient with possible lung cancer cannot be overemphasised. Clinical context is very important if the pathologist is to make the best diagnosis for the patient. Differential diagnosis will then be determined by the type and anatomical origin of the sample, and will vary depending on whether the lesion sampled is a peripheral lung mass, a central (endobronchial) tumour, a pleural lesion, in the mediastinum or in an extrathoracic location. Numerous differential considerations include primary lung *versus* metastatic carcinoma, lung amongst a range of possible other sources for an extrapulmonary lesion, malignant mesothelioma, sarcoma or lymphoma in the lung, benign lung tumours, and a wide range of reactive processes that can mimic lung cancers in various ways. If a peripheral lung sample shows lepidic-pattern growth of atypical glandular cells, the pathologist cannot distinguish between AIS and a lepidic pattern of ADC with invasion elsewhere in the lesion. Not infrequently, a bronchial biopsy shows morphologically malignant squamous epithelium but, in the absence of definite evidence of invasion, it is extremely difficult, if not impossible, to distinguish severe bronchial dysplasia or SCC *in situ* from invasive SCC; this is also an issue when cytologically malignant squamous cells are found in bronchial cytology. Some of these issues have been discussed elsewhere [67].

## Conclusion

The histological diagnosis of lung cancer is central to the proper management of patients suffering from this most common, most malignant and very varied group of tumours. The WHO classification is fundamental, combined with TNM (tumour, metastasis and node) staging [68], to a complete diagnosis of surgically resected cases. Most patients, however, have only small biopsy or cytology specimens for diagnosis, where the WHO classification cannot be applied in full and where IHC has become a key factor in predicting the likely diagnosis when tumour morphology is undifferentiated. The increasing diversity of treatments offered to patients with SCLC and to those with squamous *versus* nonsquamous NSCLC has made subtyping of NSCLC important. There is now abundant evidence that a simple IHC approach can refine this subtype diagnosis in most cases with good accuracy. Furthermore, as discussed elsewhere in this *Monograph*, subtyping of NSCLC is also required to follow current guidelines for the selection of cases for molecular pathology testing, in order to identify patients for various targeted drug therapies.

## References


1. Schwartz AM, Katayoon Rezaei M. Diagnostic surgical pathology in lung cancer diagnosis and management of lung cancer, 3rd ed: American College of Chest Physicians evidence based clinical practice guidelines. *Chest* 2013; 143: Suppl., e251S–e262S.
2. Riaz SP, Linklater KM, Page R, *et al.* Recent trends in resection rates among non-small cell lung cancer patients in England. *Thorax* 2012; 67: 811–814.
3. Rich AL, Tata LJ, Free CM, *et al.* Inequalities in outcomes for non-small cell lung cancer: the influence of clinical characteristics and features of the local lung cancer service. *Thorax* 2011; 66: 1078–1084.
4. National Cancer Intelligence Network. Recent trends in resection rates among non-small cell lung cancer patients in England. www.ncin.org.uk/publications/data_briefings/recent_trends_in_resection_rates__among_non_small_cell_lung_cancer__patients_in_england
5. Kerr KM. Pulmonary adenocarcinoma: classification and reporting. *Histopathol* 2009; 54: 12–27.
6. Travis WD, Brambilla E, Muller-Hermelink HK, *et al.* eds. World Health Organisation Classification of Tumours. Pathology and Genetics of Tumours of the Lung, Pleura, Thymus and Heart. Lyon, IARC press, 2004.

7. Travis WD, Brambilla E, Noguchi M, *et al.* International Association for the Study of Lung Cancer/American Thoracic Society/European Respiratory Society international multidisciplinary classification of lung adenocarcinoma. *J Thorac Oncol* 2011; 6: 244–285.
8. Travis WD, Brambilla E, Noguchi M, *et al.* Diagnosis of lung cancer in small biopsies and cytology: implications of the 2011 International Association for the Study of Lung Cancer/American Thoracic Society/European Respiratory Society Classification. *Arch Pathol Lab Med* 2013; 137: 668–684.
9. Kerr KM. Clinical relevance of the new IASLC/ERS/ATS adenocarcinoma classification. *J Clin Pathol* 2013; 66: 832–838.
10. Eguchi T, Kadota K, Park BJ, *et al.* The new IASLC-ATS-ERS lung adenocarcinoma classification: what the surgeon should know. *Semin Thorac Cardiovasc Surg* 2014; 26: 210–222.
11. Yatabe Y, Mitsudomi T, Takahashi T. TTF-1 expression in pulmonary adenocarcinomas. *Am J Surg Pathol* 2002; 26: 767–773.
12. Stenhouse G, Fyfe N, King G, *et al.* Thyroid transcription factor 1 in pulmonary adenocarcinoma. *J Clin Pathol* 2004; 57: 383–387.
13. Yoshizawa A, Motoi N, Riely GJ, *et al.* Impact of proposed IASLC/ATS/ERS classification of lung adenocarcinoma: prognostic subgroups and implications for further revision of staging based on analysis of 514 stage I cases. *Mod Pathol* 2011; 24: 653–664.
14. Russell PA, Wainer Z, Wright GM, *et al.* Does lung adenocarcinoma subtype predict patient survival? *J Thorac Oncol* 2011; 6: 1496–1504.
15. Warth A, Muley T, Meister M, *et al.* The novel histologic International Association for the Study of Lung Cancer/American Thoracic Society/European Respiratory Society classification system of lung adenocarcinoma is a stage-independent predictor of survival. *J Clin Oncol* 2012; 30: 1438–1446.
16. Travis WD, Colby TV, Corrin B, *et al.* eds. Histological typing of lung and pleural tumours. 3rd Edn. Berlin, Springer, 1999.
17. Noguchi M, Morokawa A, Kawasaki M, *et al.* Small adenocarcinoma of the lung. Histologic characteristics and prognosis. *Cancer* 1995; 75: 2844–2852.
18. Jones KD. Whence lepidic? The history of a Canadian neologism. *Arch Pathol Lab Med* 2013; 137: 1822–1824.
19. Yokose T, Suzuki K, Nagai K, *et al.* Favourable and unfavourable morphological prognostic factors in peripheral adenocarcinoma of the lung 3 cm or less in diameter. *Lung Cancer* 2000; 29: 179–188.
20. Sakurai H, Maeshima A, Watanabe S, *et al.* Grade of stromal invasion in small adenocarcinoma of the lung. Histopathological minimal invasion and prognosis. *Am J Surg Pathol* 2004; 28: 198–206.
21. Bishop JA, Ogawa T, Chang X, *et al.* HPV analysis in distinguishing second primary tumors from lung metastases in patients with head and neck squamous cell carcinoma. *Am J Surg Pathol* 2012; 36: 142–148.
22. Klein F, Amin Kotb WF, Petersen I. Incidence of human papilloma virus in lung cancer. *Lung Cancer* 2009; 65: 13–18.
23. Srinivasan M, Taioli E, Ragin CC. Human papillomavirus type 16 and 18 in primary lung cancers – a meta-analysis. *Carcinogenesis* 2009; 30: 1722–1728.
24. Yanagawa N, Wang A, Kohler D, *et al.* Human papilloma virus genome is rare in North American non-small cell lung carcinoma patients. *Lung Cancer* 2013; 79: 215–220.
25. Van Boerdonk RAA, Daniels JMA, Bloemena E, *et al.* High-risk human papillomavirus–positive lung cancer. Molecular evidence for a pattern of pulmonary metastasis. *J Thorac Oncol* 2013; 8: 711–718.
26. Funai K, Yokose T, Ishii G, *et al.* Clinicopathologic characteristics of peripheral squamous cell carcinoma of the lung. *Am J Surg Pathol* 2003; 27: 978–984.
27. Brambilla CG, Laffaire J, Lantuejoul S, *et al.* Lung squamous cell carcinomas with basaloid histology represent a specific molecular entity. *Clin Cancer Res* 2014; 20: 5777–5786.
28. Moro-Sibilot D, Lantuejoul S, Diab S, *et al.* Lung carcinomas with a basaloid pattern: a study of 90 cases focusing on their poor prognosis. *Eur Respir J* 2008; 31: 854–859.
29. Wang LC, Wang L, Kwauk S, *et al.* Analysis on the clinical features of 22 basaloid squamous cell carcinoma of the lung. *J Cardiothorac Surg* 2011; 6: 10–15.
30. Kim DJ, Kim KD, Shin DH, *et al.* Basaloid carcinoma of the lung: a really dismal histologic variant? *Ann Thorac Surg* 2003; 76: 1833–1837.
31. Thunnissen E, Noguchi M, Aisner S, *et al.* Reproducibility of histopathological diagnosis in poorly differentiated NSCLC. An international multiobserver study. *J Thorac Oncol* 2014; 9: 1354–1362.
32. Seidel D, Zander T, Heukamp LC, *et al.* A genomics-based classification of human lung tumors. *Sci Transl Med* 2013; 5: 209ra153.
33. Rekhtman N, Tafe LJ, Chaft JE, *et al.* Distinct profile of driver mutations and clinical features in immunomarker-defined subsets of pulmonary large-cell carcinoma. *Mod Pathol* 2013; 26: 511–522.
34. Hwang DH, Szeto DP, Perry AS, *et al.* Pulmonary large cell carcinoma lacking squamous differentiation is clinicopathologically indistinguishable from solid-subtype adenocarcinoma. *Arch Pathol Lab Med* 2014; 138: 626–635.

35. Rossi G, Mengoli MC, Cavazza A, *et al.* Large cell carcinoma of the lung: clinically oriented classification integrating immunohistochemistry and molecular biology. *Virchows Arch* 2014; 464: 61–78.
36. Chaft JE, Sima CS, Ginsberg MS, *et al.* Clinical outcomes with perioperative chemotherapy in sarcomatoid carcinomas of the lung. *J Thorac Oncol* 2012; 7: 1400–1405.
37. Cortot AB, Janne PA. Molecular mechanisms of resistance in epidermal growth factor receptor-mutant lung adenocarcinomas. *Eur Respir Rev* 2014; 23: 356–366.
38. Jones MH, Virtanen C, Honjoh D, *et al.* Two prognostically significant subtypes of high-grade lung neuroendocrine tumours independent of small-cell and large-cell neuroendocrine carcinomas identified by gene expression profiles. *Lancet* 2004; 363: 775–781.
39. Fernandez-Cuesta L, Peifer M, Lu X, *et al.* Frequent mutations in chromatin-remodelling genes in pulmonary carcinoids. *Nat Commun* 2014; 5: 3518.
40. French CA, Kutok JL, Faquin WC, *et al.* Midline carcinoma of children and young adults with NUT rearrangement. *J Clin Oncol* 2004; 22: 4135–4139.
41. The National Lung Cancer Audit Project Team. National Lung Cancer Audit Report. www.hscic.gov.uk/catalogue/PUB12719/clin-audi-supp-prog-lung-nlca-2013-rep.pdf Date last updated: 2013.
42. Scagliotti GV, Parikh P, Pawel JV, *et al.* Phase III study comparing cisplatin plus gemcitabine with cisplatin plus pemetrexed in chemotherapy-naïve patients with advanced-stage non-small-cell lung cancer. *J Clin Oncol* 2008; 26: 1–10.
43. Pao W, Iafrate AJ, Su Z. Genetically informed lung cancer medicine. *J Pathol* 2011; 223: 230–240.
44. Pao W, Girard N. New driver mutations in non-small-cell-lung cancer. *Lancet Oncol* 2011; 12: 175–180.
45. Kris MG, Johnson BE, Berry LD, *et al.* Using multiplexed assays of oncogenic drivers in lung cancers to select targeted drugs. *JAMA* 2014; 311: 1998–2006.
46. Kerr KM, Bubendorf L, Edelman MJ, *et al.* 2nd ESMO Consensus Conference on Lung Cancer: pathology and molecular biomarkers for non-small-cell lung cancer. *Ann Oncol* 2014; 25: 1681–1690.
47. Johnson DH, Fehrenbacher L, Novotny WF, *et al.* Randomized phase II trial comparing bevacizumab plus carboplatin and paclitaxel with carboplatin and paclitaxel alone in previously untreated locally advanced or metastatic non-small cell lung cancer. *J Clin Oncol* 2004; 22: 2184–2191.
48. Collins BT, Chen AC, Wang JF, *et al.* Improved laboratory resource utilization and patient care with the use of rapid on-site evaluation for endobronchial ultrasound fine needle aspiration biopsy. *Cancer Cytopathol* 2013; 121: 544–551.
49. Rossi ED, Martini M, Straccia P, *et al.* The potential of liquid-based cytology in lymph node cytological evaluation: the role of morphology and the aid of ancillary techniques. *Cytopathology* 2014 [In press DOI: 10.1111/cyt.12229].
50. Hecht SA, McCormack M. Comparison of three cell block techniques for detection of low frequency abnormal cells. *Pathol Lab Med Int* 2013; 5: 1–7.
51. Sanz-Santos J, Serra P, Andreo F, *et al.* Contribution of cell blocks obtained through endobronchial ultrasound-guided transbronchial needle aspiration to the diagnosis of lung cancer. *BMC Cancer* 2012; 12: 34–38.
52. Schreiber G, McCrory DC. Performance characteristics of different modalities for diagnosis of suspected lung cancer: summary of published evidence. *Chest* 2003; 123: 115–128.
53. Rivera M, Mehta AC, Wahidi MM. Establishing the diagnosis of lung cancer diagnosis and management of lung cancer, 3rd ed: American College of Chest Physicians evidence-based clinical practice guidelines. *Chest* 2013; 143: Suppl., e142S–e165S.
54. Wang-Memoli JS, Nietert PJ, Silvestri GA. Meta-analysis of guided bronchoscopy for evaluation of the pulmonary nodule. *Chest* 2012; 142: 385–393.
55. Van der Laan PA, Wang HH, Majid A, *et al.* Endobronchial ultrasound-guided transbronchial needle aspiration (EBUS-TBNA): an overview and update for the cytopathologist. *Cancer Cytopathol* 2014; 122: 561–576.
56. Coghlin CL, Smith LJ, Bakar S, *et al.* Quantitative analysis of tumor in bronchial biopsy specimens. *J Thorac Oncol* 2010; 5: 448–452.
57. Edwards SL, Roberts C, McKean ME, *et al.* Preoperative histological classification of primary lung cancer: accuracy of diagnosis and use of the non-small cell category. *J Clin Pathol* 2000; 53: 537–540.
58. Chuang MT, Marchevsky A, Teirstein AS, *et al.* Diagnosis of lung cancer by fibreoptic bronchoscopy: problems in the histological classification of non-small cell carcinomas. *Thorax* 1984; 39: 175–178.
59. Thomas JS, Lamb D, Ashcroft T, *et al.* How reliable is the diagnosis of lung cancer using small biopsy specimens? Report of a UKCCCR Lung Cancer Working Party. *Thorax* 1993; 48: 1135–1139.
60. Wallace WA, Rassl DM. Accuracy of cell typing in nonsmall cell lung cancer by EBUS/EUS-FNA cytological samples. *Eur Respir J* 2011; 38: 911–917.
61. Loo PS, Thomas SC, Nicolson MC, *et al.* Subtyping of undifferentiated non-small cell carcinomas in bronchial biopsy specimens. *J Thorac Oncol* 2010; 5: 442–447.
62. Mukhopadhyay S, Katzenstein AL. Subclassification of non-small cell lung carcinomas lacking morphologic differentiation on biopsy specimens: utility of an immunohistochemical panel containing TTF-1, napsin A, p63, and CK5/6. *Am J Surg Pathol* 2011; 35: 15–25.

63. Terry J, Leung S, Laskin J, *et al.* Optimal immunohistochemical markers for distinguishing lung adenocarcinomas from squamous cell carcinomas in small tumor samples. *Am J Surg Pathol* 2010; 34: 1805–1811.
64. Righi L, Graziano P, Fornari A, *et al.* Immunohistochemical subtyping of nonsmall cell lung cancer not otherwise specified in fine-needle aspiration cytology: a retrospective study of 103 cases with surgical correlation. *Cancer* 2011; 117: 3416–3423.
65. Kret A, Clark C, Scott P, *et al.* Mutation analysis and association with TTF1 expression in lung non-squamous NSCLC. *Lung Cancer* 2015; 87: Suppl. 1, s16.
66. Thunnissen E, Boers E, Heideman DAM, *et al.* Correlation of immunohistochemical staining p63 and TTF-1 with EGFR and K-ras mutational spectrum and diagnostic reproducibility in non small cell lung carcinoma. *Virchows Arch* 2012; 461: 629–638.
67. Kerr KM, Popper HH. Differential diagnosis of pre-invasive lung lesions. *In*: Timens WPopper HH, eds. Pathology of the Lung: Recent Advances in Clinical and Experimental Pathology. *ERS Monogr* 2007; 12: 37–62.
68. Goldstraw P, Crowley J, Chansky K, *et al.* The IASLC lung cancer staging project: proposals for the revision of the TNM stage groupings in the forthcoming (seventh) edition of the TNM classification of malignant tumours. *J Thorac Oncol* 2007; 2: 706–714.

---

Disclosures: None declared.

Chapter 7

# The current and future roles of genomics

Kwun M. Fong[1,2], Marissa Daniels[1,2], Felicia Goh[2], Ian A. Yang[1,2] and Rayleen V. Bowman[1,2]

Lung cancer research has been positively informed by genetic and now genomic technologies and discoveries. In the last few years, we have seen the emergence of cancer genomic data in the public arena; information that is challenging long-held theories of cancer mutational biology and changing how clinicians are thinking about a future with genomics-based lung cancer care. Lung cancer mutation catalogues will continue to expand, giving rise to an appreciation of tumour biology beyond the classic clinical–pathological standpoint. This will lead to new considerations, including how best to exploit this data for diagnostics and therapeutics. Research is needed to characterise the vast and complex cancer mutations, distinguish drivers from passengers, and validate and functionally characterise cancer genomes in order to generate information that can meaningfully alter clinical management in a cost-effective manner. International research collaborations represent an encouraging model for engaging, sharing insights and learning how to best use and contribute to clinical applications of cancer genomics.

Much work has been undertaken to understand the molecular basis of lung cancer, particularly that involving classic oncogenes and tumour suppressor genes (TSGs or recessive oncogenes). With modern technologies, the pace of research has rapidly accelerated, bringing with it knowledge of the place of genetics, genomics and epigenetics in lung cancer pathogenesis. The current model suggests that human tumours, such as lung cancer, arise as a result of the accumulation of multiple molecular events which target critical cellular pathways in key cells, events that are distinct from random background genetic damage occurring during tumour progression. Specific oncogenes and TSGs are the likely targets of somatic aberrations resulting from the genotoxicity of tobacco smoke carcinogens.

Rapid technological advances in the background of the Human Genome Project have led to an explosion of knowledge about cancer genomics, including lung cancer, a common and most deadly cancer. Cancer genomics, the study of the cancer cell's DNA, has come a long way since pivotal DNA sequencing technologies were introduced in the mid-1970s [1, 2]. After discovery of the first human tumourigenic somatic mutation in 1982 [3] and elucidation of the human reference genome [4, 5], impressive technological advances

[1]Dept of Thoracic Medicine, The Prince Charles Hospital, Brisbane, Australia. [2]University of Queensland Thoracic Research Centre, Brisbane, Australia

Correspondence: Kwun M. Fong, Dept of Thoracic Medicine, The Prince Charles Hospital, Rode Road, Chermside, Brisbane 4032, Australia. E-mail: kwun.fong@health.qld.gov.au

 Print ISBN: 978-1-84984-061-3. Online ISBN: 978-1-84984-062-0. Print ISSN: 2312-508X. Online ISSN: 2312-5098.

enabled the first human cancer genome to be sequenced a few years later [6]. The relative speed and scalability of modern sequencing technologies is quickly improving our ability to explore the cancer genome, and is exponentially advancing our understanding of lung cancer pathogenesis and management [7–10].

The current and future potential roles of lung cancer genomics for improving actual health outcomes for our patients will be explored in this chapter.

## Lung carcinogenesis

Knowledge of the molecular changes occurring in lung cancer is rapidly increasing. The molecular pathology and clinical implications are covered in detail in other chapters of this *Monograph*. Table 1 shows selected common somatic cancer aberrations, and individual affected genes are catalogued in large publicly available databases such as the Catalogue of Somatic Mutations in Cancer (COSMIC, http://cancer.sanger.ac.uk/cosmic/). The drive behind molecular cancer research stems from its ability to contribute substantial new knowledge of carcinogenesis, and to translate actionable molecular biomarkers into co-dependent therapies, which result in improved health outcomes for people with the disease subtype. Examples include sensitising EGFR mutations and ALK fusion genes [11].

Table 1. Examples of molecular aberrations in lung cancer

| | SCLC | NSCLC |
|---|---|---|
| **Oncogenes** | | |
| RAS mutation | <1% | ~15–20% |
| MYC amplification/overexpression | ~15–30% | ~5–10% |
| EGFR mutation | Rare | ~10% (higher in Asians, nonsmokers, ADC, females) |
| EML4/ALK fusion | | ~1–5% |
| ROS1 fusion | | ~1–2% |
| LKB1 mutation | | 39% |
| HER2 mutation/amplification | | ~2–4% |
| PIK3CA mutation/amplification | | ~2–18% |
| TTF1 amplification | | ~15% |
| BRAF alterations | | ~2–3% |
| MET mutation/amplification | ? rare | ~1–20% |
| FGFR1 amplification | | ~22% SCC |
| SOX2 amplification | | ~23% |
| Autocrine loops | GRP/GRPR, SCF/KIT | HGF/MET, neuregulin/ERBB |
| **Tumour suppressor genes** | | |
| CDKN2A mutation | <1% | ~10–40% |
| TP53 mutation | ~75–100% | ~50% |
| 17p LOH | ~80–90% | ~70% |
| Absent RB1 expression | ~90% | ~15–30% |
| 13q LOH | ~75% | ~40–60% |
| 3p allele loss | >90% | ~50–80% |
| 9p LOH | ~20–50% | ~50–75% |

GRP: gastrin-releasing peptide; GRPR: GRP receptor; SCF: stem cell factor; LOH: loss of heterozygosity.

Prior to the development of massively parallel sequencing (MPS, commonly called "next-generation"), understanding of the molecular pathology of lung cancer was based on methods such as PCR, capillary electrophoresis-based Sanger sequencing of candidate genes [12], single nucleotide polymorphism (SNP) arrays [13], array-based genome-wide analysis of amplifications and deletions [14], and gene expression arrays [15] to find genomic drivers of cancer [13, 16, 17] and novel therapeutic targets [17, 18].

High throughput sequencing enabled comprehensive examination of the lung cancer exome [19] and genome [20, 21]. MPS is able to generate sequence data orders of magnitude more quickly, and at lower cost, than traditional techniques [7, 22]. MPS applications [23] include: whole genome sequencing (WGS) and whole exome sequencing (WES) to find novel mutations [24]; paired-end and mate-pair sequencing to identify structural variations [25]; targeted resequencing for mutation discovery and validation [26]; transcriptome sequencing for quantification of gene expression and discovery of transcribed mutations [27]; small RNA sequencing for microRNA profiling [28]; large-scale analysis of DNA methylation [29]; and chromatin immunoprecipitation for genomic mapping of DNA–protein interactions [30]. MPS can identify the major somatic alterations in cancer, including nucleotide substitutions, small insertions and deletions (indels), copy number alterations, chromosomal rearrangements and microbial infections. In addition, mutational profiles can be identified, including *kataegis* (foci of localised substation hypermutation implicating the APOBEC enzyme family) [31], *chromothripsis* (chromosomal shattering, a catastrophic event with multiple rearrangements typically in one or a few chromosomes) [32] and chromosomal chains [33, 34].

An important and key global collaborative approach to cancer MPS is led by the International Cancer Genome Consortium (ICGC) and The Cancer Genome Atlas (TCGA) [35, 36], whose endeavours included evaluation of the two major subtypes of lung cancer, ADC and SCC. These long and careful cancer genomic research projects provide knowledge of the complete genome of cancer cells, which can now be exploited for modern therapeutics [10, 37].

Initial large-scale sequencing projects aimed to identify genes that contain "driver" somatic mutations in tumour samples compared with "passenger" mutations that do not contribute to carcinogenesis [38]. In one study, >1000 somatic mutations were found in 274 megabases of DNA corresponding with the coding exons of 518 protein kinase genes in 210 diverse human cancers, of which perhaps 120 genes were thought to harbour driver mutations [39]. Interestingly, a novel analysis combining MPS with conventional epidemiology suggested that three sequential mutations are required to develop lung ADC, fewer than previously thought [40].

An earlier study in lung cancer used SNP arrays to identify homozygous deletions and chromosome amplifications in primary lung carcinoma and cell lines. Two homozygous deletion regions were identified: one near PTPRD (protein tyrosine phosphatase, receptor type, D) on 9p23; and another in 3q25. High-level amplifications were identified within 8q12–13 in two SCLC specimens, 12p11 in two NSCLC specimens, and 22q11 in four NSCLC specimens. Tyrosine kinase genes showing high-level amplification included EGFR (three NSCLC), FGFR1 (two NSCLC), ERBB2 (one NSCLC) and MET (one NSCLC) [41].

Earlier studies focussed on candidate cancer genes: DNA sequencing of 623 candidates in 188 lung ADCs revealed >1000 somatic mutations, including in 26 genes that are mutated at high frequencies, such as tyrosine kinase genes, ephrin receptor genes, VEGFR kinase domain receptor and neurotrophic tyrosine kinase receptor genes. These studies in primary lung ADC also provided evidence of somatic mutations in tumour-suppressor genes implicated in other cancers, including NF1 (neurofibromin 1), APC (adenomatous polyposis coli), RB1 (retinoblastoma 1) and ATM (ataxia telangiectasia mutated), and of sequence changes in PTPRD, as well as the frequently deleted gene LRP1B (low density lipoprotein receptor-related protein 1B) [12]. Another study searched for somatic mutations in 1507 coding genes from 441 tumours (breast, lung, ovarian and prostate), and discovered 2576 mutations, with heterogeneity in mutation rates and affected genes across tumour types and subtypes. The 77 statistically significantly mutated genes included protein kinases and G-protein-coupled receptors, such as GRM8 (glutamate receptor metabotropic 8), BAI3 (brain-specific angiogenesis inhibitor 3), AGTRL1 and LPHN3 (latrophilin 3). Another 35 altered genes, including GNAS (GNAS complex locus), were identified by integrated evaluation of somatic mutations and copy number alterations [42].

## Lung cancer genome studies

The current lung cancer MPS studies are summarised in table 2. The genomes of two lung cancer cell lines (neuroendocrine and SCLC) were published in 2008 [25], followed by another SCLC cell line [43]. The SCLC line NCI-H209 demonstrated 22910 somatic substitutions, including 134 in coding exons, evidence of different mutation signatures, and a tandem duplication affecting CHD7 (chromodomain helicase DNA binding protein 7) [43]. WGS studies of primary tumours paired with normal lung soon followed [20, 21], notably the WGS by Imielinski *et al.* [44] of 36 pulmonary ADCs/normal lung pairs, coupled with WES of another 92 pairs, with mean coverages of 69x and 91x, respectively. Using an optimal combination of four bioinformatics strategies, this study identified 25 significantly mutated genes. Following this, TCGA published their large-scale analysis of SCC with 178 WES and 19 WGS on paired SCC/germline DNA, and whole transcriptome profiling using integrated RNA sequencing and microarray data [45]. Gene expression subtype signatures were described that classified tumours in terms of gene overexpression relative to other subtypes, according to functional themes [60]. Subsequently, TCGA's study of ADC was published [49]. The field is rapidly progressing, with the most striking findings including identification of novel lung cancer genes, increasing recognition of actionable mutations in ADC [49], and emerging molecular themes in cancers arising in different organs [61, 62].

WGS has also been used, in association with whole transcriptome sequencing, to study genomic differences between NSCLC in smokers and never-smokers. Govindan *et al.* [47] performed paired-end WGS sequencing on 17 tumour/normal lung pairs, including 16 ADCs and a single large cell carcinoma, with mean haploid coverage of 30x. In addition to the influence of known carcinogens and inherited predisposition, recent analysis suggests that much of the lifetime risk of cancer may be due to random mutations occurring during DNA replication in normal, non-cancerous stem cells [63].

## TCGA contribution

TCGA's contribution to cancer genomic research has been significant, and we have been fortunate enough to contribute tumour biospecimens to the lung SCC and ADC categories of

Table 2. Genomic studies of lung cancer

| First author/study group [ref.] | Year | Design | Findings |
|---|---|---|---|
| **Campbell [25]** | 2008 | WGS of one SCLC cell line and one neuroendocrine lung cancer cell line. | 103 somatic rearrangements predominantly in heavily amplified regions, including tandem duplications, inverted duplication creating *PVT-CHD7* fusion gene. 8q24 amplification with 35-fold *MYC* amplification. |
| **Pleasance [43]** | 2010 | WGS of single SCLC cell line integrated with Affymetrix U133A microarray. | 22 910 somatic substitutions, including 134 in coding regions, 65 indels, 334 CNVs and 58 SVs. *RB1*, *TP53* and *MLL2* mutations; *PVT-CHD7* fusion gene. Signatures of DNA repair and tobacco-associated mutation observed. |
| **Lee [21]** | 2010 | WGS of single NSCLC/normal lung pair integrated with Agilent Human Genome CGH 244A microarray and Affymetrix SNP 6.0 array. | 17.7 mutations per megabase. >50 000 SNVs, 392 in coding regions; 43 structural variants. Evidence of selective pressures within tumour environment observed. |
| **Ju [20]** | 2012 | Integrated analysis of WGS and transcriptome sequencing of single NSCLC liver metastasis/normal lung pair. | Novel *KIF5B-RET* fusion gene identified as candidate driver variant. 10 724 SNVs, 334 coding region indels and 70 large deletions, including 10 nonsynonymous somatic mutations identified. 52 fusion genes. |
| **Imielinski [44]** | 2012 | 183 ADC and matched normal tissue; 159 WES, 23 WES plus WGS, one WGS. | 12.0 somatic mutations/megabase. Novel recurrently mutated genes: *ARID1A*, *RBM10*, *U2AF1*. In-frame exonic SVs in *EGFR* and *SIK2*. |
| **Caner Genome Atlas Research Network [45]** | 2012 | Integrated analysis of 178 SCCs and matched germline: 178 WES, 19 WGS, 178 array-based copy number assessment, 178 RNA sequencing, 121 Agilent 224 K gene expression microarray, 158 miRNA sequencing, 178 DNA methylation array. | Novel mutation in HLA-A. Significantly altered pathways: *NFE2L2/KEAP1* (34%), squamous differentiation (44%), *PI3K/AKT* (47%), *CDKN2A/RB1* (72%). |
| **Peifer [46]** | 2012 | Integrated analysis of WES of 27 SCLC tumour/normal pairs, WES of two SCLC cell line/normal pairs, WGS of two SCLC tumour/normal pairs with transcriptome sequencing 15 SCLC. | High mutation rate: 7.4±1 nonsynonymous mutations/megabase; universal *TP53* and *RB1* inactivation; recurrent mutations in histone modifiers *CREBBP*, *EP300*, and *MLL*. |
| **Govindan [47]** | 2012 | Integrated analysis of WGS of 16 ADC/normal pairs and WGS of one large cell carcinoma/normal pair, with RNA sequencing of all 17 tumours. | Novel mutations in chromatin modification and DNA repair pathways; 14 fusions, including *ROS*, *ALK* and metabolic enzymes. Possible roles of *EGFR* and *KRAS* as tumour initiators. |

Continued

Table 2. Continued

| First author/study group [ref.] | Year | Design | Findings |
|---|---|---|---|
| **Yin [48]** | 2014 | WES of nine NSCLC/normal tissue pairs from Chinese patients. | Significant intertumoural variation; mean numbers of nonsynonymous, synonymous and intergenic/intronic mutations per case were 132, 40 and 229, respectively. 93 indels and 301 deleterious CNV events. Significantly altered pathways: DNA repair, NF-κB, *JAK/STAT* signalling and chromatin modification. Recurrent mutations in histone-lysine methyltransferase gene *MLL2*. |
| **Cancer Genome Atlas Research Network [49]** | 2014 | WES, SNP array copy number analysis, low coverage WGS (average 5.6x), mRNA sequencing, reverse phase protein array, methylation profiling and miRNA sequencing of 230 ADC with matched constitutional DNA. | Six molecular subtypes identified. Significantly altered genes included oncogenes (*TP53* 46%, *KRAS* 33%, *EGFR* 14%, *BRAF* 10%, *PIK3CA* 7%, *MET* 7%, *RIT1* 2%), tumour suppressor genes (*STK11* 17%, *KEAP1* 17%, *NF1* 11%, *RB1* 4%, *CDKN2A* 4%), chromatin-modifying genes (*WETD2* 9%, *ARID1A* 7%, *SMARCA4* 6%) and RNA-splicing genes (*RBM10* 8%, *U2AF1* 3%). Novel amplification of *CCND3*. Chromothripsis in six out of 93. Recurrent abnormalities in RTK/RAS/RAF (76%), PI(3)K-mTOR (25%), p53 pathway alteration (63%), cell cycle regulators (64%), oxidative stress (22%), chromatin and RNA splicing (49%). |
| **Zhang [50]** | 2014 | Multiregion WES of 11 ADC (48 regions) with paired normal. | Branched evolution observed. Copy number alterations and mutation in known cancer genes acquired early in tumour development. 76% of mutations identified in all regions within a tumour. Imprint of different mutational processes at different tumour developmental stages. Tumour recurrence after resection may be associated with increasing subclonal fraction. |
| **de Bruin [51]** | 2014 | Multiregion WES of seven NSCLC (25 regions) with paired normal; WGS of two regions. | Branched evolution observed. Median 30% mutations heterogeneously distributed; both truncal and branch mutations and CNVs observed. ITH of SVs observed. Significant shifts of mutational patterns during tumour evolution. |
| **Cancer Genome Atlas Research Network [52]** | 2013 | Analysis of 5074 tumour samples from 12 different tumour types, including lung SCC and ADC. 93% assessed for genomic, epigenomic, gene expression and protein analysis on at least one platform. | The Pan-Cancer project aimed to identify patterns of genomic change across the spectrum of these 12 human tumour types, investigate the number of samples required for accurate analysis and assess for actionable targets. |

Continued

Table 2. Continued

| First author/study group [ref.] | Year | Design | Findings |
|---|---|---|---|
| Ciriello [53] | 2013 | Hierarchical classification of genetic (WES and SNP) array, and epigenetic (methylation array) events in 3229 tumours of 12 cancer types, including 229 lung ADC and 182 SCC. | ADC are characterised either by mutations or copy number alterations; SCC are primarily characterised by copy number alterations. |
| Lawrence [54] | 2013 | WGS and WES of 3083 tumours of 12 cancer types, including 514 lung cancers: 179 SCC (14 WGS and 165 WES) and 335 ADC (WES). | Lung ADC and SCC have high rates of somatic mutations relative to other tumours; C→A mutations predominate. |
| Zack [55] | 2013 | SCNA profiling of 357 ADC and 344 SCC using SNP array and WGS. | Lung ADC and SCC have high rates of whole genome duplication relative to other tumour types (59% ADC and 64% SCC); recurrent focal SCNAs seen in lung SCC and head and neck SCC. |
| Kandoth [56] | 2013 | Mutation analysis of 3281 tumours from 12 cancer types, including 230 lung ADC and 178 SCC. | The highest mutation rates of all cancers studied were seen in lung ADC and SCC. This was related to *TP53* mutations. *KEAP1* mutations predominate in lung ADC and SCC. *EPHA*, *SETBP1* and *STK11* mutations predominate in lung ADC. |
| Tamborero [57] | 2013 | Mutational analysis of 3205 tumours from 12 tumour types, including 226 ADC and 174 SCC. | Lung ADC and SCC have high rates of protein-activating mutations in high confidence driver mutations relative to other tumour types (median of nine per tumour). |
| Gonzalez-Perez [58] | 2013 | Resequencing data from 4623 exomes from 13 tumour types, including 390 ADC, 31 NSCLC, 174 SCC and 69 SCLC. | IntOGen-mutations platform is a web-based analysis pipeline, which is able to summarise genomic data systematically. |
| Lawrence [59] | 2014 | Predominantly WES of 405 ADC tumour-normal pairs and 178 SCC tumour-normal pairs. | Estimates suggest the number of driver mutations detected in SCC may more than double given sufficient sample size. In excess of 3000 tumour-normal pairs required to detect alterations in 90% of genes mutated at 2% above background with 90% power. |

WGS: whole genome sequencing; CNV: copy number variation; SV: structural variation; SNV: single nucleotide variation; WES: whole exome sequencing; HLA-A: human leukocyte antigen A; miRNA: micro RNA; NF-κB: nuclear factor-κB; SNP: single nucleotide polymorphism; ITH: intratumoural heterogeneity; SCNA: somatic copy number alteration.

this large-scale collaboration. TCGA began as a pilot in 2006 when the US National Cancer Institute (NCI) and National Human Genome Research Institute (NHGRI) created a network of research and technology, underpinned by infrastructure, to make data publicly accessible. The entire process was carefully quality assured to ensure that the highest quality data was achieved from paired tumour and non-tumour control samples (over 500 specimens per tumour type), which had to meet strict clinical criteria to avoid misclassification and confounders, coupled with stringent quality standards for nucleotide sequencing and mutation calling. Extracted DNA and RNA data from TCGA are publically available to the international community to facilitate further data analysis and validation of discoveries [12].

## Challenges for lung cancer genomics

### *Technical and bioinformatic*

MPS technologies offer significant advantages but are not free of technical limitations. Traditional Sanger sequencing is widely available; meticulous, but time-consuming, it generally delivers reads of ~1000 bp with raw accuracy of 99.999% [23]. Newer MPS techniques generate large numbers of relatively short reads using techniques vulnerable to systematic error when applied to comprehensive genomic analysis [64]. Indeed, each sequencing platform has a unique profile of strengths and weaknesses [65]. Short sequence read lengths can be troublesome to assemble, and can create a biased aligned read that is insensitive to repeat content, hindering systematic exploration of the genetic basis of disease. Even the "complete reference" is reported to contain up to 350 gaps [64]. Regions of the genome rich in repeats, such as those in proximity with centromeres and telomeres, are particularly challenging to map with small read lengths. Long sequences of repeated bases, degraded or damaged DNA, and C-G rich regions are problematic [64]. Sanger sequencing remains the method of choice for characterising regions where NGS is suboptimal [66].

Cancer genomics requires massive advances in both experimental and computational bioinformatics technology. The extremely large MPS datasets demand effective strategies to optimally store, analyse and handle the "big data". Assembly programmes are essential for sequence alignment and mapping, but, like the sequencing platforms themselves, they also have the potential to confound results [67]. A variety of sample preparation technologies are now available to help eliminate the need for template amplification and to generate reads of sufficient length to bridge repeat regions. After generating and aligning sequencing data, MPS bioinformaticians face the intricate complexity of the mutational profile of lung cancer as they attempt to discriminate between driver and passenger mutations. There are multiple MPS data variant callers with differing characteristics [68]. Common strategies include the selection of biologically relevant, recurrent mutations; however, the definition of "recurrent" can be inconsistent [44, 69].

A tiered approach to mutation classification has been suggested [70]. Tier 1 mutations include changes in the coding regions of annotated exons, consensus splice-site regions, and RNA genes (including miRNA). Tier 2 features changes in conserved regions of the genome or those with regulatory potential. Tier 3 is characterised by mutations in the non-repetitive part of the genome not included in Tier 2. The remainder of the genome is allocated to Tier 4.

### *Clinical translation challenges*

Investigators are now focussing on efforts to synthesise the vast data from MPS into evidence-based clinical strategies and recommendations using open access, open source knowledge commons [71, 72]. A typical cancer genomics workflow that has clinical utility will require analytical and clinical validity, underpinned by consideration of the whole process, from genome sequencing to reporting. Critical steps include standardised production of tumour short sequence reads, alignment to a reference genome, application of mutation detection algorithms, filtering, review, validation and annotation, with application of functional prediction algorithms, leading to a clinically meaningful report. Validation may be complex given the large number of potential variants likely to be identified [73]. We need to better understand how MPS will perform in comparison to current diagnostic reference standards [74]. In order to understand the clinical utility of mutations identified by MPS, cross-referencing to current literature (such as PubMed), drug–gene interaction databases (*e.g.* the Drug Gene Interaction Database (DGIdb)), relevant clinical trials and known clinical actionability databases will be needed.

Lung cancers are well known to be relatively difficult to biopsy given their location within the thorax and the frequent associated comorbidities in patients with the disease. Typically, only a small biopsy sample (by bronchoscopy or fine-needle aspiration) can be submitted, and these limited samples pose problems for complete and unbiased MPS interrogation of the whole genome. Given that most of the current data has been generated from high-quality DNA from carefully selected (frequently fresh frozen) biospecimens, uncertainties exist regarding the performance of MPS with routine lung cancer samples [73]. Nonetheless, targeted approaches to actionable panels using MPS technology are increasingly reported [75]. Most genomic studies to date are from cell lines and primary cancers, so gaps exist for pre-neoplastic lung lesions as well as metastatic lesions. Also, to understand the natural history of cancer genomics, serial samples require testing.

## Intra-tumoural heterogeneity

The concept of intra-tumoural heterogeneity is not new to the clonal model of cancer [76]. Second-generation sequencing studies of geographical regions (multiregion sequencing) within a single tumour have provided new insights that enable the study of both spatial and temporal variation within cancer genomes (table 2). The visual representation of tumour growth as a Darwinian tree, with the trunk representing ubiquitous mutations and the branches representing heterogeneous mutations, provides a conceptual framework for tumour clonal development [77, 78]. Two recent analyses by Zhang *et al.* [50] and de Bruin *et al.* [51] report evidence of branched evolution of NSCLC. The presence of subclonal driver variants, observed with both geographic and temporal variation, and the intra-tumoural differences in mutational patterns suggest that these tumours may develop in response to local influences that evolve over time. In fact, de Bruin *et al.* [51] observed that smoking-related mutations may be acquired decades prior to the development of clinically evident disease. As suggested by Govindan [79], ongoing research is required to understand the processes of regional and temporal tumour evolution, and their influence on the natural history of lung cancer.

Intra-tumoural heterogeneity is postulated to contribute to treatment resistance by enabling drug resistance to develop in subclones during the course of treatment. Alternatively, subclones may have resistance mutations, such as EGFR T790M. Consequently, strategies to address the genomics of the major and relevant subclones may prove valuable, and should certainly be considered in the design of clinical trials. This also has implications for sampling tumours, as current biopsy techniques may provide data on some, but not all, subclones. A full understanding of the geographical and temporal heterogeneity in nonsurgical lung cancer may be restricted by practical constraints if repeated biopsies are needed [80]. In future, single-cell sequencing (from circulating tumour cells, for example) may shed light on the plasticity of the tumour genome and allow monitoring of clonal responses to therapeutics [34, 81–83].

## Lung cancer susceptibility: candidate and genome-wide association studies

Despite the fact that tobacco smoke is implicated in most cases of lung cancer, only a proportion of smokers develop lung cancer. Clearly, there are other important factors operating apart from the simple inhalation of tobacco smoke. It has been postulated that individuals may exhibit genetic polymorphisms in carcinogen metabolising pathways, leading to inherited differences in the risk of lung cancer associated with tobacco smoking. The relationships of human lung cancer to polymorphisms of phase I pro-carcinogen-activating and phase II-deactivating enzymes and intermediate biomarkers of DNA mutation (such as DNA adducts, oncogene and tumour suppressor gene mutation) and polymorphisms have been compiled [84]. In evaluation of cancer risk conferred by a genetic variant, the genome-wide association study (GWAS) methodology uses an association testing approach on a genome-wide scale, testing large numbers of SNPs using standard microarray platforms [6]. The key advantage of this approach is that it enables testing of SNPs across the entire genome without needing a prior hypothesis about the identity of causal genes (as in traditional genetic association approaches, such as linkage studies and candidate gene approaches) [6]. Disadvantages include lack of coverage of rare variants and the inability to analyse gene–gene interactions, gene–environment interactions, epigenomics or other principles that can explain variance in heritability.

A number of lung cancer GWAS have now been published (table 3). The most frequent genetic association for lung cancer in smokers was observed with SNPs in chromosomal region 15q25 containing the genes for the neuronal nicotinic acetylcholine receptor subunits (*CHRNA3* and *CHRNA5* (cholinergic receptor, nicotinic, α3 and α 5)). This chromosomal region has also been associated with smoking behaviour and intensity *e.g.* cigarettes per day, in several GWAS. Whilst the association of smoking behaviour with nicotine receptor SNPs could partly explain the relationship with lung cancer, many of the GWAS and subsequent validation studies have adjusted for measures of smoking intensity [106]. With this adjustment, the association with nicotine receptor SNPs has remained positive in many studies. The mechanism postulated is that variation in the nicotine receptor pathway, due to genetic variation, contributes directly to lung cancer susceptibility, in addition to or independent from smoking intensity. Another chromosomal region, at 13q, has been associated with lung cancer in never-smokers [95].

Overall, it would seem that the more common putative susceptibility variants are associated with a relatively small increased risk of disease, and in the case of smoking-related lung cancer, risk is clearly influenced by the gene–environment (tobacco carcinogens) interaction. Further recent work suggests a significant component of chance in human cancer development [63]. Nevertheless, research is still expected to suggest novel future diagnostics and biomarkers, with diverse applications ranging from risk prediction for CT screening programmes to prediction of toxicities and response to medicines (pharmacogenomics).

Table 3. Genome-wide association studies for lung cancer susceptibility

| First author [ref.] | Year | Lung cancer cases (discovery set)# | Controls (discovery set) | Arrays (SNPs n) | Chromosomal regions and main associated genes |
|---|---|---|---|---|---|
| **Spinola [85]** | 2007 | 335 smokers | 338 smokers | Affymetrix (116 204) | 10p *KLF6* |
| **Amos [86]** | 2008 | 1154 smokers | 1137 smokers | Illumina (317 498) | 15q *CHRNA3* |
| **Hung [87]** | 2008 | 1989 smokers | 2625 smokers | Illumina (317 139) | 15q *CHRNA3*, *CHRNA5* |
| **Liu [88]** | 2008 | 194 with familial lung cancer | 219 smokers and nonsmokers | Affymetrix (500 568 and 906 703) | 15q various genes |
| **Thorgeirsson [89]** | 2008 | 1024 smokers | 32 244 | Illumina (306 207) | 15q *CHRNA3* |
| **McKay [90]** | 2008 | 3259 smokers | 4159 smokers | Illumina (315 194) | 5p *TERT-CLPTM1L*, 15q *CHRNA3* |
| **Wang [91]** | 2008 | 1952 smokers | 1438 smokers | Illumina (511 919) | 5p *CLPTM1L*, 6p *BAT3-MSH5*, 15q *CHRNA3* |
| **Broderick [92]** | 2009 | 1978 smokers and meta-analysis | 1438 smokers and meta-analysis | Meta-analysis | 5p *TERT-CLPTM1L*, 6p *BAT3-MSH5*, *TNXB*, 15q *CHRNA3* |
| **Landi [93]** | 2009 | 5739 smokers | 5848 smokers | Illumina (515 922) | 5p *TERT-CLPTM1L*, 15q *CHRNA3* |
| **Hsiung [94]** | 2010 | 584 cases (never-smoking females with lung ADC) | 585 (never-smoking females) | Illumina (610 901) | 5p15 *TERT-CLPTM1L* |
| **Li [95]** | 2010 | 377 never-smokers | 377 never-smokers | Illumina (373 397 and 592 532) | 13q31.3 *GPC5* |
| **Miki [96]** | 2010 | 1004 with lung ADC | 1900 | Illumina (610 901) | 3q28 *TP63*, 5p15 *TERT* |
| **Yoon [97]** | 2010 | 621 cases (smokers and never-smokers) | 1541 (smokers and never-smokers) | Affymetrix (500 568) | 3q29 *C3orf21*, 5p *TERT-CLPTM1L* |
| **Hu [98]** | 2011 | 2331 cases (smokers and never-smokers) | 3077 (smokers and never-smokers) | Affymetrix (906 703) | 3q28 *TP63*, 5p15 *TERT-CLPTM1L*, 13q12 *MIPEP-TNFRSF19*, 22q12 *MTMR3-HORMAD2-LIF* |
| **Ahn [99]** | 2012 | 446 never-smokers | 497 | Affymetrix (906 703 | 18p11 *FAM38B* |
| **Dong [100]** | 2012 | 833 cases with SCC | 3094 | Affymetrix (906 703 | 12q23 *SLC17A8-NR1H4* |
| **Lan [101]** | 2012 | 5510 never-smoking female lung cancer cases | 4544 | Various | 3q28 *TP63*, 5p15, 6p21 *HLA*, 6q22 *ROS1*, *DCBLD1*, 10q25 *VTI1A*, 17q24 *BPTF* |
| **Shiraishi [102]** | 2012 | 1722 cases (smokers and never-smokers) | 5846 (smokers and never-smokers) | Illumina (709 857) | 3q28 *TP63*, 5p15 *TERT*, 6p21 *BTNL2*, 17q24 *BPTF* |
| **Timofeeva [103]** | 2012 | Meta-analysis: 14 900 cases (smokers and never-smokers) | 29 485 (smokers and never-smokers) | Various | 5p15, 6p21, 15q25 for NSCLC; 9p21 for SCC |
| **Kim [104]** | 2013 | 285 female never-smokers with lung cancer | 1455 | Affymetrix (440 794) | 2p16 *NRXN1* |
| **Wang [105]** | 2014 | 11 348 cases | 15 861 | Illumina (various), meta-analysis | *BRCA2* p.Lys3326X (rs11571833) and CHEK2 p.Ile157Thr (rs17879961) with SCC, 3q28 (*TP63*, rs13314271) with ADC |

SNP: single-nucleotide polymorphism; SCC: squamous cell carcinoma. #: replication study samples sizes have not been included. For details, see www.genome.gov/gwastudies.

## Conclusion

The Human Genome Project and associated efforts have brought much hope for lung cancer medicine, given the potential of cancer genomics to provide hitherto unavailable insight into the spectrum of somatic cancer derangements. Future studies are set to provide deeper understanding of genetic lung cancer susceptibility, and thus pave the way to better prevention and early detection strategies. Comparison of mutational spectra across human cancers has provided new insights into the diversity and commonalities in somatic mutational patterns and profiles, improving understanding of carcinogenesis and molecular epidemiology [31].

These modern genetic/genomic, epigenetic/epigenomic techniques, coupled with the emergence of proteomics, should not only improve our knowledge of cellular transformation, progression and prognosis, but should also lead to novel genomic-based interventions for the prevention, early detection, monitoring of response/resistance, and treatment of lung cancer [107]. New therapeutics *e.g.* TKIs, are already in routine clinical use and the new paradigm of specifically targeted therapies [108] may be associated with relatively short timeframes from discovery to the bedside, as exemplified by ALK inhibitor treatment for sensitive ALK fusion tumours. Nonetheless, given the fundamental differences afforded by the "new" second- and future-generation sequencing-based genomics, there will be many challenges to be addressed in order for the full potential of cancer genomics to be realised by lung cancer multidisciplinary teams currently accustomed to single biomarker evidence-based medicine paradigms. As cost-effective platforms with short turn-around times are implemented and become readily available, the accumulation, secure storage and analysis of massive amounts of genomic information, including constitutional data, will tax prevailing clinical data and information systems. Important health service delivery considerations will include the optimal incorporation of lung cancer genomics investigations into the design and performance of clinical trials, and provision of evidence to adequately inform future clinical, regulatory and reimbursement perspectives [109, 110].

The fruits of hard and thoughtful genomics research efforts are clearly evident for lung and other human cancers. Taking into account the unique methodological requirements of genomic research, ongoing effort is required to bring about the clinical application of cancer genomics [111]. With careful planning and integration with conventional surgical, radiation and systemic/immunological therapies, the future paradigm of care can safely and optimistically be predicted to change for people at risk of or with lung cancer [112, 113]. Meanwhile, cataloguing all cancer mutations (especially low-frequency mutations, which require a large sample size) from initiation to metastases, and understanding the relevance of individual mutations to cellular pathways and systems biology, remain key to fully exploiting cancer genomics in the clinic [34].

## References

1. Sanger F, Coulson AR. A rapid method for determining sequences in DNA by primed synthesis with DNA polymerase. *J Mol Biol* 1975; 94: 441–448.
2. Maxim AM, Gilbert W. A new method for sequencing DNA. *Proc Natl Acad Sci USA* 1977; 74: 560–564.
3. Reddy EP, Reynolds RK, Santos E, *et al.* A point mutation is responsible for the acquisition of transforming properties by the T24 human bladder carcinoma oncogene. *Nature* 1982; 300: 149–152.
4. International Human Genome Sequencing Consortium. Finishing the euchromatic sequence of the human genome. *Nature* 2004; 431: 931–945.

5. Lander ES, Linton LM, Birren B, *et al.* Initial sequencing and analysis of the human genome. *Nature* 2001; 409: 860–920.
6. Ley TJ, Mardis ER, Ding L, *et al.* DNA sequencing of a cytogenetically normal acute myeloid leukaemia genome. *Nature* 2008; 456: 66–72.
7. Ross JS, Cronin M. Whole cancer genome sequencing by next-generation methods. *Am J Clin Pathol* 2011; 136: 527–539.
8. Mardis ER. A decade's perspective on DNA sequencing technology. *Nature* 2011; 470: 198–203.
9. Lander ES. Initial impact of the sequencing of the human genome. *Nature* 2011; 470: 187–197.
10. Meyerson M, Gabriel S, Getz G. Advances in understanding cancer genomes through second-generation sequencing. *Nat Rev Genet* 2010; 11: 685–696.
11. Reck M, Heigener DF, Mok T, *et al.* Management of non-small-cell lung cancer: recent developments. *Lancet* 2013; 382: 709–719.
12. Ding L, Getz G, Wheeler DA, *et al.* Somatic mutations affect key pathways in lung adenocarcinoma. *Nature* 2008; 455: 1069–1075.
13. Weir BA, Woo MS, Getz G, *et al.* Characterizing the cancer genome in lung adenocarcinoma. *Nature* 2007; 450: 893–898.
14. Beroukhim R, Mermel CH, Porter D, *et al.* The landscape of somatic copy-number alteration across human cancers. *Nature* 2010; 463: 899–905.
15. Tomlins SA, Rhodes DR, Perner S, *et al.* Recurrent fusion of TMPRSS2 and ETS transcription factor genes in prostate cancer. *Science* 2005; 310: 644–648.
16. Soda M, Choi YL, Enomoto M, *et al.* Identification of the transforming EML4-ALK fusion gene in non-small-cell lung cancer. *Nature* 2007; 448: 561–566.
17. Paez JG, Jänne PA, Lee JC, *et al.* EGFR mutations in lung cancer: correlation with clinical response to gefitinib therapy. *Science* 2004; 304: 1497–1500.
18. Kwak E, Bang YJ, Camidge DR, *et al.* Anaplastic lymphoma kinase inhibition in non-small-cell lung cancer. *N Engl J Med* 2010; 363: 1693–1703.
19. Liu P, Morrison C, Wang L, *et al.* Identification of somatic mutations in non-small cell lung carcinomas using whole-exome sequencing. *Carcinogenesis* 2012; 33: 1270–1276.
20. Ju YS, Lee WC, Shin JY, *et al.* A transforming KIF5B and RET gene fusion in lung adenocarcinoma revealed from whole-genome and transcriptome sequencing. *Genome Res* 2012; 22: 436–445.
21. Lee W, Jiang Z, Liu J, *et al.* The mutation spectrum revealed by paired genome sequences from a lung cancer patient. *Nature* 2010; 465: 473–477.
22. Daniels M, Goh F, Wright CM, *et al.* Whole genome sequencing for lung cancer. *J Thorac Dis* 2012; 4: 155–163.
23. Shendure J, Ji H. Next-generation DNA sequencing. *Nat Biotechnol* 2008; 26: 1135–1145.
24. Wheeler DA, Srinivasan M, Egholm M, *et al.* The complete genome of an individual by massively parallel DNA sequencing. *Nature* 2008; 452: 872–876.
25. Campbell PJ, Stephens PJ, Pleasance ED, *et al.* Identification of somatically acquired rearrangements in cancer using genome-wide massively parallel paired-end sequencing. *Nat Genet* 2008; 40: 722–729.
26. Hodges E, Xuan Z, Balija V, *et al.* Genome-wide in situ exon capture for selective resequencing. *Nat Genet* 2007; 39: 1522–1527.
27. Sugarbaker DJ, Richards WG, Gordon GJ, *et al.* Transcriptome sequencing of malignant pleural mesothelioma tumors. *Proc Natl Acad Sci USA* 2008; 105: 3521–3526.
28. Morin RD, O'Connor MD, Griffith M, *et al.* Application of massively parallel sequencing to microRNA profiling and discovery in human embryonic stem cells. *Genome Res* 2008; 18: 610–621.
29. Ordway JM, Budiman MA, Korshunova Y, *et al.* Identification of novel high-frequency DNA methylation changes in breast cancer. *PLoS One* 2007; 2: e1314.
30. Robertson G, Hirst M, Bainbridge M, *et al.* Genome-wide profiles of STAT1 DNA association using chromatin immunoprecipitation and massively parallel sequencing. *Nat Methods* 2007; 4: 651–657.
31. Alexandrov LB, Nik-Zainal S, Wedge DC, *et al.* Deciphering signatures of mutational processes operative in human cancer. *Cell Rep* 2013; 3: 246–259.
32. Stephens PJ, Greenman CD, Fu B, *et al.* Massive genomic rearrangement acquired in a single catastrophic event during cancer development. *Cell* 2011; 144: 27–40.
33. Berger MF, Lawrence MS, Demichelis F, *et al.* The genomic complexity of primary human prostate cancer. *Nature* 2011; 470: 214–220.
34. Garraway LA, Lander ES. Lessons from the cancer genome. *Cell* 2013; 153: 17–37.
35. Wu K, Huang RS, House L, *et al.* Next-generation sequencing for lung cancer. *Future Oncol* 2013; 9: 1323–1336.
36. International Cancer Genome Consortium,Hudson TJ, Anderson W, *et al.* International network of cancer genome projects. *Nature* 2010; 464: 993–998.
37. Stratton MR, Campbell PJ, Futreal PA. The cancer genome. *Nature* 2009; 458: 719–724.
38. Greaves M, Maley CC. Clonal evolution in cancer. *Nature* 2012; 481: 306–313.

39. Greenman C, Stephens P, Smith R, *et al.* Patterns of somatic mutation in human cancer genomes. *Nature* 2007; 446: 153–158.
40. Tomasetti C, Marchionni L, Nowak MA, *et al.* Only three driver gene mutations are required for the development of lung and colorectal cancers. *Proc Natl Acad Sci USA* 2015; 112: 118–123.
41. Zhao X, Weir BA, LaFramboise T, *et al.* Homozygous deletions and chromosome amplifications in human lung carcinomas revealed by single nucleotide polymorphism array analysis. *Cancer Res* 2005; 65: 5561–5570.
42. Kan Z, Jaiswal BS, Stinson J, *et al.* Diverse somatic mutation patterns and pathway alterations in human cancers. *Nature* 2010; 466: 869–873.
43. Pleasance ED, Stephens PJ, O'Meara S, *et al.* A small-cell lung cancer genome with complex signatures of tobacco exposure. *Nature* 2010; 463: 184–190.
44. Imielinski M, Berger AH, Hammerman PS, *et al.* Mapping the hallmarks of lung adenocarcinoma with massively parallel sequencing. *Cell* 2012; 150: 1107–1120.
45. Cancer Genome Atlas Research Network. Comprehensive genomic characterization of squamous cell lung cancers. *Nature* 2012; 489: 519–525.
46. Peifer M, Fernández-Cuesta L, Sos ML, *et al.* Integrative genome analyses identify key somatic driver mutations of small-cell lung cancer. *Nat Genet* 2012; 44: 1104–1110.
47. Govindan R, Ding L, Griffith M, *et al.* Genomic landscape of non-small cell lung cancer in smokers and never-smokers. *Cell* 2012; 150: 1121–1134.
48. Yin S, Yang J, Lin B, *et al.* Exome sequencing identifies frequent mutation of MLL2 in non-small cell lung carcinoma from Chinese patients. *Sci Rep* 2014; 4: 6036.
49. Cancer Genome Atlas Research Network. Comprehensive molecular profiling of lung adenocarcinoma. *Nature* 2014; 511: 543–550.
50. Zhang J, Fujimoto J, Zhang J, *et al.* Intratumor heterogeneity in localized lung adenocarcinomas delineated by multiregion sequencing. *Science* 2014; 346: 256–259.
51. de Bruin EC, McGranahan N, Mitter R, *et al.* Spatial and temporal diversity in genomic instability processes defines lung cancer evolution. *Science* 2014; 346: 251–256.
52. Cancer Genome Atlas Research Network,Weinstein JN, Collisson EA, *et al.* The Cancer Genome Atlas Pan-Cancer analysis project. *Nat Genet* 2013; 45: 1113–1120.
53. Ciriello G, Miller ML, Aksoy BA, *et al.* Emerging landscape of oncogenic signatures across human cancers. *Nat Genet* 2013; 45: 1127–1133.
54. Lawrence MS, Stojanov P, Polak P, *et al.* Mutational heterogeneity in cancer and the search for new cancer-associated genes. *Nature* 2013; 499: 214–218.
55. Zack TI, Schumacher SE, Carter SL, *et al.* Pan-cancer patterns of somatic copy number alteration. *Nat Genet* 2013; 45: 1134–1140.
56. Kandoth C, McLellan MD, Vandin F, *et al.* Mutational landscape and significance across 12 major cancer types. *Nature* 2013; 502: 333–339.
57. Tamborero D, Gonzalez-Perez A, Perez-Llamas C, *et al.* Comprehensive identification of mutational cancer driver genes across 12 tumor types. *Sci Rep* 2013; 3: 2650.
58. Gonzalez-Perez A, Perez-Llamas C, Deu-Pons J, *et al.* IntOGen-mutations identifies cancer drivers across tumor types. *Nat Methods* 2013; 10: 1081–1084.
59. Lawrence MS, Stojanov P, Mermel CH, *et al.* Discovery and saturation analysis of cancer genes across 21 tumour types. *Nature* 2014; 505: 495–501.
60. Wilkerson MD, Yin X, Hoadley KA, *et al.* Lung squamous cell carcinoma mRNA expression subtypes are reproducible, clinically important, and correspond to normal cell types. *Clin Cancer Res* 2010; 16: 4864–4875.
61. Martínez E, Yoshihara K, Kim H, *et al.* Comparison of gene expression patterns across 12 tumor types identifies a cancer supercluster characterized by TP53 mutations and cell cycle defects. *Oncogene* 2014; [In press DOI: 10.1083/onc.2014.216].
62. Hoadley KA, Yau C, Wolf DM, *et al.* Multiplatform analysis of 12 cancer types reveals molecular classification within and across tissues of origin. *Cell* 2014; 158: 929–944.
63. Tomasetti C, Vogelstein B. Cancer etiology. Variation in cancer risk among tissues can be explained by the number of stem cell divisions. *Science* 2015; 347: 78–81.
64. Marx V. The genome jigsaw. *Nature* 2013; 501: 263–268.
65. Quail MA, Smith M, Coupland P, *et al.*. A tale of three next generation sequencing platforms: comparison of Ion Torrent, Pacific Biosciences and Illumina MiSeq sequencers. *BMC Genomics* 2012; 13: 341.
66. Kirby A, Gnirke A, Jaffe DB, *et al.* Mutations causing medullary cystic kidney disease type 1 lie in a large VNTR in MUC1 missed by massively parallel sequencing. *Nat Genet* 2013; 45: 299–303.
67. Kim D, Kim WY, Lee SY, *et al.* Revising a personal genome by comparing and combining data from two different sequencing platforms. *PLoS One* 2013; 8: e60585.
68. Liu X, Han S, Wang Z, *et al.* Variant callers for next-generation sequencing data: a comparison study. *PLoS One* 2013; 8: e75619.

69. Vignot S, Frampton GM, Soria JC, *et al.* Next-generation sequencing reveals high concordance of recurrent somatic alterations between primary tumor and metastases from patients with non-small-cell lung cancer. *J Clin Oncol* 2013; 31: 2167–2172.
70. Mardis ER, Ding L, Dooling DJ, *et al.* Recurring mutations found by sequencing an acute myeloid leukemia genome. *N Engl J Med* 2009; 361: 1058–1066.
71. Dienstmann R, Dong F, Borger D, *et al.* Standardized decision support in next generation sequencing reports of somatic cancer variants. *Mol Oncol* 2014; 8: 859–873.
72. Good BM, Ainscough BJ, McMichael JF, *et al.* Organizing knowledge to enable personalization of medicine in cancer. *Genome Biol* 2014; 15: 438.
73. Salto-Tellez M, Gonzalez de Castro D. Next-generation sequencing: a change of paradigm in molecular diagnostic validation. *J Pathol* 2014; 234: 5–10.
74. McCourt CM, McArt DG, Mills K, *et al.* Validation of next generation sequencing technologies in comparison to current diagnostic gold standards for BRAF, EGFR and KRAS mutational analysis. *PLoS One* 2013; 8: e69604.
75. Karnes HE, Duncavage EJ, Bernadt CT. Targeted next-generation sequencing using fine-needle aspirates from adenocarcinomas of the lung. *Cancer Cytopathol* 2014; 122: 104–113.
76. Nowell PC. The clonal evolution of tumor cell populations. *Science* 1976; 194: 23–28.
77. Yap TA, Gerlinger M, Futreal PA, *et al.* Intratumor heterogeneity: seeing the wood for the trees. *Sci Transl Med* 2012; 4: 127ps10.
78. Gerlinger M, Rowan AJ, Horswell S, *et al.* Intratumor heterogeneity and branched evolution revealed by multiregion sequencing. *N Engl J Med* 2012; 366: 883–892.
79. Govindan. Cancer. Attack of the clones. *Science* 2014; 346: 169–170.
80. Bedard PL, Hansen AR, Ratain MJ, *et al.* Tumour heterogeneity in the clinic. *Nature* 2013; 501: 355–364.
81. Navin N, Hicks J. Future medical applications of single-cell sequencing in cancer. *Genome Med* 2011; 3: 31.
82. Navin N, Kendall J, Troge J, *et al.* Tumour evolution inferred by single-cell sequencing. *Nature* 2011; 472: 90–94.
83. Fox EJ, Loeb LA. Cancer: one cell at a time. *Nature* 2014; 512: 143–144.
84. Spivack SD, Fasco MJ, Walker VE, *et al.* The molecular epidemiology of lung cancer. *Crit Rev Toxicol* 1997; 27: 319–365.
85. Spinola M, Leoni VP, Galvan A, *et al.* Genome-wide single nucleotide polymorphism analysis of lung cancer risk detects the KLF6 gene. *Cancer Lett* 2007; 251: 311–316.
86. Amos CI, Wu X, Broderick P, *et al.* Genome-wide association scan of tag SNPs identifies a susceptibility locus for lung cancer at 15q25.1. *Nat Genet* 2008; 40: 616–622.
87. Hung RJ, McKay JD, Gaborieau V, *et al.* A susceptibility locus for lung cancer maps to nicotinic acetylcholine receptor subunit genes on 15q25. *Nature* 2008; 452: 633–637.
88. Liu P, Vikis HG, Wang D, *et al.* Familial aggregation of common sequence variants on 15q24–25.1 in lung cancer. *J Natl Cancer Inst* 2008; 100: 1326–1330.
89. Thorgeirsson TE, Geller F, Sulem P, *et al.* A variant associated with nicotine dependence, lung cancer and peripheral arterial disease. *Nature* 2008; 452: 638–642.
90. McKay JD, Hung RJ, Gaborieau V, *et al.* Lung cancer susceptibility locus at 5p15.33. *Nat Genet* 2008; 40: 1404–1406.
91. Wang Y, Broderick P, Webb E, *et al.* Common 5p15.33 and 6p21.33 variants influence lung cancer risk. *Nat Genet* 2008; 40: 1407–1409.
92. Broderick P, Wang Y, Vijayakrishnan J, *et al.* Deciphering the impact of common genetic variation on lung cancer risk: a genome-wide association study. *Cancer Res* 2009; 69: 6633–6641.
93. Landi MT, Chatterjee N, Yu K, *et al.* A genome-wide association study of lung cancer identifies a region of chromosome 5p15 associated with risk for adenocarcinoma. *Am J Hum Genet* 2009; 85: 679–691.
94. Hsiung CA, Lan Q, Hong YC, *et al.* The 5p15.33 locus is associated with risk of lung adenocarcinoma in never-smoking females in Asia. *PLoS Genet* 2010; 6: e1001051.
95. Li Y, Sheu CC, Ye Y, *et al.* Genetic variants and risk of lung cancer in never smokers: a genome-wide association study. *Lancet Oncol* 2010; 11: 321–330.
96. Miki D, Kubo M, Takahashi A, *et al.* Variation in TP63 is associated with lung adenocarcinoma susceptibility in Japanese and Korean populations. *Nat Genet* 2010; 42: 893–896.
97. Yoon K.-A, Park JH, Han J, *et al.* A genome-wide association study reveals susceptibility variants for non-small cell lung cancer in the Korean population. *Hum Mol Genet* 2010; 19: 4948–4954.
98. Hu Z, Wu C, Shi Y, *et al.* A genome-wide association study identifies two new lung cancer susceptibility loci at 13q12.12 and 22q12.2 in Han Chinese. *Nat Genet* 2011; 43: 792–796.
99. Ahn M.-J, Won HH, Lee J, *et al.* The 18p11.22 locus is associated with never smoker non-small cell lung cancer susceptibility in Korean populations. *Hum Genet* 2012; 131: 365–372.
100. Dong J, Jin G, Wu C, *et al.* Genome-wide association study identifies a novel susceptibility locus at 12q23.1 for lung squamous cell carcinoma in Han Chinese. *PLoS Genet* 2013; 9: e1003190.

101. Lan Q, Hsiung CA, Matsuo K, *et al.* Genome-wide association analysis identifies new lung cancer susceptibility loci in never-smoking women in Asia. *Nat Genet* 2012; 44: 1330–1335.
102. Shiraishi K, Kunitoh H, Daigo Y, *et al.* A genome-wide association study identifies two new susceptibility loci for lung adenocarcinoma in the Japanese population. *Nat Genet* 2012; 44: 900–903.
103. Timofeeva MN, Hung RJ, Rafnar T, *et al.* Influence of common genetic variation on lung cancer risk: meta-analysis of 14 900 cases and 29 485 controls. *Hum Mol Genet* 2012; 21: 4980–4995.
104. Kim JH, Park K, Yim SH, *et al.* Genome-wide association study of lung cancer in Korean non-smoking women. *J Korean Med Sci* 2013; 28: 840–847.
105. Wang Y, McKay JD, Rafnar T, *et al.* Rare variants of large effect in BRCA2 and CHEK2 affect risk of lung cancer. *Nat Genet* 2014; 46: 736–741.
106. Truong T, Hung RJ, Amos CI, *et al.* Replication of lung cancer susceptibility loci at chromosomes 15q25, 5p15, and 6p21: a pooled analysis from the International Lung Cancer Consortium. *J Natl Cancer Inst* 2010; 102: 959–971.
107. McDermott U, Downing JR, Stratton MR. Genomics and the continuum of cancer care. *N Engl J Med* 2011; 364: 340–350.
108. Cardarella S, Johnson BE. The impact of genomic changes on treatment of lung cancer. *Am J Respir Crit Care Med* 2013; 188: 770–775.
109. Institute of Medicine. Genome-based diagnostics: demonstrating clinical utility in oncology. Workshop summary. Washington, National Academies Press, 2013.
110. Institute of Medicine. Assessing genomic sequencing information for health care decision making: workshop summary. Washington, National Academies Press, 2014.
111. Mwenifumbo JC, Marra MA. Cancer genome-sequencing study design. *Nat Rev Genet* 2013; 14: 321–332.
112. Garraway LA. Genomics-driven oncology: framework for an emerging paradigm. *J Clin Oncol* 2013; 31: 1806–1814.
113. Tran B, Dancey JE, Kamel-Reid S, *et al.* Cancer genomics: technology, discovery, and translation. *J Clin Oncol* 2012; 30: 647–660.

---

Support statement: This work was supported by: a National Health and Medical Research Council (NHMRC) project grant (K.M. Fong); a NHMRC Practitioner Fellowship (K.M. Fong); a NHMRC Career Development Fellowship (I.A. Yang); a NHMRC PhD Scholarship (M. Daniels); a Cancer Council Queensland (CCQ) Senior Research Fellowship (K.M. Fong); a CCQ PhD Scholarship (M. Daniels); CCQ project grants; Health and Medical Research project grants; and The Prince Charles Hospital Foundation.

Disclosures: None declared.

Chapter 8

# Molecular pathology

Florian Laenger[1], Nicolas Dickgreber[2] and Ulrich Lehmann[1]

The discovery of druggable molecular targets in NSCLC has led to a shift from the former "one size fits all" chemotherapy approach to treatment selection based on tumour biology. Recent work has demonstrated that most known driving mutations are homogeneously distributed in NSCLCs, allowing meaningful molecular analysis and therapy based on small tissue samples. Although currently, a mix of methods is necessary to analyse NSCLCs, NGS techniques will allow the simultaneous analysis of most relevant mutations and translocations in NSCLCs in the near future. At the moment, approved drugs are available for patients with tumours revealing *EGFR* mutations and *ALK* translocations, although there are ongoing clinical trials for many more targets and patients showing secondary resistance mechanisms. Thus, comprehensive profiling of all NSCLCs before and during treatment will become the standard of care for NSCLC patients.

Lung cancer has been classified by conventional morphology into SCLC and NSCLC, with NSCLC further subdivided into ADC, SCC and large cell lung carcinoma (LCLC) [1]. Even this very basic classification scheme has been shown to be valuable for treatment decisions regarding safety and efficacy, for example, the use of pemetrexed [2] and bevacizumab [3] has been restricted to non-SCC.

As the currently applicable World Health Organization classification is based primarily on conventional morphology, proper typing in small biopsies is not possible in up to 40% of cases and had to be refined by integrating IHC (figs 1 and 2) [4]. By using a small panel of antibodies, a rate of <10% of unclassifiable NSCLCs can and should be achieved [5–7].

This rather descriptive taxonomy of lung cancer has been both strengthened and challenged by the recognition of numerous somatic genetic alterations in the last decade [8–11]. While the histotype and genotype of ADCs and SCCs show considerable concordance, there is substantial transcriptional similarity between the morphologically separate entities of SCLC and LCNEC [10, 12]. Moreover, in most cases, LCLCs group with either ADC or SCC on a molecular level, challenging the conventional classification scheme [10, 12].

Of all altered genes, currently, 54 are identified as driving genetic alterations that actively control cell survival and proliferation, and may thus serve as potential therapeutic targets [13].

[1]Institute of Pathology, Medical School Hannover, Hannover, Germany. [2]Dept of Pneumology, Thoracic Oncology and Respiratory Care Medicine, Mathias Spital Rheine, Rheine, Germany.

Correspondence: Florian Laenger, Institute of Pathology, Medical School Hannover, Carl-Neuberg-Str. 1, 30625 Hannover, Germany. E-mail: laenger.florian@mh-hannover.de

 Print ISBN: 978-1-84984-061-3. Online ISBN: 978-1-84984-062-0. Print ISSN: 2312-508X. Online ISSN: 2312-5098.

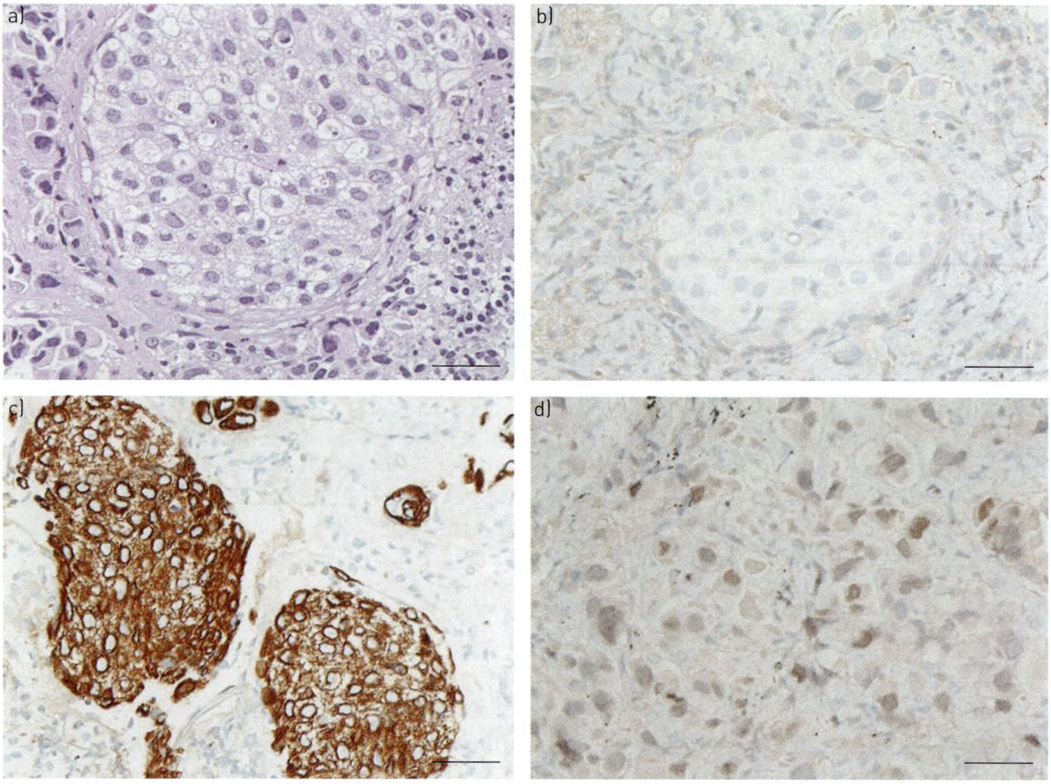


Figure 1. Biopsy of poorly differentiated bronchial ADC with solid growth shows characteristic coexpression of cytokeratin (CK)7 and thyroid transcription factor (TTF)1 without detectable expression of p40. a) Haematoxylin and eosin stain (scale bar=50 μm); b) p40 (scale bar=150 μm); c) CK7 (scale bar=150 μm); d) TTF1 (scale bar=150 μm).

There is an ongoing effort by basic scientists and clinicians to characterise further the lung cancer genome, and discover therapeutic targets, which is supported by newly developed molecular techniques (table 1) [44]. Thus, currently histotype and genotype complement information for the clinician.

## Comprehensive molecular profiling of lung cancer and its subtypes

Lung cancer shows a high mutation burden, as demonstrated by absolute numbers of >20 000 mutations/tumour and up to 12 mutations per megabase (Mb) compared with three mutations per Mb in colorectal cancer or one mutation per Mb in breast cancer [9, 10, 13]. This is due to exogenous stimuli such as smoking as well as consecutive errors of replicative DNA polymerases and repair mechanisms [45, 46]. Recently, ADCs [8, 10, 14, 47], SCCs [9, 10, 47], LCLCs [10] and LCNECs [10] have been comprehensively analysed by NGS, elucidating their molecular oncogenesis.

### Adenocarcinoma

Analysis of 412 whole-exome sequenced ADCs identified 18 statistically significantly mutated driver genes (fig. 3) [11]. These occurred in the well-known oncogenes *KRAS* (Kirsten rat

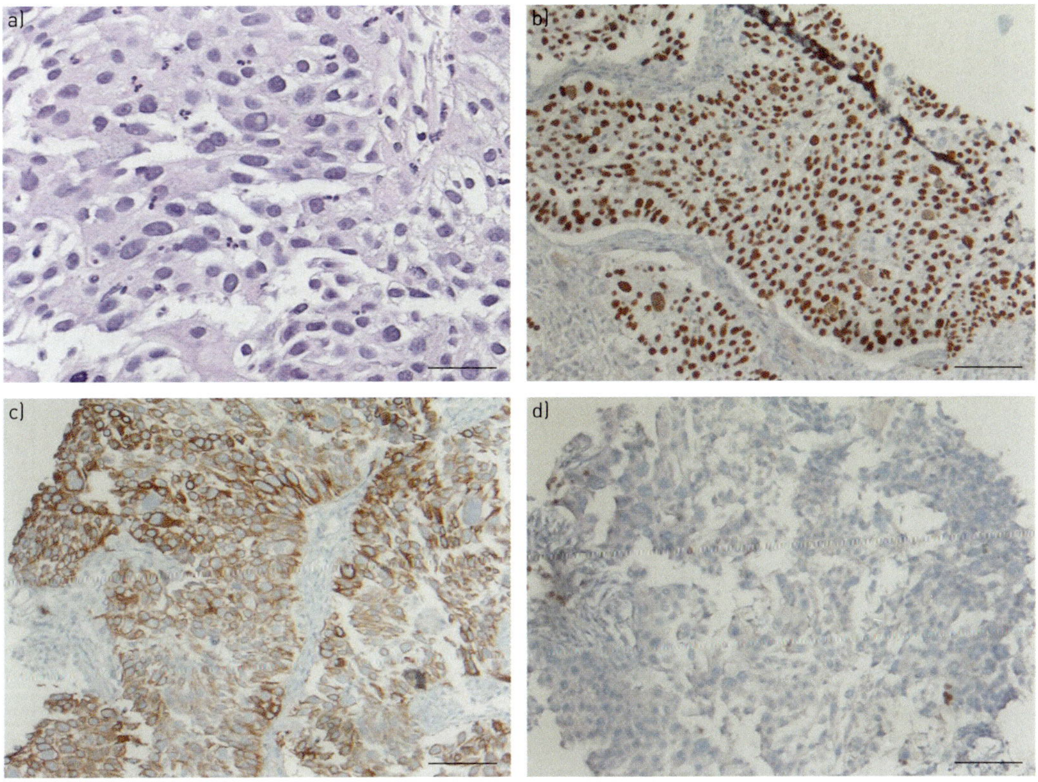


Figure 2. Biopsy of poorly differentiated SCC without obvious keratinisation reveals typical expression of p40, with moderate coexpression of cytokeratin (CK)7 and lack of thyroid transcription factor (TTF)1. a) Haematoxylin and eosin stain (scale bar=50 µm); b) p40 (scale bar=50 µm); c) CK7 (scale bar=50 µm); d) TTF1 (scale bar=50 µm).

sarcoma viral oncogene homologue) (33%), *EGFR* (14%), *BRAF* (B-Raf) (10%), *PIK3CA* (phosphatidylinositol-4,5-bisphosphate 3-kinase (PI3K), catalytic subunit α) (7%) and *MET* (Met) (7%), as well as in in chromatin-modifying genes (*SETD2* (huntingtin-interacting protein 1)), *ARID1A* (encoding an AT-rich interactive domain-containing protein) and SMARCA4 (a SWI/SNF-related, matrix-associated, actin-dependent regulator of chromatin), RNA-splicing genes (*RBM10* (an RNA-binding motif protein 10)) and *U2AF* (a U2 small nuclear RNA auxiliary factor) and tumour suppressor genes (*TP53* (p53), *STK11* (a serine/threonine kinase), *KEAP1* (a Kelch-like, ECH-associated protein), *NF1* (neurofibromin 1), *RB1* (retinoblastoma protein) and *CDKN2A* (Arf)) [11]. Other common genetic alterations included fusions involving *ALK*, *ROS1* (c-ros), *RET* (Ret) and *MET* (Met) [11]. Using comprehensive genomic analyses, >90% of lung cancers diagnosed as ADC by conventional histology are aggregated into a genomic cluster distinct from all other lung cancers [10, 12]. In all, 62% [11] to 64% [15] of ADCs harbour currently known activating mutations. Nevertheless, there remains a subset of ⩾25% of ADCs with no known driving mutation [15]. Moreover, in recent work, only 6% of ADCs had alterations assigned to all six classic hallmarks of cancer [14]. These data underline our still significant lack of understanding of the molecular basis of lung cancer carcinogenesis, as genetic alterations affecting proliferation, invasion or metastases are detectable only in a minority of cases.

Table 1. Summary of clinicopathological characteristics of drugable mutations in ADCs

| Alteration [ref.] | Prevalence % | Ethnicity | Sex/age | Smoking history | Histology | Drug |
|---|---|---|---|---|---|---|
| ***KRAS* [8, 10, 11, 14–19]** | 25–33 | Caucasian | Not distinctive | Smokers | ADC, mucinous | Selumetinib |
| ***EGFR* (only studies with Caucasian patients) [8, 10, 11, 14–17, 20–22]** | 10–23 | Asian | Female/ younger | Nonsmokers | ADC, nonmucinous | Gefitinib, erlotinib, afatinib, dacomitinib, neratinib |
| ***ALK* [10, 15–17, 23–26]** | 3–8 | Not distinctive | Female/ younger | Light/ never-smokers | ADC, solid or cribriform mucinous with signet ring cells | Crizotinib |
| ***BRAF* [10, 11, 14, 15, 27–30]** | 2–10 | Caucasian | Not distinctive | Smokers | ADC, papillary, micropapillary | Vemurafenib, dabrafenib, selumetinib |
| ***ROS1* [31–34]** | 1–2 | Not distinctive | Female/ younger | Light/ never-smokers | ADC, solid or cribriform mucinous with signet ring cells | Crizotinib |
| ***RET* [31, 35–37]** | 1–2 | Not distinctive | Younger | Nonsmokers | ADC, solid or cribriform mucinous with signet ring cells | Vandetanib, cabozantinib |
| ***PIK3CA* [10, 15–17, 38, 39]** | 1–7 | Not distinctive | Not distinctive | Not distinctive | ADC, SCC | Everolimus, tensirolimus |
| ***HER2* [10, 15, 40–42]** | 23 | Asian | Female/ younger | Nonsmokers | Not distinctive | Trastuzumab, pertuzumab, lapatanib |
| ***MET* [43]** | 8 | Not distinctive | Not distinctive | Not distinctive | ADC, SCC | Vandetanib, cabozantinib |

*KRAS*: Kirsten rat sarcoma viral oncogene homologue; *BRAF*: B-Raf; *ROS1*: c-ros; *RET*: Ret; *PIK3CA*; phosphatidylinositol-4,5-bisphosphate 3-kinase, catalytic subunit $\alpha$; *MET*: Met.

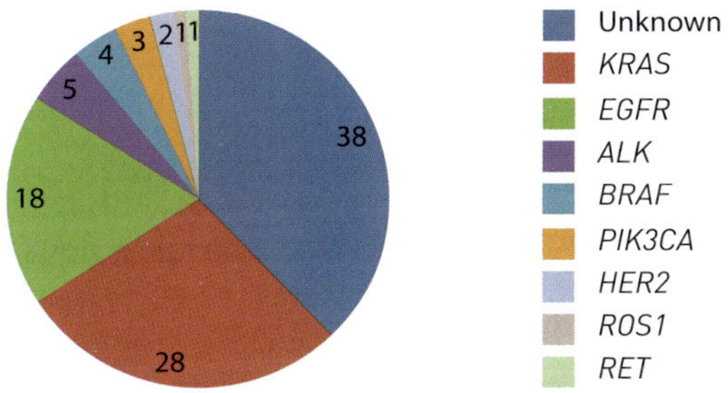


Figure 3. Distribution of potentially drugable mutations in ADCs: *EGFR* [8, 10, 11, 14–17, 20–22], *KRAS* (Kirsten rat sarcoma viral oncogene homologue) [8, 10, 11, 14–19], *BRAF* (B-Raf) [10, 11, 14, 15, 27–30], *ALK* [10, 15–17, 23–26], *HER2* [10, 15, 40–42], *RET* (Ret) [31, 35–37], *ROS1* (c-ros) [31–34] and *PIK3CA* (phosphatidylinositol-4,5-bisphosphate 3-kinase, catalytic subunit α) [10, 15–17, 38, 39]. Numbers represent percentages of molecular alterations.

## Squamous cell carcinoma

Data for SCCs are less extensively documented but also show mutated genes occurring in oncogenes such as *DDR2* (encoding a discoidin domain receptor tyrosine kinase) (5%), *PIK3CA* (16%) and *NOTCH1* (8%), as well as in antioxidants (*NFE2L2*, an NFE2-related factor) and in tumour suppressor genes (*TP53*, *CDKN2A*, *PTEN* (phosphatase and tensin homologue), *KEAP1* and *RB1*) (fig. 4) [9, 47]. Moreover, amplifications of *SOX2*, *FGFR1* and *TP63* (p63) have been described in SCCs [9]. Thus, pathways controlling the cell cycle, response to oxidative stress, apoptotic signalling and squamous differentiation are involved [9]. Histologically defined SCCs cluster together in ~80% of all molecularly analysed cases [10]. Of interest is the overlap of genetic alterations with non-human-papilloma-virus-related SCCs of other locations, especially the head and neck, underlying their shared pathogenesis and implying common therapeutic accessibility [47].

## Large cell lung carcinoma

Most cases histologically defined as LCLC show molecular traits of either ADC or SCC, recapitulating former results using IHC [10]. Only rare cases defy clustering with other well-defined entities of NSCLC. Thus, retaining LCLC as a separately defined entity of lung cancer is currently under discussion [48].

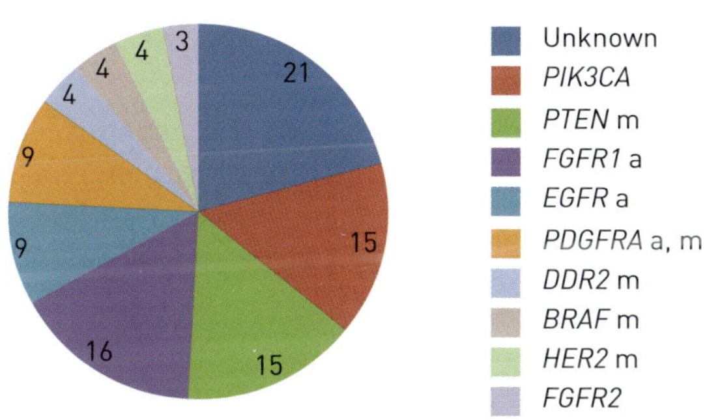


Figure 4. Distribution of potentially drugable molecular alterations in SCCs [10]: *PIK3CA* (phosphatidylinositol-4,5-bisphosphate 3-kinase, catalytic subunit α), *PTEN* (phosphatase and tensin homologue), *FGFR1*, *EGFR*, *PDGFRA* (platelet-derived growth factor receptor α), *DDR2* (discoidin domain receptor tyrosine kinase 2), *BRAF* (B-Raf), *HER2* and *FGFR2*. m: mutation; a: amplification. Numbers represent percentages of molecular alterations.

### Small cell lung cancer

In contrast to the aforementioned forms of lung cancer, SCLC is not associated with specific somatic mutations [49, 50]. Mutations of the tumour suppressor genes *TP53* and *RB1* are the most frequent and early events in carcinogenesis [51]. Mutations of other suppressor genes (*SLIT2*, *PTEN*, *STK11*, *KEAP1* and *FHIT*), histone acetylases (*EP300* (p300) and *CREBBP* (CREB-binding protein)), methyltransferases (*MLL*) and some potential driving genes (*EGFR*, *ROS1*, *PIK3CA* and *MET*) have been described less frequently [49, 50, 52]. Moreover, translocations of members of the *MYC* family, *SOX2* and *FGFR1* occur at frequencies <10% [51].

## Intra-tumoural heterogeneity of lung cancer

Heterogeneity on a morphological level has long been recognised in lung cancer by pathologists. Heterogeneity on the genetic level regarding the major oncologic drivers would make molecular testing and targeted therapy highly problematic [53–56]. Reports about the intra-tumoural distribution of *EGFR* mutations in lung cancer have been rather contradictory, as summarised recently [57]. Employing more sensitive assays, most true driver mutations could be demonstrated as clonal and homogeneous in all tumour specimens examined [54–56, 58].

Nevertheless, in up to 30% of cases, heterogeneously distributed, nonsilent mutations often developing late during oncogenesis have been detected, indicating a branched evolution into distinct subclones [54–56]. These subclonal molecular alterations only very rarely include additional driver mutations; mostly affected are *BRAF* and *PIK3CA* mutations in addition to pre-existing clonal *EGFR*, *ALK* or *KRAS* mutations [13, 17, 28, 54]. Even nondriving mutations may confer survival advantages regarding the local micromilieu or drug resistance. This has been shown for the evolution of T790M-mutated subclones following TKI treatment and secondary *ALK*-mutated tumour cells following crizotinib therapy [59, 60].

Regarding discrepancies of the molecular makeup between the primary tumour and metastases, a high concordance has been shown for both *EGFR* and *ALK* [58, 61].

## Methodology and general recommendations for testing of lung cancer

As tumour tissue is often sparse, molecular testing still expensive and time-consuming, a diligent choice of testing platforms, samples and targets is mandatory. Numerous guidelines from national and international professional organisations address the most important issues for molecular testing in routine clinical practice, some of which are summarised in table 2 and the following paragraphs [62, 65–71].

### Methodology of molecular testing

Traditionally, point mutations as well as small to medium-sized insertions and/or deletions have been detected by Sanger sequencing of PCR products generated in individual reactions [73]. In particular, the low sensitivity and limited throughput of this method led to the introduction of other techniques, which are briefly introduced in table 3 [73–77].

Table 2. Recommendations and guidelines for molecular testing of NSCLC

| | Pre-selection for molecular testing | Testing method |
|---|---|---|
| **ESMO [63]** | All nonsquamous tumours, selected SCCs from patients with minimal or remote smoking history should strongly be considered | *EGFR*: any methodology with a wide coverage of mutations<br>*ALK*: definite assessment is determined by FISH, IHC may be employed for screening |
| **SEOM, SEAP [64]** | Nonsquamous tumours, all NSCLCs of nonsmokers irrespective of histological type | *EGFR*: Sanger sequencing only if high tumour content (>50%), a highly sensitive method (sensitivity threshold <5% tumour contents) should be ideally used<br>*ALK*: FISH and IHC are both applicable, though only FISH is FDA approved |
| **NCCN [65]** | Mutational testing is strongly recommended in all NSCLCs favouring ADC | *EGFR*: no recommendation<br>*ALK*: FISH is the standard testing method, IHC can be used for rapid prescreening |
| **Australia National Working Group [66]** | Nonsquamous tumours, for SCCs in small samples molecular testing may still be considered, if suggested by clinicopathological characteristics (young age, no smoking history) | *ALK*: FISH assay as a confirmation tool following screening by IHC |
| **CAP, IASLC, AMP [67]** | Resection specimen: all ADCs and tumours with an ADC component (pure SCC or LCLC should not be tested)<br>Biopsy/cytology: all NSCLCs, where an ADC component cannot be completely excluded (even SCLC or SCC, if young of age or lack of smoking history) | *EGFR*: any validated testing method fulfilling the criteria (methods with detection threshold of 50% tumour cell content should be used, more sensitive tests with threshold of 10% tumour cell content strongly recommended)<br>*ALK*: FISH assay should be used, carefully validated IHC may be considered as screening technology<br>RT-PCR not recommended |
| **ASCO [68]** | See above | See above |
| **AIOM, SIAPEC-IAP [69]** | ADCs, LCLCs, tumours with an ADC component and NSCLC, NOS | *ALK*: FISH assay the elective method, carefully validated IHC may be considered as screening technology |
| **Thunissen *et al.* [70]** | No specific recommendation | *ALK*: FISH as gold standard, IHC as screening method |

Continued

Table 2. Continued

| | Pre-selection for molecular testing | Testing method |
|---|---|---|
| **INCa [71]** | ADCs (*KRAS* wildtype) | *EGFR*: no recommendation<br>*ALK*: IHC as screening tool, FISH as confirmation test and for doubtful cases |
| **NICE [72]** | Testing should be carried out on all eligible patients (stage IV NSCLC) irrespective of their sex, ethnicity and smoking status | *EGFR*: for Cobas EGFR Mutation Test (Roche Molecular Diagnostics, Rotkreuz, Switzerland) and for Sanger sequencing-based methods, an equivalent evidence base exists, and therefore these tests and the Therascreen EGFR PCR Kit (QIAGEN, Venlo, the Netherlands) can be considered clinically effective and cost effective, for other testing methods the evidence was insufficient to allow any recommendations to be made on their use |

ESMO: European Society for Medical Oncology; SEOM: Spanish Society of Medical Oncology; SEAP: Spanish Society of Pathology; NCCN: National Comprehensive Cancer Network; CAP: College of American Pathologists; IASLC: International Association for the Study of Lung Cancer; AMP: Association of Molecular Pathology; ASCO: American Association of Clinical Oncology; AIOM: Italian Association of Medical Oncology; SIAPEC-IAP: Italian Society of Anatomic Pathology and Diagnostic Cytopathology; INCa: National Cancer Institute; NICE: National Institute for Health and Care Excellence; FDA: Food and Drug Administration; LCLC: large cell lung carcinoma; RT-PCR: reverse transcriptase PCR; NOS: not otherwise specified.

Gene translocations with multiple possible fusion partners (*e.g.* *ALK* and *ROS1*) are difficult to detect comprehensively by conventional sequencing-based methods. For these types of genetic alterations, FISH and/or IHC (table 4) show better sensitivities, especially in small samples, and are currently the established testing methods. Especially in the USA, specific testing platforms (*e.g.* FISH for detection of *ALK* translocations) have been made mandatory as companion diagnostics. Due to the short period between biomarker discovery and drug approval as well as different companies introducing different testing procedures for the same biomarker protein, this kind of stipulation will probably have to be abandoned in the near future [78, 79].

The currently used mix of sequencing and FISH or IHC-based methods necessary to detect the most relevant mutations is time- and tissue-consuming as well as expensive. NGS methods are currently implemented in many laboratories as a testing standard and promise to detect point mutations, small and large insertions and deletions (indels), copy number alterations, and chromosomal rearrangements in a single experiment. NGS manages to simultaneously sequence thousands to millions of short nucleic acid sequences in a massively parallel way [77]. Thus, larger regions of the genome can be analysed at a lower

Table 3. Comparison of characteristics of molecular techniques

| Method | Amount of DNA | Sensitivity % mutated clone necessary | Specification of detected mutation | Detection only of known sequences | Adaptable to include new targets | Sample throughput | Costs per exon |
|---|---|---|---|---|---|---|---|
| **Sanger sequencing [73]** | High | 15–20 | Yes | No | Yes | Low | High |
| **Pyrosequencing [74]** | High | 5–10 | Yes | No | Yes | Low | Low |
| **High-resolution melting [75]** | High | 1–10 | No | No | Yes | Medium | Low |
| **Allele-specific PCR [76]** | High | 1–5 | Not always | Yes | No | Medium | High |
| **NGS [77]** | Low | 1–5 | Yes | No | Yes | Very high | Low |

price and higher sensitivity. Several commercial platforms are currently available that use different approaches. Semiconductor sequencing measures the incorporation of nucleotides by detecting proton release, which causes a pH shift. Therefore, this approach does not rely on modified nucleotides. The templates for sequencing are prepared by clonal amplification of single target molecules by emulsion PCR [80]. Sequencing by synthesis uses the reversible adherence of fluorescently labelled nucleotides on immobilised DNA templates. The immobilised templates are photodocumented after each synthesis step before removal of the fluorescence label and the start of the next extension cycle [81]. Sequencing by oligonucleotide ligation and detection (SOLiD; Applied Biosystems, Waltham, MA, USA) combines elements of both methods. After clonal amplification by emulsion PCR, the sequence under study is interrogated by hybridisation and ligation of fluorescence-labelled probes. Only perfectly matching probes can be ligated. After imaging of the incorporated probes, the fluorescent labels are cleaved off and a new cycle begins. The 454 technology (Roche Life Science, Mannheim, Germany) [82], based on massively parallel pyrosequencing in picolitre reactors [83] and distinguished from all three methods described so far by a superior read length, is now discontinued by the current owner of the technology.

Direct sequencing of single molecules has not yet reached the routine diagnostic laboratory; however, it may revolutionise the field in the near future [84].

Table 4. IHC of drugable mutations [14, 66, 67]

| Target clone | Provider | Specificity % | Sensitivity % |
|---|---|---|---|
| ***EGFR*** | | | |
| Exon 19 | Cell Signaling Technology, Danvers, MA, USA | 85–100 | 40–100 |
| Exon 21 | Cell Signaling Technology | 91–99 | 36–95 |
| ***ALK*** | | | |
| D5F3 | Cell Signaling Technology | 87–100 | 93–97 |
| 5A4 | Novocastra, Newcastle, UK | 88–98 | 100 |
| *ALK1* M7195 | Dako, Carpinteria, CA, USA | 91–99 | 64–100 |
| ***BRAF*** | | | |
| V600 clone VE1 | Ventana Medical Systems, Tucson, AZ, USA | 100 | 74–91 |
| D4D6 | Cell Signaling Technology | 30–92 | 94 |

*BRAF*: B-Raf.

So far, affordable benchtop machines with moderate capacity but improved turnaround time suitable for routine diagnostic applications are available only for semiconductor sequencing and sequencing by synthesis (Ion Torrent PGM (Thermo Fisher Scientific, Waltham, MA, USA) and MiSequ (Illumina, San Diego, CA, USA), respectively).

These benchtop machines allow rapid (5–24 h) analysis with high accuracy and sensitivity. The major bottleneck of any NGS approach is still the data evaluation, which requires time-consuming manual curation by highly experienced personnel.

Regardless of the technical platform, rigorous internal and external quality testing, standardisation of the protocols, and cross-validation of the findings are mandatory [85, 86].

## Selection and handling of material for molecular testing

The amount of tumour tissue rather than the type of tissue sample or fixation is usually the major obstacle for successful testing [8, 35]. Resection specimens, biopsies and cytological preparations are suitable. Blood-based testing of free tumour DNA is an emerging approach that is particularly suited for sequential testing of patients under treatment [87].

Conventional stains and IHC to establish the diagnosis and typing should be used judiciously and sparingly. Cutting a predefined number of sections in one session for conventional histology (haematoxylin and eosin or per-iodic acid–Schiff staining), IHC (thyroid transcription factor (TTF)1 or p40) and molecular processing as well as FISH analysis has proven to be the most efficient use of biopsy material, and is recommended by the European Society of Medical Oncology consensus conference [7, 63].

As driver mutations are distributed homogeneously [54–56, 58, 88], the most easily accessible tumour site, whether primary or metastasis, can be biopsied, as outlined by the College of American Pathologists/International Association for the Study of Lung Cancer (IASLC)/Association of Molecular Pathology guidelines [67]. If multiple, apparently separate primary tumours are observed, testing these lesions individually according to the American Association of Clinical Oncology (ASCO) recommendations is an option, as divergent driver mutations are possible [68]. Sequential testing during therapy should also be considered, as the detection of secondary mutations (*e.g.* T790M) may alter the treatment regimen [67].

## Clinical pre-selection for molecular testing

Pre-selection criteria have been used to "enrich" patient cohorts for the detection of actionable mutations. Clinical parameters such as ethnicity, sex or smoking status should not be used for pre-selection though, as, for example, >25% of all *EGFR* mutations are detected in males or (ex)smokers [15]. Excluding SCC diagnosed in small biopsies from testing for *EGFR* and *ALK* should also be regarded critically, as mutations can be found in tumours with mixed histology and typing in small biopsies has been shown to be either unreliable or not fully representative of the whole tumour [63]. The existing guidelines and recommendations all suggest testing nonsquamous NSCLCs; moreover, other histologies (SCCs and SCLCs) should also be included, if special clinicopathological characteristics exist (young age and no smoking history) (table 2) [63, 67].

As newer NGS techniques can simultaneously test for a large number of molecular alterations, including translocations using small amounts of tumour, in the near future, lung cancer panels customised for these platforms will most probably abrogate the need for any kind of pre-selection.

## *EGFR* mutations

### Type and incidence of molecular alterations of the *EGFR* gene

Although most NSCLCs overexpress EGFR protein on the cell surface and high copy numbers can be observed in 10–30% of NSCLCs, activating mutations in exons 18–21 of the tyrosine-kinase domain of EGFR have been shown to be the best and most robust predictors for response to anti-EGFR therapy [89–92].

EGFR is a transmembrane tyrosine kinase receptor encoded by a gene located on chromosome 7p11.2 containing 28 exons. Physiologically, ligand binding in the human EGFR family causes homo- or heterodimerisation of the transmembrane receptor molecules with subsequent phosphorylation, activation and triggering of the PI3Kα/AKT1/MTOR or RAS/RAF1/MAP2K1 pathways regulating cell proliferation, angiogenesis and inhibition of apoptosis [88, 93]. The most common in-frame deletions of exon 19 (delE746–A750) and point mutations of exon 21 (L858R) comprise ~90% of all *EGFR* gene mutations and target key structures around the ATP-binding cleft of the receptor molecule, thus continuously activating the kinase function [94, 95].

The incidence of *EGFR* mutations shows a well-documented bias toward patients of Asian descent (40–55%), never-smokers (42%), females (22%) and ADCs (15–20%) [8, 19, 22]. Without any further pre-selection, the incidence of *EGFR* mutations in NSCLCs of Caucasian patients is close to 10% [20], whereas in ADCs of Caucasian patients frequencies of 10% [20] to 23.1% [16] are documented. In SCC, originally, frequencies of up to 15% were reported [20, 96], although in recent studies with high stringency of the histological criteria, mutations were either undetectable or extremely rare [9, 17, 20, 22, 96, 97]. Double mutations of *EGFR* and *KRAS* are seen in up to 1.6% of all NSCLCs [38], although comutation rates in American and European patients have been lower [17].

Response rates of 56–83% with a mean PFS of 9.2–13.1 months have been documented for TKI therapy in lung cancers with activating mutations [62, 98–103], recently reviewed by Melosky [104]. Despite the crossover design of all studies, a survival advantage was also recently demonstrated [105]. Exon 19 deletions may show a better response to TKI therapy than exon 21 deletions [106], while rarer activating missense mutations of exons 18–21 often show rather worse response rates [88, 107].

### Resistance mechanisms to EGFR-TKIs

Primary resistance to TKI therapy is seen in 4–10% of patients and is associated with incompletely defined host factors, such as smoking and polymorphism of the pro-apoptotic *BIM* gene (encoding a BCL2-like protein), as well as some rarer insertion mutations in exon 18 and 20 [108, 109]. Moreover, loss of *PTEN* and somatic mutations of *KRAS* and *PIK3CA* have also been implicated [59, 110].

Even after an initially good response to EGFR-TKI therapy, progress due to acquired resistance mechanisms will eventually occur [111–114]. There are two basic mechanisms involved: genetic alterations of the target molecule (by point mutations or amplifications) or activation of bypass signalling.

Most important is the exon 20 point mutation T790M, which functions as a gatekeeper and significantly reduces the potency of TKIs [114]. Using Sanger sequencing, only ~2% of the tumours show this mutation pre-treatment, though by employing more sensitive assays, low-level mutations are seen in 35–65% of all *EGFR*-mutated tumours [108, 115]. As these rates are comparable to T790M mutation rates after TKI treatment of 49% [112], 62% [113] and 68% [116], it seems reasonable to assume that most or all T790M mutations are already present prior to therapy, and "surface" by clonal evolution and surpassing the technical detection threshold during therapy with TKIs [55, 56].

Detection of T790M pre-treatment is associated with worse primary response rates and shorter mean time to progression, making the choice of a third-generation TKI preferable [111–113]; secondary resistance due to T790M mutations is associated with longer PFS than non-T790M mechanisms [116]. Recently, *de novo* detection of T790M in cell-free tumour DNA from plasma samples has been described as associated with tumour progression and therapy failure [87].

Other secondary resistance mechanisms include activation of bypass signalling through *MET* amplification (5–22%), *PIK3CA* mutation (3%), *BRAF* mutation (1%), *AXL* (encoding a receptor tyrosine kinase) overexpression and *HER2* amplification (13%) [110–113, 117, 118]. In a subset of patients, neuroendocrine dedifferentiation to SCLC can be demonstrated (2–14%) [111–113]. In most of these cases, additional molecular alterations such as *RB1* mutations, *MET* amplifications or *PIK3CA* mutations can be shown [112–116].

### Specific recommendations for *EGFR* testing

According to existing guidelines and recommendations, any validated method with sufficient performance characteristics may be used for the detection of *EGFR* mutations (table 3). The guidelines from IASLC and ASCO highly recommend assays reaching sensitivities of >90%, especially for use in small biopsies [44, 67, 68]. Moreover, the tests employed should detect all published individual mutations with an incidence of >1%. For the detection of resistance-associated T790M mutations, methods with a sensitivity of ⩾95% should be used. Using IHC or *EGFR* amplification analyses as selection criteria for EGFR TKI therapy is not recommended [67, 68].

## *ALK* translocations

### Type and incidence of molecular alterations of the *ALK* gene

*ALK* fusion-positive lung cancers have gained clinical interest due to the discovery of ALK-targeting TKIs showing objective response rates of 57–65% and a median PFS of 7.7–10 months in second-line therapy [119–122].

ALK is a transmembrane tyrosine kinase receptor, encoded by the *ALK* gene on chromosome 2p23. Following ligand binding and homodimerisation, autophosphorylation ensues with subsequent activation of such divergent pathways as PI3Kα/AKT1/MTOR or RAS/RAF1/MAP2K1. Following the initial description of activating *ALK* alterations in anaplastic non-Hodgkin's lymphoma, low-frequency alterations have been described in other epithelial, mesenchymal and melanocytic tumours, as recently reviewed by Shackelford *et al.* [123]. Soda *et al.* [124] and Rikova *et al.* [125] described *ALK* translocations involving 6.7% and 4.4% of bronchial ADCs respectively. By an inversion within the short arm of chromosome 2, involving *EML4* or a translocation and fusion with various other genetic partners, a chimaeric protein is encoded, leading to constitutive activation with potent oncogenic activity [124].The specific fusion partner influences *ALK* expression level, protein stability and response to TKIs [123]. Although mostly mutually exclusive, in rare cases, double mutations with *EGFR* have been documented [126].

The reported incidence of *ALK* fusion-positive NSCLCs in unselected Caucasian populations ranges between 1.8% and 7.5% with an average of 3.7% [16, 23–26, 127, 128]. According to a recent meta-analysis, patients tend to be female (7.6% *versus* 4.8% male patients), younger (median of 55 years) and light or never-smokers (8.6% *versus* 3.6% in smokers) [129]. Regarding histology, most *ALK*-positive lung cancers have a least a partial ADC component, and a solid or mucinous, cribriform morphology with signet ring cells is very often present [31, 130].

## Resistance mechanisms to ALK-TKIs

All patients with *ALK*-fusion positive lung cancers will eventually relapse, after a response to TKIs typically lasting for 8–10 months [119–121]. In contrast to the acquired resistance to *EGFR*, mutations altering the drug target (*e.g.* L1196M and C1156Y) are observed only in a minority of cases (22–36%) with a higher heterogeneity of alterations, which complicates possible mechanisms to overcome resistance [131, 132]. Bypass signalling includes activation of *EGFR* signals, *KIT* (Kit) amplifications, *KRAS* mutations and loss of *ALK* mutation [131]. Unfortunately, a combination of resistance mechanisms, such as the combination of gatekeeper mutations with *EGFR* activation, has been found in both cell lines and tumour samples [60]. Second-generation TKIs are effective even in cases with gatekeeper mutations [133, 134], although acquired mutations affecting even the efficacy of these new drugs have already been documented [135].

## Specific recommendations for *ALK* testing

Since the introduction of crizotinib, *ALK* mutation testing has been recommended for stage IV NSCLCs in small biopsies and ADCs in resection specimens (table 2) [63, 67, 68, 70]. The molecular heterogeneity of *ALK* alterations makes RT-PCR-based sequencing techniques cumbersome [123]. Thus, FISH analysis is currently the gold standard, as it is sensitive and independent of the involved breakpoint [63, 67, 68, 123]. Nevertheless, it does not identify specific fusion partners, has a high cost and its specificity is very operator dependent [44, 123]. Therefore, IHC has been established as a valuable adjunct to diagnosis. Overcoming the low level of protein expression using new antibody clones and detection systems, a very high sensitivity (93–97%) and specificity (87–100%) could be achieved [70, 136–138]. Nevertheless, false-negative results in the range of 3–7% are to be expected, making its use as a pre-screening method questionable [136, 139]. Routine testing for secondary mutations associated with acquired resistance is currently not recommended [132].

## Rare oncogenic mutations in lung cancer

### *BRAF* mutations

Although the discovery of *BRAF* mutations antedates the identification of *ALK* translocations in NSCLCs, few clinical studies are available, and most clinical data refer to malignant melanomas and other neoplasms with higher frequencies of *BRAF* mutations [140, 141].

*BRAF* encodes a member of the Raf kinase family and is located on chromosome 7q34. It lies downstream from *KRAS*, and regulates cell proliferation and survival. Mutations can be demonstrated in malignant melanomas (40–70%), thyroid cancer (36–53%), colorectal cancer (5–22%) and ovarian serous carcinoma (20%) [142–144]. The most common mutation is V600E, resulting in constitutive activation [27, 143].

*BRAF* mutations have been shown in 2–10% of NSCLCs [10, 11, 14, 15, 27–30]. V600E mutations (50%) are the most common, followed by G469A mutations in 39% and D594G in 11% [28]. Recently, a double mutation rate of 16% with co-occurring mutations of *EGFR*, *PIK3CA*, *KRAS* and *ALK* has been shown, implying that *BRAF* mutations may not always be the predominant oncogenic driver [27].

*BRAF* mutations occur almost exclusively in ADCs and cases often show a predominant papillary or micropapillary pattern [27]. The clinical characteristics are rather unique, as most patients are Caucasians who are either current or ex-smokers [27].

It is of interest that there are major differences in the response to anti-B-Raf therapy in tumours of divergent locations, implying unidentified cofactors modifying the efficacy of targeted B-Raf therapy [145]. The published data indicate an efficacy of second-generation anti-B-Raf therapy, such as vemurafenib and dabrafenib, against ADCs with V600E mutations with an objective response rate of 54%, although the efficacy of these drugs against non-V600E mutations was nil [28, 29].

PCR-based sequencing methods are the current gold standard for testing; IHC, although rather specific, shows low sensitivities even for V600E mutations of only 74% and even less for non-V600E mutations [146].

### *ROS1* mutations

For patients with lung cancers showing *ROS1* rearrangements, an objective response rate to crizotinib therapy of 72% with a median PFS of 19.2 months has recently been reported [147]. Resistance to crizotinib eventually develops, resulting from either secondary mutations preventing drug binding or EGFR activation, although next-generation ALK inhibitors may be effective even in this context [133, 147].

The *ROS1* gene on chromosome 6q22 encodes a receptor tyrosine kinase with unknown ligands and physiological function. Ros is closely related to ALK, sharing 80% of the amino acid sequence and its binding affinity for crizotinib [125]. Rearrangements with ⩾12 different genetic partners cause constitutive activation of downstream signalling in pathways controlling cell cycling, cell proliferation and survival [148].

The incidence lies between 1% and 2% of all lung cancer, and *ROS1* alterations are almost always mutually exclusively with *KRAS*, *EGFR* and *ALK* mutations [34, 147]. Thus, in a "triple negative" cohort (*ALK*, *KRAS* and *EGFR* wild type), *ROS1* mutations are discovered in 7% of tumours analysed [149].

The clinicopathological profile closely resembles *ALK*-mutated tumours, as mostly ADCs of patients with no or only a light smoking history without sex or age preference reveal *ROS1* alterations [31–33, 150]. Histologically, most tumours are TTF1-positive ADCs showing at least partially solid and mucinous cribriform patterns with signet ring cells [31, 33, 35, 149].

Analogous to testing for *ALK* mutations, FISH is currently the gold standard [31, 147, 149, 150]. IHC shows a good sensitivity (94%) but is hampered by a low specificity, as up to 30% of lung cancers show upregulation of *ROS1*, which reduces its usability as a pre-screening tool [33, 149, 150].

### *RET* mutations

As Ret kinase activity can be targeted by a number of TKIs, such as sunitinib, sorafenib, cabozantinib and vandetanib, *RET* appears as a new actionable mutation in NSCLC, which is mutually exclusive with *KRAS*, *EGFR*, *ALK* and *BRAF* [36].

*RET* (rearranged during transfection) is a receptor tyrosine kinase gene mapping to chromosome 10q11.2, and is involved in cell proliferation, migration and differentiation [36]. Germline and sporadic mutations of *RET* cause multiple endocrine neoplasia type 2 syndrome, sporadic medullary carcinoma, as well as sporadic and radiation-induced papillary thyroid cancer [37]. Recently, novel gene fusions of *RET* partnered with either *KIF5B* (kinesin family member 5B), *CCDC6* (encoding a coiled-coil domain-containing protein) or *NCOA4* (nuclear receptor coactivator 4) have been described in NSCLC [138, 139]. Irrespective of its fusion partner, these translocations induce receptor dimerisation with constitutive activation, similar to *ALK*.

The overall incidence lies between 0.9% and 1.7% in all examined lung cancers, although in triple-negative ADCs, up to 16% *RET*-mutated tumours can be demonstrated [11, 31, 35, 37].

The clinicopathological characteristics show a preferential occurrence of *RET* mutations in younger patients (median 55–58 years) and never-smokers, with no detectable sex preference [35–37]. All mutated cases are TTF1-positive ADCs or mixed adenosquamous carcinomas with a solid or mucinous cribriform architecture containing variable numbers of signet ring cells [35–37]. *RET*-mutated ADCs tend to be small (pT1) with involvement of N2 lymph nodes [37].

Analogous to *ALK* testing, RT-PCR, FISH and IHC are available, although established antibody clones for IHC seem rather insensitive (54–67%) and unspecific (86%); therefore, FISH is currently the most effective diagnostic technology [36, 37].

### *PIK3CA* mutations

PI3K is an intracellular, membrane-bound kinase. The catalytic α-subunit is encoded by *PIK3CA*, which is located on chromosome 3q26.3, regulates cell growth, proliferation and survival, and is negatively regulated by *PTEN* [39]. Mutations (and amplifications) of

*PIK3CA* occur in 3–16% of NSCLC patients [16, 38, 39], with a predominance in SCCs (3.9–16%) [9, 17, 39] compared to ADCs (1.0–6.9%) [11, 15–17, 38, 39]. *PIK3CA* mutations cause aberrant signalling in the PI3Kα/AKT1/MTOR pathway and in 46–70% of lung cancers coexist with other oncogenic drivers, such as *EGFR* (3.2–3.5% of all *EGFR* mutations), *BRAF* (7.7% of all *BRAF* mutations), *KRAS* (2.3–6% of all *KRAS* mutations) or *ALK* [16, 38]. As *PIK3CA* mutations have been shown to be one of the few heterogeneously distributed driver mutations in NSCLC, *PIK3CA* is probably primarily a cofactor and not the predominant oncogenic driver [54]. There is no documented correlation between mutation incidence and sex, smoking history, tumour history or stage [38, 39]. PCR-based sequencing methods are the gold standard for testing.

### *HER2* alterations

*HER2*-mutated tumours show a resistance to anti-EGFR therapy, but good response rates of 50% and disease control rates of 80% have been described for anti-HER2 therapy, such as trastuzumab and lapatinib, as well as pan-ErbB inhibitors, such as neratinib or afatinib [40, 151].

HER2 is encoded by a gene on chromosome 17q12. It belongs to the EGFR family and is the favoured dimerisation partner of the other EGFRs [152]. Whether protein expression, gene amplification or mutations are the best predictors for anti-HER2 therapy in NSCLCs is still under discussion, which is reminiscent of the situation for EGFR some years ago.

*HER2* overexpression has been shown in up to 35% of NSCLCs. It has been associated with a worse prognosis, and implicated as a resistance factor for chemotherapy and radiation. Moreover, it was not associated with a consistent response to EGFR-TKI or anti-HER2 therapy [153, 154].

*HER2* amplifications occur at a frequency of up to 10% and have been implicated as a possible mechanism for secondary EGFR-TKI resistance, as already discussed [113].

*HER2* mutations have been described in 1–4% of all NSCLCs, with a preferential occurrence in ADCs [40–42]. In triple-negative ADC, frequencies can reach 6% [40]. Type and location of the documented mutations differ between NSCLCs, breast and colorectal cancers, suggesting different functional mechanisms [155]. The clinicopathological characteristics resemble those in patients with *EGFR*-mutated tumours, since tumours from patients of Asian ethnicity, female sex, never-smoking status and ADC histology preferentially show *HER2* mutations [42, 155].

### *MET* mutations

Several antibodies against Met and its ligand HGF have been developed and tested in phase 2 and 3 studies, with mixed results favouring subgroups defined by *MET* or *HGF* overexpression [156, 157].

The proto-oncogene *MET* (named for its involvement in mesenchymal–epithelial transition) is located on chromosome 7q31 and encodes a receptor tyrosine-kinase. Upon binding to its only known ligand, HGF, it propagates many physiological processes, including cell growth, proliferation, migration and angiogenesis, during organogenesis and wound healing [158, 159]. Overexpression, amplification and mutations of *MET* can enhance normal signalling, and occur in numerous forms of cancer including NSCLC, and breast, colon, stomach, and head and neck cancer [159].

Met protein overexpression has been detected in 22–77% of NSCLC samples with nonsquamous histology and in 1–57% of NSCLC samples with squamous histology, as reviewed by Scagliotti *et al.* [158]. So far, the lack of standardisation regarding the antibody clones and scoring method employed severely hampers the comparability of clinical studies, although mostly, a moderate expression by ⩾50% of the tumour cells is used to define high Met expression [156].

*MET* amplification occurs in 2–21% of all NSCLCs and is described in up to 4% of chemotherapy-naïve ADCs. It has been associated with a poor prognosis and is a known mechanism of acquired EGFR resistance [11, 111–113]. The dual inhibition of EGFR and Met by TKIs has failed in a recent trial, although molecular analyses are pending [157].

*MET* activating mutations have been described in sporadic and hereditary renal cancer and paediatric liver cancer. In NSCLCs, it has been described in 5% of a Caucasian and 12% of

Table 5. Summary of recommendations for routine clinical practice [67, 68, 70]

| | |
|---|---|
| **Which patient specimens should be tested?** | Non squamous NSCLCs<br>In small biopsies, other histologies may also be considered (if patients are young or never smokers) |
| **When should patient specimens be tested?** | At the time of diagnosis, all stage IV NSCLCs that are suitable for therapy<br>Previously, earlier stages at the time of relapse or tumour progress |
| **What types of patient specimen should be tested?** | Cytological and histological specimens are both suitable<br>The amount of tumour content is the most important aspect<br>Primary tumour or metastases are equally suited |
| **What are the requirements for the testing laboratory?** | Laboratories should have accreditation and continuously participate in internal and external quality programmes, use a standardised reporting format, and guarantee a turnaround time of <10 working days |
| **Which molecular alterations should be tested for?** | Testing for *EGFR* and *ALK* should be prioritised<br>*EGFR/ALK*-negative tumours may be considered for testing for *ROS1/RET/BRAF* or other markers, preferably in clinical studies<br>Routine testing for markers predictive for cytotoxic chemotherapy (*ERCC1*, *TYMS* or *RRM1*) is not recommended |
| **What methods should be used?** | Any validated testing method is suitable for *EGFR* testing<br>All mutations occurring with a frequency of ⩾1% should be detected<br>*EGFR* testing should at least detect mutations in specimens with a 50% tumour content<br>Methods achieving a detection threshold of 10% are strongly encouraged<br>For *ALK*, FISH testing remains the gold standard<br>IHC may be used as a pre-screening tool |

*ROS1*: c-ros; *RET*: Ret; *BRAF*: B-Raf; *ERCC1*: excision repair cross-complementation group 1; *TYMS*: thymidylate synthetase; *RRM1*: ribonucleotide reductase M1.

an Asian cohort [43]. There is a preferential occurrence in males, smokers and tumours with squamous histology [43]. So far, no data regarding the association of *MET* mutations and anti-Met therapy are available.

## Summary of recommendations for routine clinical practice

A summary of recommendations for routine clinical practice is presented in table 5.

## Outlook

Historically, NSCLC was treated as a single disease entity with limited response rates and poor survival. The discovery of potentially druggable molecular alterations gave rise to a new class of targeted therapies, with approved drugs for *EGFR*- and ALK-mutated NSCLCs becoming available. Currently, up to 64% of ADCs [15] and SCCs [9] have been shown to carry druggable molecular alterations. Further progress is hampered, though, as many of these alterations affect only a minority of cases, and routine molecular testing has been performed for *EGFR* and *ALK* mutations only, mostly for reasons of tissue availability and economy. Thus, recruiting patients with NSCLCs with rare molecular alterations for clinical trials has been cumbersome. In the very near future, NGS techniques with standardised kits for mutations and translocations suitable for testing small biopsies with small amounts of tumour will abrogate this diagnostic bottleneck. This comprehensive molecular characterisation of NSCLCs and other tumours will allow so-called basket trials [160], where solid tumours with identical mutations are treated with the same compounds regardless of their location. Another approach will be stratified biomarker-driven trials, such as the Lung Cancer Master Protocol trial for SCCs, where tumours from all enrolled patients are comprehensively analysed and, for each set of abnormalities, standard chemotherapy will be matched with a new targeted approach [161].

## References

1. Travis WD, Brambilla E, Muller-Hermelink HK, *et al.* Pathology and Genetics of Tumours of the Lung, Pleura, Thymus and Heart IARC WHO Classification of Tumours. Lyon, International Agency for Research on Cancer Press, 2004.
2. Scagliotti GV, Parikh P, von Pawel J, *et al.* Phase III study comparing cisplatin plus gemcitabine with cisplatin plus pemetrexed in chemotherapy-naive patients with advanced-stage non-small-cell lung cancer. *J Clin Oncol* 2008; 26: 3543–3551.
3. Johnson DH, Fehrenbacher L, Novotny WF, *et al.* Randomized phase II trial comparing bevacizumab plus carboplatin and paclitaxel with carboplatin and paclitaxel alone in previously untreated locally advanced or metastatic non-small-cell lung cancer. *J Clin Oncol* 2004; 22: 2184–2191.
4. Travis WD, Brambilla E, Noguchi M, *et al.* International Association for the Study of Lung Cancer/American Thoracic Society/European Respiratory Society international multidisciplinary classification of lung adenocarcinoma. *J Thorac Oncol* 2011; 6: 244–285.
5. Rossi G, Pelosi G, Barbareschi M, *et al.* Subtyping non-small cell lung cancer: relevant issues and operative recommendations for the best pathology practice. *Int J Surg Pathol* 2013; 21: 326–336.
6. Travis WD, Brambilla E, Noguchi M, *et al.* Diagnosis of lung cancer in small biopsies and cytology: implications of the 2011 International Association for the Study of Lung Cancer/American Thoracic Society/European Respiratory Society classification. *Arch Pathol Lab Med* 2013; 137: 668–684.
7. Thunnissen E, Kerr KM, Herth FJ, *et al.* The challenge of NSCLC diagnosis and predictive analysis on small samples. Practical approach of a working group. *Lung Cancer* 2012; 76: 1–18.
8. Ding L, Getz G, Wheeler DA, *et al.* Somatic mutations affect key pathways in lung adenocarcinoma. *Nature* 2008; 455: 1069–1075.

9. Genome Atlas Research Network. Comprehensive genomic characterization of squamous cell lung cancers. *Cancer Nature* 2012; 489: 519–525.
10. Clinical Lung Cancer Genome Project (CLCGP), Network Genomic Medicine (NGM). A genomics-based classification of human lung tumors. *Sci Transl Med* 2013; 5: 209ra153.
11. Cancer Genome Atlas Research Network. Comprehensive molecular profiling of lung adenocarcinoma. *Nature* 2014; 511: 543–550.
12. Rossi G, Mengoli MC, Cavazza A, *et al.* Large cell carcinoma of the lung: clinically oriented classification integrating immunohistochemistry and molecular biology. *Virchows Arch* 2014; 464: 61–68.
13. Vogelstein B, Papadopoulos N, Velculescu VE, *et al.* Cancer genome landscapes. *Science* 2013; 339: 1546–1558.
14. Imielinski M, Berger AH, Hammerman PS, *et al.* Mapping the hallmarks of lung adenocarcinoma with massively parallel sequencing. *Cell* 2012; 150: 1107–1120.
15. Kris MG, Johnson BE, Berry LD, *et al.* Using multiplexed assays of oncogenic drivers in lung cancers to select targeted drugs. *JAMA* 2014; 311: 1998–2006.
16. Chaft JE, Arcila ME, Paik PK, *et al.* Coexistence of *PIK3CA* and other oncogene mutations in lung adenocarcinoma – rationale for comprehensive mutation profiling. *Mol Cancer Ther* 2012; 11: 485–491.
17. Sequist LV, Heist RS, Shaw AT, *et al.* Implementing multiplexed genotyping of non-small-cell lung cancers into routine clinical practice. *Ann Oncol* 2011; 22: 2616–2624.
18. Sartori G, Cavazza A, Sgambato A, *et al.* EGFR and K-ras mutations along the spectrum of pulmonary epithelial tumors of the lung and elaboration of a combined clinicopathologic and molecular scoring system to predict clinical responsiveness to EGFR inhibitors. *Am J Clin Pathol* 2009; 131: 478–489.
19. Dogan S, Shen R, Ang DC, *et al.* Molecular epidemiology of *EGFR* and *KRAS* mutations in 3,026 lung adenocarcinomas: higher susceptibility of women to smoking-related *KRAS*-mutant cancers. *Clin Cancer Res* 2012; 18: 6169–6177.
20. Gahr S, Stoehr R, Geissinger E, *et al. EGFR* mutational status in a large series of Caucasian European NSCLC patients: data from daily practice. *Br J Cancer* 2013; 109: 1821–1828.
21. Rosell R, Moran T, Queralt C, *et al.* Screening for epidermal growth factor receptor mutations in lung cancer. *N Engl J Med* 2009; 361: 958–967.
22. Weber B, Hager H, Sorensen BS, *et al. EGFR* mutation frequency and effectiveness of erlotinib: a prospective observational study in Danish patients with non-small cell lung cancer. *Lung Cancer* 2014; 83: 224–230.
23. Boland JM, Erdogan S, Vasmatzis G, *et al.* Anaplastic lymphoma kinase immunoreactivity correlates with *ALK* gene rearrangement and transcriptional up-regulation in non-small cell lung carcinomas. *Hum Pathol* 2009; 40: 1152–1158.
24. Martelli MP, Sozzi G, Hernandez L, *et al. EML4–ALK* rearrangement in non-small cell lung cancer and non-tumor lung tissues. *Am J Pathol* 2009; 174: 661–670.
25. Rodig SJ, Mino-Kenudson M, Dacic S, *et al.* Unique clinicopathologic features characterize *ALK*-rearranged lung adenocarcinoma in the western population. *Clin Cancer Res* 2009; 15: 5216–5223.
26. Alì G, Proietti A, Pelliccioni S, *et al. ALK* rearrangement in a large series of consecutive non-small cell lung cancers: comparison between a new immunohistochemical approach and fluorescence *in situ* hybridization for the screening of patients eligible for crizotinib treatment. *Arch Pathol Lab Med* 2014; 138: 1449–1458.
27. Villaruz LC, Socinski MA, Abberbock S, *et al.* Clinicopathologic features and outcomes of patients with lung adenocarcinomas harboring BRAF mutations in the Lung Cancer Mutation Consortium. *Cancer* 2015; 121: 448–456.
28. Paik PK, Arcila ME, Fara M, *et al.* Clinical characteristics of patients with lung adenocarcinomas harboring *BRAF* mutations. *J Clin Oncol* 2011; 29: 2046–2051.
29. Cardarella S, Ogino A, Nishino M, *et al.* Clinical, pathologic, and biologic features associated with *BRAF* mutations in non-small cell lung cancer. *Clin Cancer Res* 2013; 19: 4532–4540.
30. Marchetti A, Felicioni L, Malatesta S, *et al.* Clinical features and outcome of patients with non-small-cell lung cancer harboring *BRAF* mutations. *J Clin Oncol* 2011; 29: 3574–3579.
31. Pan Y, Zhang Y, Li Y, *et al. ALK, ROS1* and *RET* fusions in 1139 lung adenocarcinomas: a comprehensive study of common and fusion pattern-specific clinicopathologic, histologic and cytologic features. *Lung Cancer* 2014; 84: 121–126.
32. Go H, Kim DW, Kim D, *et al.* Clinicopathologic analysis of *ROS1*-rearranged non-small-cell lung cancer and proposal of a diagnostic algorithm. *J Thorac Oncol* 2013; 8: 1445–1450.
33. Yoshida A, Kohno T, Tsuta K, *et al. ROS1*-rearranged lung cancer: a clinicopathologic and molecular study of 15 surgical cases. *Am J Surg Pathol* 2013; 37: 554–562.
34. Warth A, Muley T, Dienemann H, *et al. ROS1* expression and translocations in non-small-cell lung cancer: clinicopathological analysis of 1478 cases. *Histopathology* 2014; 65: 187–194.
35. Lee SE, Lee B, Hong M, *et al.* Comprehensive analysis of *RET* and *ROS1* rearrangement in lung adenocarcinoma. *Mod Pathol* 2015; 28: 468–479.
36. Tsuta K, Kohno T, Yoshida A, *et al. RET*-rearranged non-small-cell lung carcinoma: a clinicopathological and molecular analysis. *Br J Cancer* 2014; 110: 1571–1578.

37. Wang R, Hu H, Pan Y, *et al.* *RET* fusions define a unique molecular and clinicopathologic subtype of non-small-cell lung cancer. *J Clin Oncol* 2012; 30: 4352–4359.
38. Li S, Li L, Zhu Y, *et al.* Coexistence of *EGFR* with *KRAS*, or *BRAF*, or *PIK3CA* somatic mutations in lung cancer: a comprehensive mutation profiling from 5125 Chinese cohorts. *Br J Cancer* 2014; 110: 2812–2820.
39. Wang L, Hu H, Pan Y, *et al.* *PIK3CA* mutations frequently coexist with *EGFR/KRAS* mutations in non-small cell lung cancer and suggest poor prognosis in *EGFR/KRAS* wildtype subgroup. *PLoS One* 2014; 9: e88291.
40. Mazières J, Peters S, Lepage B, *et al.* Lung cancer that harbors an *HER2* mutation: epidemiologic characteristics and therapeutic perspectives. *J Clin Oncol* 2013; 31: 1997–2003.
41. Buttitta F, Barassi F, Fresu G, *et al.* Mutational analysis of the *HER2* gene in lung tumors from Caucasian patients: mutations are mainly present in adenocarcinomas with bronchioloalveolar features. *Int J Cancer* 2006; 119: 2586–2591.
42. Shigematsu H, Takahashi T, Nomura M, *et al.* Somatic mutations of the HER2 kinase domain in lung adenocarcinomas. *Cancer Res* 2005; 65: 1642–1646.
43. Krishnaswamy S, Kanteti R, Duke-Cohan JS, *et al.* Ethnic differences and functional analysis of *MET* mutations in lung cancer. *Clin Cancer Res* 2009; 15: 5714–5723.
44. Dacic S, Nikiforova MN. Present and future molecular testing of lung carcinoma. *Adv Anat Pathol* 2014; 21: 94–99.
45. Loeb LA. Human cancers express mutator phenotypes: origin, consequences and targeting. *Nat Rev Cancer* 2011; 11: 450–457.
46. Alexandrov LB, Nik-Zainal S, Wedge DC, *et al.* Signatures of mutational processes in human cancer. *Nature* 2013; 500: 415–421.
47. Hoadley KA, Yau C, Wolf DM, *et al.* Multiplatform analysis of 12 cancer types reveals molecular classification within and across tissues of origin. *Cell* 2014; 158: 929–944.
48. Shames DS, Wistuba II. The evolving genomic classification of lung cancer. *J Pathol* 2014; 232: 121–33.
49. Pleasance ED, Stephens PJ, O'Meara S, *et al.* A small-cell lung cancer genome with complex signatures of tobacco exposure. *Nature* 2010; 463: 184–190.
50. van Meerbeeck JP, Fennell DA, De Ruysscher DK. Small-cell lung cancer. *Lancet* 2011; 378: 1741–1755.
51. Peifer M, Fernández-Cuesta L, Sos ML, *et al.* Integrative genome analyses identify key somatic driver mutations of small-cell lung cancer. *Nat Genet* 2012; 44: 1104–1110.
52. Bordi P, Tiseo M, Barbieri F, *et al.* Gene mutations in small-cell lung cancer (SCLC): results of a panel of 6 genes in a cohort of Italian patients. *Lung Cancer* 2014; 86: 324–328.
53. Lawrence MS, Stojanov P, Polak P, *et al.* Mutational heterogeneity in cancer and the search for new cancer-associated genes. *Nature* 2013; 499: 214–218.
54. de Bruin EC, McGranahan N, Mitter R, *et al.* Spatial and temporal diversity in genomic instability processes defines lung cancer evolution. *Science* 2014; 346: 251–216.
55. Hiley C, de Bruin EC, McGranahan N, *et al.* Deciphering intratumor heterogeneity and temporal acquisition of driver events to refine precision medicine. *Genome Biol* 2014; 15: 453.
56. Zhang J, Fujimoto J, Zhang J, *et al.* Intratumor heterogeneity in localized lung adenocarcinomas delineated by multiregion sequencing. *Science* 2014; 346: 256–259.
57. Mansuet-Lupo A, Zouiti F, Alifano M, *et al.* Intratumoral distribution of *EGFR* mutations and copy number in metastatic lung cancer, what impact on the initial molecular diagnosis? *J Transl Med* 2014; 12: 131.
58. Yatabe Y, Matsuo K, Mitsudomi T. Heterogeneous distribution of *EGFR* mutations is extremely rare in lung adenocarcinoma. *J Clin Oncol* 2011; 29: 2972–2977.
59. Cortot AB, Jänne PA. Molecular mechanisms of resistance in epidermal growth factor receptor-mutant lung adenocarcinomas. *Eur Respir Rev* 2014; 23: 356–366.
60. Katayama R, Shaw AT, Khan TM, *et al.* Mechanisms of acquired crizotinib resistance in *ALK*-rearranged lung Cancers. *Sci Transl Med* 2012; 4: 120ra17.
61. Kim H, Xu X, Yoo SB, *et al.* Discordance between anaplastic lymphoma kinase status in primary non-small-cell lung cancers and their corresponding metastases. *Histopathology* 2013; 62: 305–314.
62. Mitsudomi T, Morita S, Yatabe Y, *et al.* Gefitinib *versus* cisplatin plus docetaxel in patients with non-small-cell lung cancer harbouring mutations of the epidermal growth factor receptor (WJTOG3405): an open label, randomised phase 3 trial. *Lancet Oncol* 2010; 11: 121–128.
63. Kerr KM, Bubendorf L, Edelman MJ, *et al.* Second ESMO consensus conference on lung cancer: pathology and molecular biomarkers for non-small-cell lung cancer. *Ann Oncol* 2014; 25: 1681–1690.
64. Felip E, Concha A, de Castro J, *et al.* Biomarker testing in advanced non-small-cell lung cancer: a National Consensus of the Spanish Society of Pathology and the Spanish Society of Medical Oncology. *Clin Transl Oncol* 2015; 17: 103–112.
65. National Comprehensive Cancer Network. NCCN Clinical Practice Guidelines in Oncology. Non-Small Cell Lung Cancer. Version 3.2015. www.nccn.org/professionals/physician_gls/f_guidelines.asp Date last accessed: January 02, 2015.

66. Cooper W, Fox S, O'Toole S, *et al.* National Working Group Meeting on ALK diagnostics in lung cancer. *Asia Pac J Clin Oncol* 2014; 10: Suppl. 2, 11–17.
67. Lindeman NI, Cagle PT, Beasley MB. Molecular testing guideline for selection of lung cancer patients for *EGFR* and *ALK* tyrosine kinase inhibitors: guideline from the College of American Pathologists, International Association for the Study of Lung Cancer, and Association for Molecular Pathology. *J Mol Diagn* 2013; 15: 415–453.
68. Leighl NB, Rekhtman N, Biermann WA, *et al.* Molecular testing for selection of patients with lung cancer for epidermal growth factor receptor and anaplastic lymphoma kinase tyrosine kinase inhibitors: American Society of Clinical Oncology endorsement of the College of American Pathologists/International Association for the Study of Lung Cancer/Association for Molecular Pathology guideline. *J Clin Oncol* 2014; 32: 3673–3679.
69. Marchetti A, Barberis M, Papotti M, *et al.* *ALK* rearrangement testing by FISH analysis in non-small-cell lung cancer patients: results of the first Italian external quality assurance scheme. *J Thorac Oncol* 2014; 9: 1470–1476.
70. Thunnissen E, Bubendorf L, Dietel M, *et al.* *EML4–ALK* testing in non-small cell carcinomas of the lung: a review with recommendations. *Virchows Arch* 2012; 461: 245–257.
71. McLeer-Florin A, Moro-Sibilot D, Melis A. Dual IHC and FISH testing for ALK gene rearrangement in lung adenocarcinomas in a routine practice: a French study. *J Thorac Oncol* 2012; 7: 348–354.
72. National Institute for Health and Care Excellence. NICE Guidelines Lung Cancer (CG121). www.nice.org.uk/guidance/conditions-and-diseases/cancer/lung-cancer Date last accessed: February 1, 2015.
73. França LT, Carrilho E, Kist TB. A review of DNA sequencing techniques. *Q Rev Biophys* 2002; 35: 169–200.
74. Harrington CT, Lin EI, Olson MT, *et al.* Fundamentals of pyrosequencing. *Arch Pathol Lab Med* 2013; 137: 1296–1303.
75. Erali M, Voelkerding KV, Wittwer CT. High resolution melting applications for clinical laboratory medicine. *Exp Mol Pathol* 2008; 85: 50–58.
76. Strerath M, Detmer I, Gaster J, *et al.* Modified oligonucleotides as tools for allele-specific amplification. *Methods Mol Biol* 2007; 402: 317–328.
77. Stranneheim H, Lundeberg J. Stepping stones in DNA sequencing. *Biotechnol J* 2012; 7: 1063–1073.
78. O'Brien CP, Taylor SE, O'Leary JJ, *et al.* Molecular testing in oncology: problems, pitfalls and progress. *Lung Cancer* 2014; 83: 309–315.
79. Hirsch FR, Bunn PA Jr, Herbst RS. Companion diagnostics: has their time come and gone? *Clin Cancer Res* 2014; 20: 4422–4424.
80. Pennisi E. Genomics. Semiconductors inspire new sequencing technologies. *Science* 2010; 327: 1190.
81. Shendure J, Ji H. Next-generation DNA sequencing. *Nat Biotechnol* 2008; 26: 1135–1145.
82. Margulies M, Egholm M, Altman WE, *et al.* Genome sequencing in microfabricated high-density picolitre reactors. *Nature* 2005; 437: 376–380.
83. Ronaghi M, Uhlén M, Nyrén P. A sequencing method based on real-time pyrophosphate. *Science* 1998; 281: 363–365.
84. van Dijk EL, Auger H, Jaszczyszyn Y, *et al.* Ten years of next-generation sequencing technology. *Trends Genet* 2014; 30: 418–426.
85. Cree IA, Deans Z, Ligtenberg MJ, *et al.* Guidance for laboratories performing molecular pathology for cancer patients. *J Clin Pathol* 2014; 67: 923–931.
86. van Krieken JH, Siebers AG, Normanno N, *et al.* European consensus conference for external quality assessment in molecular pathology. *Ann Oncol* 2013; 24: 1958–1963.
87. Sorensen BS, Wu L, Wei W, *et al.* Monitoring of epidermal growth factor receptor tyrosine kinase inhibitor-sensitizing and resistance mutations in the plasma DNA of patients with advanced non-small cell lung cancer during treatment with erlotinib. *Cancer* 2014; 120: 3896–3901.
88. Yatabe Y. *EGFR* mutations and the terminal respiratory unit. *Cancer Metastasis Rev* 2010; 29: 23–36.
89. Lynch TJ, Bell DW, Sordella R, *et al.* Activating mutations in the epidermal growth factor receptor underlying responsiveness of non-small-cell lung cancer to gefitinib. *N Engl J Med* 2004; 350: 2129–2139.
90. Paez JG, Jänne PA, Lee JC, *et al.* *EGFR* mutations in lung cancer: correlation with clinical response to gefitinib therapy. *Science* 2004; 304: 1497–1500.
91. Pao W, Miller V, Zakowski M, *et al.* EGF receptor gene mutations are common in lung cancers from "never smokers" and are associated with sensitivity of tumors to gefitinib and erlotinib. *Proc Natl Acad Sci USA* 2004; 101: 13306–13311.
92. Tsao MS, Sakurada A, Cutz JC, *et al.* Erlotinib in lung cancer – molecular and clinical predictors of outcome. *N Engl J Med* 2005; 353: 133–144.
93. Kosaka T, Yatabe Y, Endoh H, *et al.* Mutations of the epidermal growth factor receptor gene in lung cancer: biological and clinical implications. *Cancer Res* 2004; 64: 8919–8923.
94. Okabe T, Okamoto I, Tamura K, *et al.* Differential constitutive activation of the epidermal growth factor receptor in non-small cell lung cancer cells bearing *EGFR* gene mutation and amplification. *Cancer Res* 2007; 67: 2046–2053.
95. Herbst RS, Heymach JV, Lippman SM. Lung cancer. *N Engl J Med* 2008; 359: 1367–1380.

96. Rekhtman N, Paik PK, Arcila ME, *et al.* Clarifying the spectrum of driver oncogene mutations in biomarker-verified squamous carcinoma of lung: lack of *EGFR/KRAS* and presence of *PIK3CA/AKT1* mutations. *Clin Cancer Res* 2012; 18: 1167–1176.
97. Thunnissen E, van der Oord K, den Bakker M. Prognostic and predictive biomarkers in lung cancer. A review. *Virchows Arch* 2014; 464: 347–358.
98. Maemondo M, Inoue A, Kobayashi K, *et al.* Gefitinib or chemotherapy for non-small-cell lung cancer with mutated *EGFR*. *N Engl J Med* 2010; 362: 2380–2388.
99. Mok TS, Wu YL, Thongprasert S, *et al.* Gefitinib or carboplatin-paclitaxel in pulmonary adenocarcinoma. *N Engl J Med* 2009; 361: 947–957.
100. Rosell R, Carcereny E, Gervais R, *et al.* Erlotinib *versus* standard chemotherapy as first-line treatment for European patients with advanced *EGFR* mutation-positive non-small-cell lung cancer (EURTAC): a multicentre, open-label, randomised phase 3 trial. *Lancet Oncol* 2012; 13: 239–246.
101. Zhou C, Wu YL, Chen G, *et al.* Erlotinib *versus* chemotherapy as first-line treatment for patients with advanced *EGFR* mutation-positive non-small-cell lung cancer (OPTIMAL, CTONG-0802): a multicentre, open-label, randomised, phase 3 study. *Lancet Oncol* 2011; 12: 735–742.
102. Sequist LV, Yang JC, Yamamoto N, *et al.* Phase III study of afatinib or cisplatin plus pemetrexed in patients with metastatic lung adenocarcinoma with EGFR mutations. *J Clin Oncol* 2013; 31: 3327–3334.
103. Yang C, Schuler MH, Yamamoto N, *et al.* LUX-Lung-3: a randomized, open label, phase III study of afatinib *versus* pemetrexed and cisplatin as first line treatment for patients with advanced adenocarcinoma of the lung harboring EGFR-activating mutations. *J Clin Oncol* 2012; 30: Suppl, LBA 7500.
104. Melosky B. Review of EGFR-TKIs in Metastatic NSCLC, Including Ongoing Trials. *Front Oncol* 2014; 4: 244.
105. Yang C, Sequist LV, Schuler MH. Overall survival (OS) in patients (pts) with advanced non-small cell lung cancer (NSCLC) harboring common (Del19/L858R) epidermal growth factor receptor mutations (EGFR mut): Pooled analysis of two large open-label phase III studies (LUX-Lung 3 [LL3] and LUX-Lung 6 [LL6]) comparing afatinib with chemotherapy (CT). *J Clin Oncol* 2014; 32: Suppl. 5, abstr 8004.
106. Lee VH, Tin VP, Choy TS, *et al.* Association of exon 19 and 21 EGFR mutation patterns with treatment outcome after first-line tyrosine kinase inhibitor in metastatic non-small-cell lung cancer. *J Thorac Oncol* 2013; 8: 1148–1155.
107. Fukihara J, Watanabe N, Taniguchi H, *et al.* Clinical predictors of response to EGFR tyrosine kinase inhibitors in patients with *EGFR*-mutant non-small cell lung cancer. *Oncology* 2014; 86: 86–93.
108. Costa C, Molina MA, Drozdowskyj A, *et al.* The impact of *EGFR* T790M mutations and *BIM* mRNA expression on outcome in patients with *EGFR*-mutant NSCLC treated with erlotinib or chemotherapy in the randomized phase III EURTAC trial. *Clin Cancer Res* 2014; 20: 2001–2010.
109. Beau-Faller M, Prim N, Ruppert AM, *et al.* Rare EGFR exon 18 and exon 20 mutations in non-small-cell lung cancer on 10 117 patients: a multicentre observational study by the French ERMETIC-IFCT network. *Ann Oncol* 2014; 25: 126–131.
110. Robinson KW, Sandler AB. The role of MET receptor tyrosine kinase in non-small cell lung cancer and clinical development of targeted anti-MET agents. *Oncologist* 2013; 18: 115–22.
111. Arcila ME, Oxnard GR, Nafa K, *et al.* Rebiopsy of lung cancer patients with acquired resistance to EGFR inhibitors and enhanced detection of the T790M mutation using a locked nucleic acid-based assay. *Clin Cancer Res* 2011; 17: 1169–1180.
112. Sequist LV, Waltman BA, Dias-Santagata D, *et al.* Genotypic and histological evolution of lung cancers acquiring resistance to EGFR inhibitors. *Sci Transl Med* 2011; 3: 75ra26.
113. Yu HA, Arcila ME, Rekhtman N, *et al.* Analysis of tumor specimens at the time of acquired resistance to EGFR-TKI therapy in 155 patients with *EGFR*-mutant lung cancers. *Clin Cancer Res* 2013; 19: 2240–2247.
114. Pao W, Miller VA, Politi KA, *et al.* Acquired resistance of lung adenocarcinomas to gefitinib or erlotinib is associated with a second mutation in the EGFR kinase domain. *PLoS Med* 2005; 2: e73.
115. Rosell R, Molina MA, Costa C, *et al.* Pretreatment *EGFR* T790M mutation and *BRCA1* mRNA expression in erlotinib-treated advanced non-small-cell lung cancer patients with EGFR mutations. *Clin Cancer Res* 2011; 17: 1160–1168.
116. Kuiper JL, Heideman DA, Thunnissen E, *et al.* Incidence of T790M mutation in (sequential) rebiopsies in *EGFR*-mutated NSCLC-patients. *Lung Cancer* 2014; 85: 19–24.
117. Ohashi K, Sequist LV, Arcila ME, *et al.* Lung cancers with acquired resistance to EGFR inhibitors occasionally harbor *BRAF* gene mutations but lack mutations in *KRAS*, *NRAS*, or *MEK1*. *Proc Natl Acad Sci USA* 2012; 109: E2127–E2133.
118. Zhang Z, Lee JC, Lin L, *et al.* Activation of the AXL kinase causes resistance to EGFR-targeted therapy in lung cancer. *Nat Genet* 2012; 44: 852–860.
119. Kwak EL, Bang YJ, Camidge DR, *et al.* Anaplastic lymphoma kinase inhibition in non-small-cell lung cancer. *N Engl J Med* 2010; 363: 1693–1703.

120. Camidge DR, Bang YJ, Kwak EL, *et al.* Activity and safety of crizotinib in patients with ALK-positive non-small-cell lung cancer: updated results from a phase 1 study. *Lancet Oncol* 2012; 13: 1011–1019.
121. Shaw AT, Kim DW, Nakagawa K, *et al.* Crizotinib *versus* chemotherapy in advanced ALK-positive lung cancer. *N Engl J Med* 2013; 368: 2385–2394.
122. Shaw AT, Yeap BY, Mino-Kenudson M, *et al.* Clinical features and outcome of patients with non-small-cell lung cancer who harbor *EML4–ALK*. *J Clin Oncol* 2009; 27: 4247–4253.
123. Shackelford RE, Vora M, Mayhall K, *et al.* *ALK*-rearrangements and testing methods in non-small cell lung cancer: a review. *Genes Cancer* 2014; 5: 1–14.
124. Soda M, Choi YL, Enomoto M, *et al.* Identification of the transforming *EML4–ALK* fusion gene in non-small-cell lung cancer. *Nature* 2007; 448: 561–566.
125. Rikova K, Guo A, Zeng Q, *et al.* Global survey of phosphotyrosine signaling identifies oncogenic kinases in lung cancer. *Cell* 2007; 131: 1190–1203.
126. Santelmo C, Ravaioli A, Barzotti E, *et al.* Coexistence of *EGFR* mutation and *ALK* translocation in NSCLC: literature review and case report of response to gefitinib. *Lung Cancer* 2013; 81: 294–296.
127. Perner S, Wagner PL, Demichelis F, *et al.* *EML4–ALK* fusion lung cancer: a rare acquired event. *Neoplasia* 2008; 10: 298–302.
128. Conklin CM, Craddock KJ, Have C, *et al.* Immunohistochemistry is a reliable screening tool for identification of *ALK* rearrangement in non-small-cell lung carcinoma and is antibody dependent. *J Thorac Oncol* 2013; 8: 45–51.
129. Wang Y, Wang S, Xu S, *et al.* Clinicopathologic features of patients with non-small cell lung cancer harboring the *EML4–ALK* fusion gene: a meta-analysis. *PLoS One* 2014; 9: e110617.
130. Yoshida A, Tsuta K, Nakamura H, *et al.* Comprehensive histologic analysis of *ALK*-rearranged lung carcinomas. *Am J Surg Pathol* 2011; 35: 1226–1234.
131. Doebele RC, Pilling AB, Aisner DL, *et al.* Mechanisms of resistance to crizotinib in patients with *ALK* gene rearranged non-small cell lung cancer. *Clin Cancer Res* 2012; 18: 1472–1482.
132. Katayama R, Shaw AT, Khan TM, *et al.* Mechanisms of acquired crizotinib resistance in *ALK*-rearranged lung cancers. *Sci Transl Med* 2012; 4: 120ra17
133. Shaw AT, Engelman JA. Ceritinib in *ALK*-rearranged non-small-cell lung cancer. *N Engl J Med* 2014; 370: 2537–2539.
134. Conde E, Angulo B, Izquierdo E, *et al.* The *ALK* translocation in advanced non-small-cell lung carcinomas: preapproval testing experience at a single cancer centre. *Histopathology* 2013; 62: 609–616.
135. Katayama R, Friboulet L, Koike S, *et al.* Two novel *ALK* mutations mediate acquired resistance to the next-generation ALK inhibitor alectinib. *Clin Cancer Res* 2014; 20: 5686–5696.
136. Zwaenepoel K, Van Dongen A, Lambin S, *et al.* Detection of ALK expression in non-small-cell lung cancer with *ALK* gene rearrangements – comparison of multiple immunohistochemical methods. *Histopathology* 2014; 65: 539–548.
137. Sholl LM, Weremowicz S, Gray SW, *et al.* Combined use of ALK immunohistochemistry and FISH for optimal detection of *ALK*-rearranged lung adenocarcinomas. *J Thorac Oncol* 2013; 8: 322–328.
138. Savic S, Bode B, Diebold J, *et al.* Detection of ALK-positive non-small-cell lung cancers on cytological specimens: high accuracy of immunocytochemistry with the 5A4 clone. *J Thorac Oncol* 2013; 8: 1004–1011.
139. Paik JH, Choi CM, Kim H, *et al.* Clinicopathologic implication of *ALK* rearrangement in surgically resected lung cancer: a proposal of diagnostic algorithm for *ALK*-rearranged adenocarcinoma. *Lung Cancer* 2012; 76: 403–409.
140. Peters S, Michielin O, Zimmermann S. Dramatic response induced by vemurafenib in a *BRAF* V600E-mutated lung adenocarcinoma. *J Clin Oncol* 2013; 31: e341–344.
141. Robinson SD, O'Shaughnessy JA, Cowey CL, *et al.* *BRAF* V600E-mutated lung adenocarcinoma with metastases to the brain responding to treatment with vemurafenib. *Lung Cancer* 2014; 85: 326–330.
142. Davies H, Bignell GR, Cox C, *et al.* Futreal mutations of the *BRAF* gene in human cancer. *Nature* 2002; 417: 949–954.
143. Rahman MA, Salajegheh A, Smith RA, *et al.* B-Raf mutation: a key player in molecular biology of cancer. *Exp Mol Pathol* 2013; 95: 336–342.
144. Villaruz LC, Burns TF, Ramfidis VS, *et al.* Personalizing therapy in advanced non-small cell lung cancer. *Semin Respir Crit Care Med* 2013; 34: 822–83646.
145. Minuti G, D'Incecco A, Cappuzzo F. Targeted therapy for NSCLC with driver mutations. *Expert Opin Biol Ther* 2013; 13: 1401–1412.
146. Fisher KE, Cohen C, Siddiqui MT, *et al.* Accurate detection of *BRAF* p.V600E mutations in challenging melanoma specimens requires stringent immunohistochemistry scoring criteria or sensitive molecular assays. *Hum Pathol* 2014; 45: 2281–2293.
147. Shaw AT, Ou SH, Bang YJ, *et al.* Crizotinib in *ROS1*-rearranged non-small-cell lung cancer. *N Engl J Med* 2014; 371: 1963–1971.
148. Davies KD, Doebele RC. Molecular pathways: *ROS1* fusion proteins in cancer. *Clin Cancer Res* 2013; 19: 4040–4045.

149. Mescam-Mancini L, Lantuéjoul S, Moro-Sibilot D, *et al.* On the relevance of a testing algorithm for the detection of *ROS1*-rearranged lung adenocarcinomas. *Lung Cancer* 2014; 83: 168–173.
150. Yoshida A, Tsuta K, Wakai S, *et al.* Immunohistochemical detection of ROS1 is useful for identifying *ROS1* rearrangements in lung cancers. *Mod Pathol* 2014; 27: 711–720.
151. Ricciardi GR, Russo A, Franchina T, *et al.* NSCLC and HER2: between lights and shadows. *J Thorac Oncol* 2014; 9: 1750–1762.
152. Stephens P, Hunter C, Bignell G, *et al.* Lung cancer: intragenic ERBB2 kinase mutations in tumours. *Nature* 2004; 431: 525–526.
153. Yoshizawa A, Sumiyoshi S, Sonobe M, *et al.* *HER2* status in lung adenocarcinoma: a comparison of immunohistochemistry, fluorescence *in situ* hybridization (FISH), dual-ISH, and gene mutations. *Lung Cancer* 2014; 85: 373–378.
154. Liu L, Shao X, Gao W, *et al.* The role of human epidermal growth factor receptor 2 as a prognostic factor in lung cancer: a meta-analysis of published data. *J Thorac Oncol* 2010; 5: 1922–1932.
155. Lee JW, Soung YH, Seo SH, *et al.* Somatic mutations of ERBB2 kinase domain in gastric, colorectal, and breast carcinomas. *Clin Cancer Res* 2006; 12: 57–61.
156. Koeppen H, Yu W, Zha J, *et al.* Biomarker analyses from a placebo-controlled phase II study evaluating erlotinib ±onartuzumab in advanced non-small cell lung cancer: MET expression levels are predictive of patient benefit. *Clin Cancer Res* 2014; 20: 4488–4498.
157. Spigel DR, Edelman MJ, O'Byrne K. Onartuzumab plus erlotinib *versus* erlotinib in previously treated stage IIIb or IV NSCLC: Results from the pivotal phase III randomized, multicenter, placebo-controlled METLung (OAM4971g) global trial. *J Clin Oncol* 2014: 32: Suppl., 8000.
158. Scagliotti GV, Novello S, von Pawel J. The emerging role of MET/HGF inhibitors in oncology. *Cancer Treat Rev* 2013; 39: 793–801.
159. Yano S, Nakagawa T. The current state of molecularly targeted drugs targeting HGF/Met. *Jpn J Clin Oncol* 2014; 44: 9–12.
160. Willyard C. 'Basket studies' will hold intricate data for cancer drug approvals. *Nat Med* 2013; 19: 655.
161. Malik SM, Pazdur R, Abrams JS, *et al.* Consensus report of a joint NCI thoracic malignancies steering committee: FDA workshop on strategies for integrating biomarkers into clinical development of new therapies for lung cancer leading to the inception of "master protocols" in lung cancer. *J Thorac Oncol* 2014; 9: 1443–1448.

---

Disclosures: F. Laenger reports being an Advisory Board Member for AstraZeneca and Roche (on the topic of lung cancer). N. Dickgreber reports receiving grants, personal fees and nonfinancial support from Boehringer Ingelheim, Lilly and Roche, personal fees and nonfinancial support from BMS and Berlin Chemie, personal fees from Teva and AstraZeneca, and grants and personal fees from Novartis, outside the submitted work.

Chapter 9

# Adequate tissue for adequate diagnosis: what do we really need?

Guido M.J.M. Roemen, Axel zur Hausen and Ernst Jan M. Speel

Current state-of-the-art diagnosis of lung cancer involves an increasing number of morphological and molecular analyses on tissue, on which a multidisciplinary team of physicians base a treatment strategy. However, most lung cancer patients present with advanced disease, which may hamper sampling of sufficient tissue material for diagnosis due to fragile health and/or tumour location. Furthermore, the interval between patients seeing a specialist and the start of treatment should be limited as this may influence the prognosis.

In this chapter, we review the current practice in lung cancer diagnosis, including sampling, transportation and processing of tissue, as well as morphological, immunohistochemical and molecular analysis on resection, biopsy and cytological material. We particularly focus on factors that may affect adequate tissue quality and diagnosis (*i.e.* collection of representative tumour tissue and variables in the downstream workflow), as well as factors influencing the outcome of molecular analyses. Finally, recommendations are provided to optimise adequate tissue diagnosis and, as a consequence, clinical diagnosis and treatment.

Many chemotherapeutic drugs used for current patient treatment lack adequate specificity and efficacy. Traditionally, lung cancer is classified on the basis of histology and supplementary immunostaining, *e.g.* to discriminate SCC from ADC, for which tumour resection specimens are the tissue material of choice [1–3]. However, as only 20% of lung cancer patients are primarily treated with surgery (stage I and II patients, and patients receiving neoadjuvant treatment followed by surgery), the remaining 80% are mainly diagnosed on the basis of biopsy or cytology material, which can be very limited and even inappropriate for histopathological diagnosis. Modified tumour classification schemes have been proposed for small biopsies and cytology, *e.g.* to diagnose carcinomas based on clearly identifiable growth patterns or, if patterns are not present, to classify a tumour on the basis of special stains [3]. The increasing number of molecular tests that are currently required for therapy stratification of patients presenting with advanced (stage IIIB/IV) disease is becoming a significant bottleneck due to limited biopsy and cytology material.

Dept of Pathology, GROW – School for Oncology and Developmental Biology, Maastricht University Medical Centre, Maastricht, The Netherlands.

Correspondence: Ernst Jan M. Speel, Dept of Pathology, GROW – School for Oncology and Developmental Biology, Maastricht University Medical Centre, PO Box 5800, 6202 AZ Maastricht, The Netherlands. E-mail: ernstjan.speel@mumc.nl

 Print ISBN: 978-1-84984-061-3. Online ISBN: 978-1-84984-062-0. Print ISSN: 2312-508X. Online ISSN: 2312-5098.

These molecular tests are the result of the rapid progress that has been made in the last decade in understanding the molecular biology of cancer, in combination with the development of new nucleic acid-sequencing technologies and platforms for the accurate analysis of nucleic acids, as well as advances in automation. This has led to applications in diagnosis, prognosis and personalised therapy, such as the identification of a large number of new, clinically important and actionable tumour-driving oncogene mutations [4, 5]. In the field of lung cancer, these mutations now define molecular subsets of tumours [4]. For example, in NSCLC, activating mutations and gene rearrangements have been found in the oncogenes *KRAS* (V-KI-RAS2 Kirsten rat sarcoma viral oncogene homologue), *EGFR*, *BRAF* (V-RAF murine sarcoma viral oncogene homologue B1), *ERBB2* (Her2Neu), *ALK*, *ROS1* (V-ROS avian UR2 sarcoma virus oncogene homologue 1), *RET* (rearranged during transfection protooncogene) and *MET* (MET protooncogene, also known as HGF receptor) (amongst others), which deregulate cell signalling pathways in tumour cells and, moreover, predict for response to small molecule TKIs that are either clinically available or in clinical trial development for advanced NSCLC [6]. EGFR mutations and ALK gene rearrangements are currently the two most robust biomarkers in this respect, and guidelines for histopathology and molecular testing of these genetic alterations in NSCLC have recently been published [7, 8]. Nevertheless, general agreement is urgently needed on best practice for the use of lung tissues for adequate histopathological diagnosis and molecular testing of NSCLC. In this chapter: 1) we present an overview of the current clinical practice of lung cancer tissue sampling, processing, diagnosis and molecular analysis; 2) we analyse factors affecting adequate tissue diagnosis; and 3) we provide recommendations to establish an adequate workflow and optimal tissue diagnosis, reporting and quality control. These factors are all essential to an accurate diagnosis, on the basis of which adequate clinical decisions can be made by the oncologist.

## Current clinical practice in lung cancer tissue sampling, processing, diagnosis and molecular analysis

Figure 1 presents a scheme of the daily workflow of laboratories performing (molecular) pathology for lung cancer in the clinic, beginning with the removal of a tissue sample in the clinic and tissue processing, then on to histopathological diagnosis and molecular pathology, and ending with presentation of the report to the clinician and patient.

### Tissue sampling

If (a diagnosis of) lung cancer is suspected, tissue diagnosis is essential to confirm the disease and classify the tumour, and also to perform molecular analyses in order to guide the treatment decisions made by a multidisciplinary team of specialists [3]. Both invasive and less invasive methods can be used, the latter being preferable if enough cell material of adequate quality can be collected. As different mechanisms of resistance exist in lung cancer [9–11], tissue sampling from progressing tumours is also required to decide upon new treatments.

#### *Resection specimens*

In stage I and II tumours or tumours that have been resected after neoadjuvant treatment (20% of patients), which are often detected *via* imaging (*i.e.* CT and PET/CT), resection material can be used for diagnosis and further molecular testing. Alternatively, biopsies can be taken using different methods, such as tissue sampling of distant metastases (if present), and, under general anaesthesia, procedures including mediastinoscopy and thoracoscopy

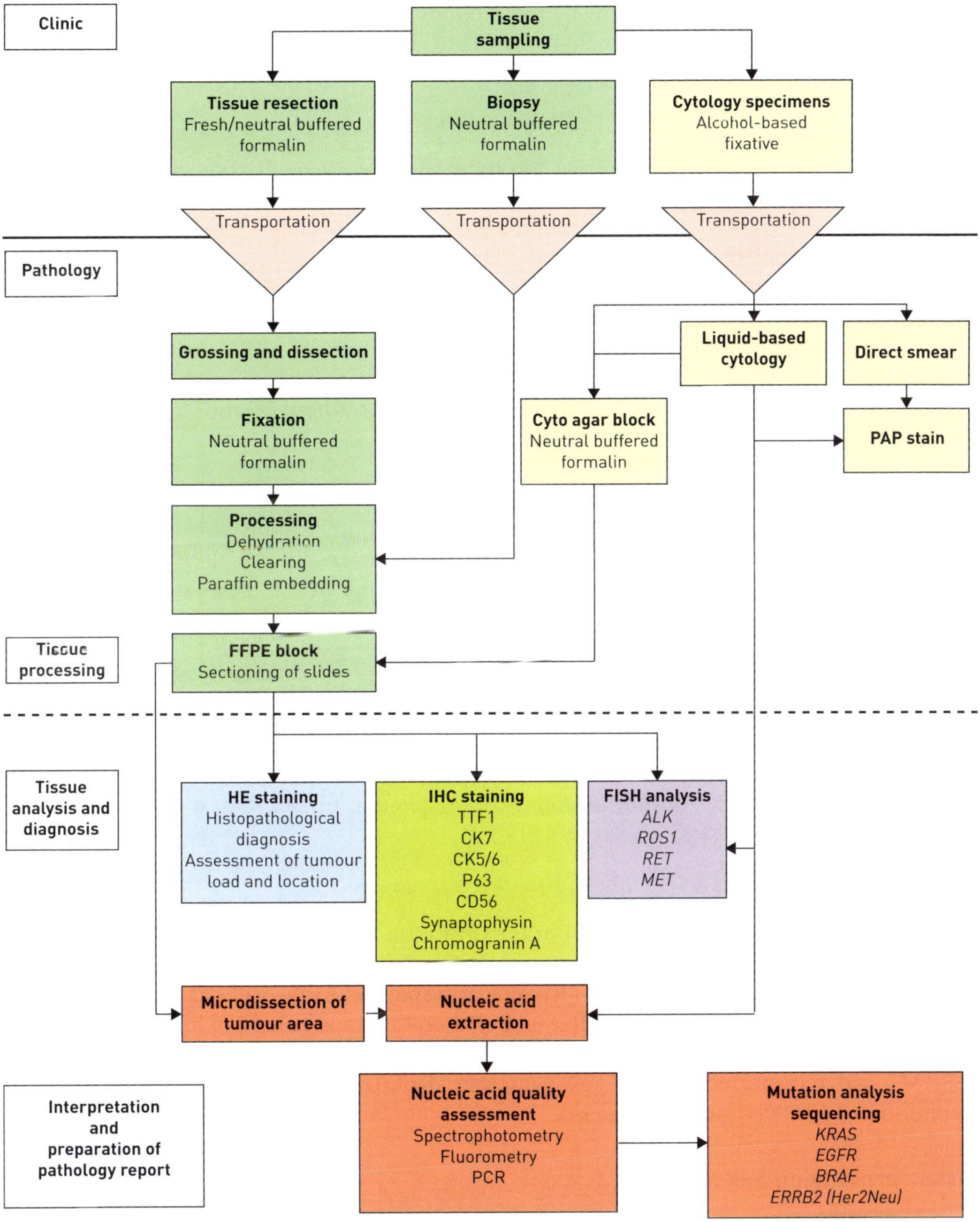


Figure 1. Workflow of laboratories performing (molecular) pathology for lung cancer in the clinic, from tissue sampling in the clinic to morphological and molecular analysis of these samples, finally leading to an integrated pathology report. FFPE: formalin-fixed, paraffin-embedded; PAP: Papanicolaou; HE: haematoxylin and eosin; TTF1: thyroid transcription factor, gene *NKX2-1* (NK2 homeobox 1); CK7: cytokeratin 7, gene *KRT7* (keratin 7); CK5/6: cytokeratins 5 and 6, genes *KRT5* (keratin 5) and *KRT6* (keratin 6); P63: protein p63, gene *TP63* (tumour protein p63); CD56: cluster of differentiation 56, gene *NCAM1* (neural cell adhesion molecule 1); *ROS1*: V-ROS avian UR2 sarcoma virus oncogene homologue 1; *RET*: rearranged during transfection protooncogene; *MET*: MET protooncogene, also known as HGF receptor; *KRAS*: V-KI-RAS2 Kirsten rat sarcoma viral oncogene homologue; BRAF: V-RAF murine sarcoma viral oncogene homologue B1.

can be used to reliably collect relatively large tumour samples of mediastinal lymph nodes (stations 1–9) or pulmonary (parenchym) lesions. Thoracoscopy may also be used to carry out wedge excisions of suspicious lung or pleural lesions [12, 13].

### *Biopsy specimens*

In patients presenting with (recurrent) advanced disease (stage III/IV), multiple biopsies rather than lung cytology (brushes or washes) are preferred for diagnostic purposes. Biopsies might be carried out using approaches such as flexible videobronchoscopy and CT-guided percutaneous needle biopsy. The former procedure might be used for endobronchial tumour biopsy with targeted diagnostic yields ⩾85% or for peripheral tumour biopsy if the imaged tumour is >2 cm and localised near an unobstructed bronchus (yield ⩾70% indicated) [14]. For enlarged or bulky lymph nodes, EBUS with transbronchial needle aspiration (21–22 gauge needle) is recommended (target diagnostic yield ⩾90%). Biopsies from lymph node stations 8 and 9, as well as the adrenal gland, left liver lobe and coeliac lymph nodes can be taken using EUS [15].

CT-guided percutaneous needle biopsy enables large and multiple tissue specimens to be taken with a single puncture as long as unnecessary complications can be avoided [16]. Diagnostic yields should be ⩾90% in tumours with a diameter ⩾1.5 cm close to the chest wall (multiple biopsies, 18–20 gauge needle). The primary tumour or the metastasis can usually be sampled with limited complications depending on local expertise and available technology.

### *Cytology specimens*

In case biopsy sampling is not possible (40–65% of patients with invasive lung carcinoma [17, 18]), cytology specimens can be used for lung cancer diagnosis, which is also less invasive for the patient. Cytological material is generally sampled using EBUS–fine-needle aspiration, bronchial cytology, pleural effusions or fine-needle aspiration from distant metastases.

## Tissue transportation

After sampling, tissue is transported from the operation room to the pathology department. Several transportation procedures are used for large surgical specimens, including placement in excess neutral buffered formalin, transport as fresh material, and transport at 4°C under vacuum conditions [19, 20]. Small diagnostic biopsies are predominantly directly immersed in excess (20–50 mL) neutral buffered formalin. Cytology samples are either collected and transported fresh to the pathology department or submersed directly in an alcohol-based fixative prior to transport.

## Tissue processing and storage

### *Formalin-fixed and paraffin-embedded tissue*

When tissue arrives at the pathology department, the subsequent processing workflow mainly consists of the fixation of tissues in a neutral-buffered 4% formaldehyde solution (10% formalin) and subsequent embedding in paraffin [21]. For large tissue specimens, grossing and dissection must be performed by the pathologist in order to select the representative tissue parts for subsequent processing and to guarantee adequate pathologic tumour node metastasis classification (pTNM) staging. Worldwide neutral-buffered formalin is still the most often used fixative in pathology laboratories. Formalin is routinely applicable, easily penetrates the tissue (at a diffusion rate of 1 $mm \cdot h^{-1}$) and is relatively cheap despite its known toxicity [22, 23]. Formalin preserves tissue morphology through the inhibition of autolysis *via* endogenous and exogenous enzymes, and the creation of crosslinks between proteins and other cellular molecules, such as glycoproteins, polysaccharides and nucleic acids. After fixation, automated tissue processing is carried out, encompassing dehydration in alcohols, clearance and paraffin impregnation. Standard practice further comprises of preparation of paraffin blocks, sectioning and haematoxylin and eosin (HE) staining to allow first-line microscopic diagnosis by the pathologist. If limited material is available, technicians should be aware not to waste a lot of material by cutting deep into a paraffin block to obtain the maximum size of the biopsy. A further advantage of formalin-fixed, paraffin-embedded (FFPE) tissue is that it can be stored for long periods of time at room temperature and contains a wealth of biological information for retrospective analysis.

#### *Fresh-frozen tissue*

If large amounts of tissue are available (*e.g.* tumour resections), additional tumour and non-neoplastic tissue can be frozen in liquid nitrogen and stored at −80°C, for example. Fresh-frozen (FF)-tissue is very appropriate for subsequent molecular analysis, because biomolecules (and especially RNA) retain their native composition due to the lack of fixatives [24]. However, FF tissue is less suitable for morphological evaluation than FFPE tissue, and storage in −80°C freezers and infrastructure is more expensive.

#### *Cytology specimens*

Fresh cytology specimens are either directly spread onto a glass slide and stained according to May–Grünwald–Giemsa or fixed using an alcohol-based fixative and smeared onto a slide and stained using a Papanicolaou test [25, 26]. Another widespread procedure is liquid-based cytology, which processes fixed cells into a monolayer on a glass slide [27, 28]. May–Grünwald–Giemsa-stained or Papanicolaou-stained slides are evaluated by the cytopathologist for diagnosis of lung cancer. The remaining material is either stored in alcohol-based fixative at −20°C or processed into paraffin agar cyto blocks preceded by short formalin fixation [29].

### Additional molecular analyses

#### *HE staining and IHC*

HE staining and a panel of diverse primary antibodies (currently amongst others directed against TTF1 (thyroid transcription factor 1), CK7, p63/p40, CK5/6 CD56, synaptophysin and chromogranin-A) are the internationally accepted and used diagnostic standard procedures on FFPE tissue for the histological diagnosis and subclassification of SCLC and NSCLC subtypes (ADCs, SCCs, LCNECs) [1, 3, 30]. IHC was the first method that allowed the assessment of expressed individual protein epitopes (antigens) in FFPE tumour tissue based on technical innovations, *e.g.* heat-induced epitope retrieval [31–34]. Nowadays, IHC is automated and standard equipment is used in a diagnostic routine pathology laboratory. Moreover, IHC allows therapy outcome to be predicted, for example, by immunostaining ALK, and more recently, ROS1 in lung ADCs [18, 35, 36]. However, IHC procedures need to be optimised in order for every single antigen to be detected, taking into consideration tissue type, fixation, antigen retrieval, primary antibodies, secondary detection conjugates and amplification systems, enzyme precipitation and visualisation systems, signal-to-noise ratio, technical controls on the same tissue section, and evaluation criteria.

### *Determination of tumour content and extraction of genomic DNA/RNA*

Molecular diagnostic analyses are currently widely implemented in clinical practice to determine gene mutations, chromosome translocations and DNA copy number variations (CNVs) (such as aneuploidy, gene amplifications and deletions) in FFPE and FF tissue, and cytology samples, including PCR-based mutation detection and sequencing methodologies and (F)ISH. Therefore, in addition to tissue sections for HE and IHC, additional material is often used in the context of precision medicine. For example, if sufficient lung ADC material of adequate quality is available, (stepwise) mutational testing for KRAS (25% of cases, which are mutually exclusive with actionable EGFR mutations), EGFR (10%), BRAF (4%) and ERBB2 (V-ERB-B2 avian erythroblastic leukaemia viral oncogene homologue 2, also known as Her2Neu (2%) is currently performed (along with additional FISH analyses; see below) (fig. 1). For this purpose, the pathologist first marks the most suitable tumour area in the slide (highest density of tumour cells) for DNA extraction. This can be the whole section or part of a section that represents the highest amount of tumour cells (⩾500–1000 tumour cells) in relation to other non-tumour cells (*e.g.* inflammatory cells). This tumour area can be adequately removed using manual macro- or microdissection (with and without the use of a microscope, respectively) [37, 38]. A minimum of 20–30% of tumour cells should be present in the material tested for genetic alterations to avoid false-negative results.

Different FFPE DNA (and RNA) extraction methods have been developed and assessed to ensure optimal nucleic acid quality for downstream analysis [20, 39–42]. DNA extractions that apply a prolonged proteinase K digestion step to reverse protein nucleic acid crosslinking, followed by a preferably automated commercial DNA purification (magnetic bead extractions) generally yield the best results [20, 43, 44]. Usually, one to five FFPE tissue sections (5–10 μm thickness) per tissue block or a volume of the cytology sample (dependent on the number and percentage of tumour cells present in the sample) is used for DNA/RNA extraction. Quantification of DNA and RNA can be performed using spectrophotometry, fluorometry or PCR [37]. Assessment of maximum DNA fragment length to predict successful molecular testing is usually measured using PCR [20, 45, 46]. Extracted DNA and RNA should be stored in labelled tubes at −20°C and −80°C, respectively.

### *Molecular analysis of actionable driver gene mutations*

The most appropriate PCR-based tests available for the analysis of actionable mutation status in DNA from FFPE and cytology material in current routine diagnostics include dideoxy (Sanger) sequencing, pyrosequencing and massive parallel sequencing (MPS)/NGS [47–51]. The former two are singleplex assays, which assess short amplified DNA fragments for the presence of mutations [52, 53]. Dideoxy sequencing is still the gold standard for mutational analysis [47], detecting substitutions, small insertions and deletions located within the examined region determined by the sequence primers. However, turnaround time (TAT) of the analysis is rather long and has only a modest detection limit (30%). Pyrosequencing is a real-time sequencing technology relying on the detection of pyrophosphate release during nucleotide incorporation. Nucleotides are added one at a time according to a predefined dispensation order depending on the sequence and the putative mutations to be analysed [54]. The detection limit (10%) and TAT are considerably lower than dideoxy sequencing and the method is extremely suitable to the detection of all possible substitutions in mutation hotspots. Pyrosequencing is, however, limited to short, predefined regions.

Because the number of actionable genes and targets for precision medicine is growing rapidly, new multiplex sequencing strategies and machines are needed that allow simultaneous mutation analysis of different targets of interest, preferably on small amounts of DNA.

Sequenom massARRAY (Sequenom, San Diego, CA, USA), SNaPShot (Life Technologies Ltd, Paisley, UK) and MPS/NGS are capable of doing so [51, 55–59]; the latter is currently being implemented on a large scale in molecular pathology laboratories. MPS/NGS has the ability to sequence millions of DNA fragments in parallel, based on clonal replication of single DNA molecules spatially separated on a solid support matrix and the use of cyclic sequencing chemistries [60]. Ion Torrent PGM (Life Technologies Ltd, Paisley, UK) and MiSeq (Illumina, San Diego, CA, USA) are the dominant MPS platforms currently in clinical practice. Both technologies use composed cancer gene panels for sequencing in molecular pathology [61–63]. The underlying biochemistry of sequence techniques differs between these platforms. Ion Torrent PGM uses a biochemistry that is similar to pyrosequencing. It detects the release of hydrogen ions during nucleotide incubation instead of pyrophosphate. The technique used by Illumina relies on a reversible terminator-based method that detects single fluorescent labelled nucleotides as they are incorporated in a DNA strand. NGS platforms require only limited amounts of input DNA (10–100 ng genomic (FFPE) DNA) of sufficient quality (⩾200 bp in length) and produce massive amounts of robust and sensitive (detection limit ~5% mutant allele) sequence data in a timeframe that is similar to that of dideoxy sequencing (4–5 working days TAT). Mutational detection is not limited to predefined positions and the platforms support sequencing of both commercially available gene panels (including third-party companies) and custom-made panels [51]. Because low frequencies of gene mutations (⩽1%) might be of importance for the prediction of tumour resistance (*e.g.* the presence of low frequencies of the EGFR T790M mutation in lung ADCs) or to monitor the patient's response to therapy (detection of gene mutations in liquid biopsies (blood)), new PCR technologies have been developed, such as digital droplet PCR [64, 65]. As for IHC, PCR and sequencing procedures (together with post-run bioinformatics) need to be optimised for the genes to be analysed and for all the variables (experiment conditions, primers, signal-to-noise ratio), and they need to be run with technical positive and negative controls.

### *Molecular analysis of translocations and CNVs by (F)ISH*

In addition to mutation analyses, FFPE and cytology preparations containing lung ADCs are also used to test for the presence of ALK, ROS1 and RET gene arrangements, and MET gene amplification to select patients for targeted therapy. For this reason, FISH is the gold standard because of its high detection sensitivity, its resolution and because it allows the possibility for combining multiple fluorochromes for the detection of multiple nucleic acid targets simultaneously in a single tissue preparation. Nevertheless, brightfield (chromogenic) ISH approaches to detect one to two targets gain more and more attention because they can be easily automated and result in permanent preparations that can be scored by brightfield microscopy and stored at room temperature (similar to IHC procedures) [8, 33, 66, 67].

FISH uses predominantly fluorescent DNA probes for sensitive and specific identification of chromosome abnormalities, including gene amplifications (such as for MET, RET and ERBB2 (Her2Neu)) in primary as well as progressing (after TKI treatment) lung ADCs and gene rearrangements. An example of the latter is FISH analysis using a dual-colour break-apart probe, which is the preferred technology in many labs for the detection of ALK gene rearrangements in NSCLC, without knowing the involved fusion partner [68, 69]. However, interpretation of FISH results is challenging and is dependent on adequately trained and experienced personnel. FISH procedures need to be optimised for every probe target to be detected, taking into consideration tissue type, fixation, target size, detection and visualisation systems, signal-to-noise ratio, technical controls and evaluation criteria. Usually, ⩾20–50 tumour cells need to be present in the cell or tissue preparations for a valid test result.

Alternatively, ALK rearrangements may be detected with IHC using the primary antibodies 5A4 or D5F3, positivity of which is highly correlated with that of ALK FISH [68–70]. A third method is reverse transcriptase-PCR, which uses mRNA to detect the presence of predetermined ALK gene fusions at a highly sensitive level of 90–100% [71, 72]. The method identifies specific ALK fusion partners (*e.g.* EML4 (echinoderm microtubule-associated protein like 4), KIF5B (kinesin family member 5B)) but is incapable of picking up unknown fusion partners. Poor-quality RNA, derived from FFPE, impedes the accurate detection of gene fusions. These problems may be overcome by using a different approach that examines the imbalance between expression levels of the 5′ and 3′ portions of ALK transcripts to detect putative gene fusions [73].

Protocols for gene rearrangement (*e.g.* ALK, ROS1, RET and neurotrophic tyrosine kinase receptor type 1 (NTRK1)) as well as CNV detection (*e.g.* MET, RET, ERBB2 (Her2Neu), PIK3CA (phosphatidylinositol-4,5-bisphophate 3-kinase, catalytic subunit $\alpha$), FGFR1–3 amplification, PTEN (phosphatase and tensin homologue) deletion and aneuploidy) in NSCLC with MPS/NGS are currently being developed and tested.

### Reporting

The final molecular test results are summarised as part of a pathology report, which needs to be understandable for the clinician [37]. An optimal report includes fixative, tumour cell content determined by an experienced pathologist, the type of micro-/macrodissection (if performed), the amount of necrosis and/or inflammation present, the limitations and uncertainties of the test (sensitivity, validation), the DNA amount and quality, the gene mutations according to the Human Genome Variation Society (HGVS) nomenclature (http://www.hgvs.org/), the single-nucleotide polymorphisms and the genetic variants of uncertain clinical significance; for (F)ISH tests, the report should also include the number of cells analysed and the number and percentage of positive events. Furthermore, inconclusive test results (caused by technical and pre-analytical issues, for example) should be reported with a possible explanation and, if possible (based on evidence of the literature), the likelihood that a cancer will respond to therapy as a result of the identified mutations. Laboratory results are filed in an up-to-date laboratory information system, in which the final pathology report will be generated and, if coupled to a hospital information system, will be available for the clinicians. If tests are carried out for another laboratory, ISO15189 accreditation requires that this be documented in a service level agreement [74]. Pathology reports are usually communicated by fax (or email) or *via* an online message system.

## Factors affecting adequate tissue diagnosis

Despite current practice of cancer tissue diagnosis, several variables during pre-analytical tissue preparation affect reliability, accuracy and success rate of downstream analysis, including sample acquisition, transportation, fixation and processing [75].

### Tissue sampling

#### *Adequate tissue for diagnosis*

Obtaining adequate tissue bearing sufficient tumour cells for subsequent molecular testing is performed using minimally invasive techniques, as described above for lung cancer.

Fragile health and difficulty of accessing the tumour location may hamper successful sample acquisition. Therefore, 40–65% of lung cancers are diagnosed by cytology without concurrent biopsy material. Cytology samples as well as biopsy samples may contain only a small number of tumour cells, and may therefore compromise tissue diagnosis and/or additional molecular analysis.

### *Ischaemia time*

The ischaemia time accounts for the timeframe between the moments that the blood circulation in tissue is stopped until tissue fixation. The ischaemia time may have a massive impact on specimen quality, and comprise the time in which tissues remain in the body at 37°C during the surgical procedures until fixation (warm ischaemia), and the time in which tissues are chilled after surgery until fixation (cold ischaemia). The ischaemia time could vary from minutes to hours and several studies have already demonstrated considerable changes in both mRNA and protein expression profiles due to differences in ischaemia time [76–80]. Ischaemia time particularly affects large surgical specimens and should be minimised using standard procedures to reduce the level of molecular degradation. In most hospitals, general guidance concerning this topic exists but exact timeframes are not yet monitored on a regular basis in the operation rooms. More attention needs to be given to the quality of surgical specimens in relation to ischaemia timeframes; this should be well documented and available in patient and specimen records [20, 78].

## Tissue transportation

Tissue transportation from the operation room to the pathology department is another factor that might have a considerable impact on overall tissue quality. Resection material should be placed in excess fixative as quickly as possible for transportation and should be incised only by a pathologist to allow optimal penetration of fixative and to guarantee appropriate reporting of the pTNM stage and R (residual tumour) classification. As formalin is toxic and potentially carcinogenic [81, 82], operation rooms are not the ideal places to work with this fixative. Many hospitals therefore transfer their surgical specimens unfixed to the pathology department, which is a good option if the pathology laboratory and the operation room are in close proximity. Pathology laboratories have dedicated areas with proper precautions for the controlled use of formalin [20]. However, tissue transportation should not be delayed. At sites where the pathology lab is situated at a distant location, fresh transport is not recommended. Immediate preservation and storage of tissue at 4°C under vacuum conditions is a good and safe option in such circumstances [23, 83]. Small diagnostic biopsies are often directly immersed in excess neutral buffered formalin, allowing rapid fixation and minimising negative effects of both ischaemic and transportation time.

## Tissue processing

### *Formalin fixation time and paraffin impregnation*

Optimal fixation should be established to ensure both good morphology and adequate conservation of protein antigenic determinants and nucleic acids (DNA, RNA), because formalin's extensive crosslinking capacities in combination with chemical modification of molecules (*e.g.* formation of methylol adducts, Schiff bases and methylene bridges [84]) may result in massive fragmentation and degradation of nucleic acids, which influences subsequent molecular analysis [85]. In general, fragment lengths of ≥200 bp of genomic

DNA are required for successful FISH, PCR and MPS/NGS analysis of FFPE material. Optimal fixation time is tissue size-dependent as neutral buffered formalin penetrates tissue with $\sim$1 mm·h$^{-1}$. In general, fixation times of 6–48 h are recommended and should be monitored to prevent under- or overfixation before proceeding to downstream dehydration and paraffinisation [86–89]. Several studies have investigated the ability of alternative fixatives to improve the conservation of biomolecules without losing the morphological properties of formalin [84, 90–95]. However, it should be noted that a change of fixative requires re-optimisation of all IHC- and (F)ISH-staining protocols in use for FFPE [19, 20].

Although subsequent tissue processing is an automated process, certain variables including time, temperature and use of vacuum or microwave heating, influence optimal paraffin impregnation and biomolecule preservation [76]. Tissue type and thickness also affect the speed of penetration during processing. Conventional vacuum infiltration processing of 6–15 h usually favours biomolecule conservation and proper paraffin infiltration [76, 96]. Modern microwave-based tissue processors speed up the infiltration process remarkably with comparable results after 1–2-h processing time [97–102]. Adequate tissue thickness (<2 mm) is an important prerequisite for proper processing using microwave-based tissue processors. Microwave-based tissue processing does not impact downstream molecular analysis [103–105].

Incomplete fixation, however, is detrimental for good tissue processing [106, 107]. A major cause for continued degradation of nucleic acids and proteins, even during long-term storage, may be the presence of remaining endogenous water, which gets trapped in tissue structures during paraffin impregnation and causes hydrolysis of molecules [96]. The same study also demonstrated that storage of FFPE slides in humid conditions negatively affected biomolecule conservation. Degradation was accelerated at higher temperatures.

Nucleic acids are generally better preserved in cytology specimens due to the use of alcohol-based fixatives; cytology smears, cytospins and liquid-based cytology have been demonstrated to be reliable sources for downstream molecular analysis [8, 27, 28, 108–111]. Optimal examination of cytology specimens demands optimal sample management by splitting the sample for all necessary tests. The construction of additional formalin-fixed cyto agar blocks, made from residual cells, enhances the diagnostic power of cytology specimens [17, 29, 112]. Slides from cell blocks may be helpful for morphological examination and IHC due to additional formalin fixation. This extra fixation step, however, might negatively affect downstream molecular analyses when using cyto agar blocks as a tissue source [111]. The biggest limitation for using cytology specimens is often the restricted availability of tumour cells in a representative tumour load. Tumour cell enrichment in cytology specimens is rather challenging. Therefore, experienced personnel should be available to ensure optimal tumour sampling. Identification of tumour cells in cytology FISH slides may also be problematic. Slides may be pre-stained and pre-screened to confirm the presence and location of atypical cells for FISH analysis [113]. The percentage and/or number of tumour cells in a cytology preparation (*e.g.* >10% for pyrosequening or NGS, and >50 tumour cells for ALK FISH) and/or the amount of DNA/RNA that can be isolated from the cells (*e.g.* 10 ng DNA for singleplex PCR analysis or 50 ng for NGS) determine whether a molecular test may be carried out.

#### *Tissue cutting in relation to required molecular analysis*

In order to use the available tissue in the optimal way, the first sections of a new tissue block should be directly used for preliminary diagnosis, or the technician should be trained to directly cut multiple (10–20) unstained sections and store them properly (<3 months) [114]. They can be used for HE staining, IHC and primary diagnosis (2–3 μm-thick sections) and, if required, for additional molecular testing (5–10 μm-thick sections) [30]. It is recommended that the algorithms for IHC and molecular testing should be defined in order to shorten TAT and preserve tissue. This can be done for stage IIIB/IV lung ADCs, for example, where sequential testing of IHC, KRAS, EGFR, BRAF, ERBB2 (Her2Neu), ALK, ROS1, RET and MET is indicated, while most of these mutations are mutually exclusive. However, this is time-consuming, and co-mutations have been observed indicating intrinsic or acquired therapy resistance.

### Assessment of tumour content

It is important that an experienced pathologist marks the tumour area with the highest percentage of tumour cells for DNA isolation, which can be manually microdissected if necessary. However, because determination of percentage tumour cells may vary considerably between different pathologists, training is recommended for this purpose [115].

## Molecular analyses

It is critically important to continuously monitor the performance of molecular diagnostic analyses. Every test is accompanied by its own defined positive and negative controls, which determine whether the test is executed successfully. Furthermore, if possible, an internal reference control should be used that directly monitors correct test performance. Variability of the test within and between different tests should also be defined. Intra-test variability can be monitored by using duplo analyses. When test results of duplo analyses are outside the range of acceptance, as defined in the standard operating procedure, the test should be repeated. This is of great importance to the identification of sequence artefacts that may be introduced during PCR amplification or due to C>U deamination, which often occurs in DNA extracted from FFPE tissue [116]. In NGS, the execution of duplo analysis is not common practice due to high analysis costs. However, sequence artefacts due to deamination may still be identified by the presence of high abundant low level C>T and G>A mutations, which should be filtered out afterwards using proper bioinformatics [44]. Inter-test variability should be evaluated through regular analysis of well-characterised samples, which should not exceed the defined acceptable variation of the test.

Participation in external quality control schemes is a premise for every diagnostic lab to monitor the sensitivity and specificity of the tests it offers. For EGFR, ALK and ROS1 testing, external quality schemes are regularly offered (*i.e.* the UK National External Quality Assessment Service (www.ukneqas-molgen.org.uk) and the European Society of Pathology (www.esp-pathology.org)) [37]. When an external quality scheme is not available for a certain test, samples may be exchanged with a partner lab on a regular basis in order to confirm the test's sensitivity and specificity.

Test results should be evaluated retrospectively over a certain period of time by comparing them to the test performance of earlier periods and the common national test performance. When results are outside the confidence limit, test performance should be questioned [37].

## Recommendations for adequate lung cancer tissue diagnosis and conclusions

The rapid advances in (targeted) treatment options for lung cancer patients, the often limited tissue material that can be sampled from patients with advanced disease and the fact that a rapid diagnosis may favourably influence the start of treatment and patient prognosis mean it is extremely important that an optimal workflow of patient care is developed in the clinic. The challenge for pathology laboratories is that they fit into this workflow with optimal tissue handling as well as reliable methods and processes that result in timely and accurate tissue diagnosis. In this chapter, we have reviewed the current practice of tissue sampling and diagnosis as well as factors that may influence this process. Based on these results, we have made recommendations to further optimise the workflow between the clinic and the (molecular) pathology laboratory (table 1). In this respect, it is important that all

Table 1. Recommendations for the establishment of an optimal workflow between the clinic and the (molecular) pathology laboratory for adequate histological and molecular diagnosis of lung cancer tissue

**General**

In patients suspected of having lung cancer, as well as patients with recurrent or progressing tumours, a histopathological and/or cytopathological diagnosis should be obtained.

Each patient should be discussed in a multidisciplinary team of specialists for optimal diagnostic and therapeutic management.

An optimal, lean workflow should be created to optimise time of diagnosis.

Standard operating procedures should be established for all aspects of the workflow, including procedures and analyses performed for tissue sampling, transport, processing and histological/cytological and molecular diagnosis. Standard operating procedures should also be prepared for secretarial handling of request forms from clinicians (including those from other hospitals) regarding both freshly sampled and already fixed tissue material, as well as for handling pathological reports to be sent out to them.

The pathology laboratory performing the tissue diagnosis should be accredited (ISO15189 or national equivalent) and participate in internal quality control schemes (internal audits) as well as (inter)national external quality assessment schemes to ensure reliable service.

**Tissue sampling**

Enough tissue should be sampled to enable diagnosis and molecular analysis of lung cancer, preferably using the least invasive procedure for biopsying and separate containers for each biopsy for transportation.

For endobronchial/transbronchial sampling, multiple (at least five) biopsies should be taken to ensure enough tumour material for histopathological diagnosis, IHC and molecular analysis.

For EBUS/EUS needle aspirations, multiple (at least four) samples should be taken per target lesion.

For percutaneous core needle biopsies (18 gauge needle), at least two samples should be taken per target lesion.

Ischaemia time between sampling and fixation should be minimised, and ischaemia timeframes should be registered in specimen and pathology records.

Although it is not preferable, cytology (lung brushes or washes, for example) samples can be used in supporting diagnosis, as well as for IHC and molecular analysis, if enough tumour cells are present (≥20–30% tumour cells are preferred).

The workflow should be secured in a standard operating procedure, including the transportation time of tissues and biopsies to the pathology department.

Optionally, blood should be sampled (liquid biopsy), if possible, at diagnosis and fixed time points during and after patient treatment, to allow the effect of therapeutic treatments to be monitored as well as the possible development of drug resistance [65].

Continued

Table 1. Continued

**Tissue processing**

Optimal formalin fixation (between 6–48 h) should be performed.

Optimal paraffin impregnation by vacuum infiltration (6–15 h) or microwave-based (1–2 h) processing should be performed.

Where there is limited tissue, multiple tissue sections should be directly cut to avoid tissue waste.

The most appropriate tumour area should be selected in a tissue section for DNA/RNA extraction and molecular analyses by consulting an experienced pathologist. For tests performed for other hospitals, their pathologists may provide digital images of tissue sections with annotated tumour areas to be used for extraction of nucleic acids.

**Molecular analyses**

Algorithms for IHC and molecular analyses should be defined and agreed upon by the multidisciplinary team, to shorten turnaround time and prevent tissue waste.

For resection material (multiple formalin-fixed, paraffin-embedded blocks) or both biopsy and cytology material of a patient, the most appropriate block/specimen should be selected for molecular analysis.

IHC, FISH and PCR-based sequencing methods should be applicable to cytology material (cell blocks, cell smears, cytospins, liquid-based cytology), but IHC and (F)ISH require other pre-treatment protocols on paraffin cell blocks and alcohol-based cytology samples.

When choosing a new molecular test and/or platform, factors to consider include: sensitivity (false negatives), specificity (false positives), reproducibility, limit of detection, turnaround time, ease of interpretation and cost (including instrument, reagent and tech time) [53].

The performance and variability of molecular analyses should be continuously monitored.

**Reporting**

Critical pre-analytical factors as well as molecular test results should be integrated into the pathology reports and discussed with a multidisciplinary team of specialists.

Molecular results should be reported according to established (inter)national guidelines and consensus systems, and should also be translated for common usage.

---

processes and analyses are described in standard operating procedures, the laboratory is ISO15189 (or national equivalent) accredited and participates in internal and external quality control schemes, and that a multidisciplinary team of specialists (tumour board) is responsible for diagnostic and therapeutic management.

## References


1. Travis WD, Brambilla E, Müller-Mermelink HK, *et al.*, eds. World Health Organization Classification of Tumours: Pathology and Genetics of Tumours of the Lung, Pleura, Thyumus and Heart. Lyon, IARC Press, 2004.
2. Travis WD. Pathology of lung cancer. *Clin Chest Med* 2011; 32: 669–692.
3. Travis WD, Brambilla E, Noguchi M, *et al.* International Association for the Study of Lung Cancer/American Thoracic Society/European Respiratory Society international multidisciplinary classification of lung adenocarcinoma. *J Thorac Oncol* 2011; 6: 244–285.
4. Shames DS, Wistuba II. The evolving genomic classification of lung cancer. *J Pathol* 2014; 232: 121–133.
5. Clinical Lung Cancer Genome Project (CLCGP), Network Genomic Medicine (NGM). A genomics-based classification of human lung tumors. *Sci Transl Med* 2013; 5: 209ra153.
6. Gerber DE, Gandhi L, Costa DB. Management and future directions in non-small cell lung cancer with known activating mutations. *Am Soc Clin Oncol Educ Book* 2014; e353–e365.
7. Kerr KM, Bubendorf L, Edelman MJ, *et al.* Second ESMO consensus conference on lung cancer: pathology and molecular biomarkers for non-small-cell lung cancer. *Ann Oncol* 2014; 25: 1681–1690.
8. Lindeman NI, Cagle PT, Beasley MB, *et al.* Molecular testing guideline for selection of lung cancer patients for EGFR and ALK tyrosine kinase inhibitors: guideline from the College of American Pathologists, International Association for the Study of Lung Cancer, and Association for Molecular Patho. *J Thorac Oncol* 2013; 8: 823–859.

9. Yu HA, Riely GJ, Lovly CM. Therapeutic strategies utilized in the setting of acquired resistance to EGFR tyrosine kinase inhibitors. *Clin Cancer Res* 2014; 20: 5898–5907.
10. Esfahani K, Agulnik JS, Cohen V. A systemic review of resistance mechanisms and ongoing clinical trials in ALK-rearranged non-small cell lung cancer. *Front Oncol* 2014; 4: 174.
11. Garraway LA, Jänne PA. Circumventing cancer drug resistance in the era of personalized medicine. *Cancer Discov* 2012; 2: 214–226.
12. Annema JT, van Meerbeeck JP, Rintoul RC, *et al.* Mediastinoscopy *vs* endosonography for mediastinal nodal staging of lung cancer: a randomized trial. *JAMA* 2010; 304: 2245–2252.
13. De Leyn P, Dooms C, Kuzdzal J, *et al.* Revised ESTS guidelines for preoperative mediastinal lymph node staging for non-small-cell lung cancer. *Eur J Cardiothorac Surg* 2014; 45: 787–798.
14. Hetzel J, Eberhardt R, Herth FJF, *et al.* Cryobiopsy increases the diagnostic yield of endobronchial biopsy: a multicentre trial. *Eur Respir J* 2012; 39: 685–690.
15. Dooms C, Muylle I, Yserbyt J, *et al.* Endobronchial ultrasound in the management of nonsmall cell lung cancer. *Eur Respir Rev* 2013; 22: 169–177.
16. Wu CC, Maher MM, Shepard J-AO. CT-guided percutaneous needle biopsy of the chest: preprocedural evaluation and technique. *AJR Am J Roentgenol* 2011; 196: W511–W514.
17. Sulpher JA, Owen SP, Hon H, *et al.* Factors influencing a specific pathologic diagnosis of non-small-cell lung carcinoma. *Clin Lung Cancer* 2013; 14: 238–244.
18. Tsao MS, Hirsch FR, Yatabe Y, eds. IASLC Atlas of ALK Testing in Lung Cancer. First IASL. Aurora, IASLC Press, 2013.
19. Groenen PJTA, Blokx WAM, Diepenbroek C, *et al.* Preparing pathology for personalized medicine: possibilities for improvement of the pre-analytical phase. *Histopathology* 2011; 59: 1–7.
20. Bonin S, Stanta G. Nucleic acid extraction methods from fixed and paraffin-embedded tissues in cancer diagnostics. *Expert Rev Mol Diagn* 2013; 13: 271–282.
21. Fox CH, Johnson FB, Whiting J, *et al.* Formaldehyde fixation. *J Histochem Cytochem* 1985; 33: 845–853.
22. Frankel A. Formalin fixation in the "-omics" era: a primer for the surgeon-scientist. *ANZ J Surg* 2012; 82: 395–402.
23. Comanescu M, Annaratone L, D'Armento G, *et al.* Critical steps in tissue processing in histopathology. *Recent Pat DNA Gene Seq* 2012; 6: 22–32.
24. Micke P, Ohshima M, Tahmasebpoor S, *et al.* Biobanking of fresh frozen tissue: RNA is stable in nonfixed surgical specimens. *Lab Invest* 2006; 86: 202–211.
25. Lopes Cardozo P. Atlas of clinical cytology a contribution to precise cytodiagnosis and cytological differential diagnosis with. 1976.
26. Yang GC, Alvarez II. Ultrafast Papanicolaou stain. An alternative preparation for fine needle aspiration cytology. *Acta Cytol* 1995; 39: 55–60.
27. Bellevicine C, Malapelle U, Vigliar E, *et al.* Epidermal growth factor receptor test performed on liquid-based cytology lung samples: experience of an academic referral center. *Acta Cytol* 2014; 58: 589–594.
28. Minca EC, Lanigan CP, Reynolds JP, *et al.* ALK status testing in non-small-cell lung carcinoma by FISH on ThinPrep slides with cytology material. *J Thorac Oncol* 2014; 9: 464–468.
29. Collins GR, Thomas J, Joshi N, *et al.* The diagnostic value of cell block as an adjunct to liquid-based cytology of bronchial washing specimens in the diagnosis and subclassification of pulmonary neoplasms. *Cancer Cytopathol* 2012; 120: 134–141.
30. Conde E, Angulo B, Izquierdo E, *et al.* Lung adenocarcinoma in the era of targeted therapies: histological classification, sample prioritization, and predictive biomarkers. *Clin Transl Oncol* 2013; 15: 503–508.
31. Shi S-R, Shi Y, Taylor CR. Antigen retrieval immunohistochemistry: review and future prospects in research and diagnosis over two decades. *J Histochem Cytochem* 2011; 59: 13–32.
32. Taylor CR, Rudbeck L, eds. Educational Guide: Immunhistochemical Staining Methods. 6th Edn. Glostrup, Dako Denmark, 2013.
33. Speel EJ. Robert Feulgen Prize Lecture 1999. Detection and amplification systems for sensitive, multiple-target DNA and RNA *in situ* hybridization: looking inside cells with a spectrum of colors. *Histochem Cell Biol* 1999; 112: 89–113.
34. Van der Loos CM. Multiple immunoenzyme staining: methods and visualizations for the observation with spectral imaging. *J Histochem Cytochem* 2008; 56: 313–328.
35. Cha YJ, Lee JS, Kim HR, *et al.* Screening of ROS1 rearrangements in lung adenocarcinoma by immunohistochemistry and comparison with ALK rearrangements. *PLoS One* 2014; 9: e103333.
36. Shan L, Lian F, Guo L, *et al.* Detection of ROS1 gene rearrangement in lung adenocarcinoma: comparison of IHC, FISH and real-time RT-PCR. *PLoS One* 2015; 10: e0120422.
37. Cree IA, Deans Z, Ligtenberg MJL, *et al.* Guidance for laboratories performing molecular pathology for cancer patients. *J Clin Pathol* 2014; 67: 923–931.
38. Dietel M, Jöhrens K, Laffert M, *et al.* Predictive molecular pathology and its role in targeted cancer therapy: a review focussing on clinical relevance. *Cancer Gene Ther* 2013; 20: 211–221.

39. Bonin S, Hlubek F, Benhattar J, *et al.* Multicentre validation study of nucleic acids extraction from FFPE tissues. *Virchows Arch* 2010; 457: 309–317.
40. Huijsmans CJ, Damen J, van der Linden JC, *et al.* Comparative analysis of four methods to extract DNA from paraffin-embedded tissues: effect on downstream molecular applications. *BMC Res Notes* 2010; 3: 239.
41. Snow AN, Stence AA, Pruessner JA, *et al.* A simple and cost-effective method of DNA extraction from small formalin-fixed paraffin-embedded tissue for molecular oncologic testing. *BMC Clin Pathol* 2014; 14: 30.
42. Sengüven B, Baris E, Oygur T, *et al.* Comparison of methods for the extraction of DNA from formalin-fixed, paraffin-embedded archival tissues. *Int J Med Sci* 2014; 11: 494–499.
43. Funabashi KS, Barcelos D, Visoná I, *et al.* DNA extraction and molecular analysis of non-tumoral liver, spleen, and brain from autopsy samples: the effect of formalin fixation and paraffin embedding. *Pathol Res Pract* 2012; 208: 584–591.
44. Heydt C, Fassunke J, Künstlinger H, *et al.* Comparison of pre-analytical FFPE sample preparation methods and their impact on massively parallel sequencing in routine diagnostics. *PLoS One* 2014; 9: e104566.
45. Van Dongen JJM, Langerak AW, Brüggemann M, *et al.* Design and standardization of PCR primers and protocols for detection of clonal immunoglobulin and T-cell receptor gene recombinations in suspect lymphoproliferations: report of the BIOMED-2 Concerted Action BMH4-CT98-3936. *Leukemia* 2003; 17: 2257–2317.
46. Sah S, Chen L, Houghton J, *et al.* Functional DNA quantification guides accurate next-generation sequencing mutation detection in formalin-fixed, paraffin-embedded tumor biopsies. *Genome Med* 2013; 5: 77.
47. Patton S, Normanno N, Blackhall F, *et al.* Assessing standardization of molecular testing for non-small-cell lung cancer: results of a worldwide external quality assessment (EQA) scheme for EGFR mutation testing. *Br J Cancer* 2014; 111: 413–420.
48. Deans ZC, Bilbe N, O'Sullivan B, *et al.* Improvement in the quality of molecular analysis of EGFR in non-small-cell lung cancer detected by three rounds of external quality assessment. *J Clin Pathol* 2013; 66: 319–325.
49. Dijkstra JR, Heideman DAM, Meijer GA, *et al.* KRAS mutation analysis on low percentage of colon cancer cells: the importance of quality assurance. *Virchows Arch* 2013; 462: 39–46
50. Dijkstra JR, Opdam FJM, Boonyaratanakornkit J, *et al.* Implementation of formalin-fixed, paraffin-embedded cell line pellets as high-quality process controls in quality assessment programs for KRAS mutation analysis. *J Mol Diagn* 2012; 14: 187–191.
51. Dubbink HJ, Deans ZC, Tops BBJ, *et al.* Next generation diagnostic molecular pathology: critical appraisal of quality assurance in Europe. *Mol Oncol* 2014; 8: 830–839.
52. Jancik S, Drabek J, Berkovcova J, *et al.* A comparison of direct sequencing, pyrosequencing, high resolution melting analysis, TheraScreen DxS, and the K-ras StripAssay for detecting KRAS mutations in non small cell lung carcinomas. *J Exp Clin Cancer Res* 2012; 31: 79.
53. Tsiatis AC, Norris-Kirby A, Rich RG, *et al.* Comparison of Sanger sequencing, pyrosequencing, and melting curve analysis for the detection of KRAS mutations: diagnostic and clinical implications. *J Mol Diagn* 2010; 12: 425–432.
54. Ronaghi M, Uhlén M, Nyrén P. A sequencing method based on real-time pyrophosphate. *Science* 1998; 281: 363–365.
55. MacConaill LE, Campbell CD, Kehoe SM, *et al.* Profiling critical cancer gene mutations in clinical tumor samples. *PLoS One* 2009; 4: e7887.
56. Fumagalli D, Gavin PG, Taniyama Y, *et al.* A rapid, sensitive, reproducible and cost-effective method for mutation profiling of colon cancer and metastatic lymph nodes. *BMC Cancer* 2010; 10: 101.
57. Dias-Santagata D, Akhavanfard S, David SS, *et al.* Rapid targeted mutational analysis of human tumours: a clinical platform to guide personalized cancer medicine. *EMBO Mol Med* 2010; 2: 146–158.
58. Su Z, Dias-Santagata D, Duke M, *et al.* A platform for rapid detection of multiple oncogenic mutations with relevance to targeted therapy in non-small-cell lung cancer. *J Mol Diagn* 2011; 13: 74–84.
59. McCourt CM, McArt DG, Mills K, *et al.* Validation of next generation sequencing technologies in comparison to current diagnostic gold standards for BRAF, EGFR and KRAS mutational analysis. *PLoS One* 2013; 8: e69604.
60. Meldrum C, Doyle MA, Tothill RW. Next-generation sequencing for cancer diagnostics: a practical perspective. *Clin Biochem Rev* 2011; 32: 177–195.
61. Singh RR, Patel KP, Routbort MJ, *et al.* Clinical validation of a next-generation sequencing screen for mutational hotspots in 46 cancer-related genes. *J Mol Diagn* 2013; 15: 607–622.
62. Sie D, Snijders PJF, Meijer GA, *et al.* Performance of amplicon-based next generation DNA sequencing for diagnostic gene mutation profiling in oncopathology. *Cell Oncol (Dordr)* 2014; 37: 353–361.
63. Nikiforov YE, Carty SE, Chiosea SI, *et al.* Highly accurate diagnosis of cancer in thyroid nodules with follicular neoplasm/suspicious for a follicular neoplasm cytology by ThyroSeq v2 next-generation sequencing assay. *Cancer* 2014; 120: 3627–3634.
64. Day E, Dear PH, McCaughan F. Digital PCR strategies in the development and analysis of molecular biomarkers for personalized medicine. *Methods* 2013; 59: 101–107.
65. Oxnard GR, Paweletz CP, Kuang Y, *et al.* Noninvasive detection of response and resistance in EGFR-mutant lung cancer using quantitative next-generation genotyping of cell-free plasma DNA. *Clin Cancer Res* 2014; 20: 1698–1705.

66. Jurmeister P, Lenze D, Berg E, *et al.* Parallel screening for ALK, MET and ROS1 alterations in non-small cell lung cancer with implications for daily routine testing. *Lung Cancer* 2015; 87: 122–129.
67. Gainor JF, Shaw AT. Novel targets in non-small cell lung cancer: ROS1 and RET fusions. *Oncologist* 2013; 18: 865–875.
68. Thunnissen E, Bubendorf L, Dietel M, *et al.* EML4-ALK testing in non-small cell carcinomas of the lung: a review with recommendations. *Virchows Arch* 2012; 461: 245–257.
69. Weickhardt AJ, Aisner DL, Franklin WA, *et al.* Diagnostic assays for identification of anaplastic lymphoma kinase-positive non-small cell lung cancer. *Cancer* 2013; 119: 1467–1477.
70. Blackhall FH, Peters S, Bubendorf L, *et al.* Prevalence and clinical outcomes for patients with ALK-positive resected stage I to III adenocarcinoma: results from the European Thoracic Oncology Platform Lungscape Project. *J Clin Oncol* 2014; 32: 2780–2787.
71. Fu S, Wang F, Shao Q, *et al.* Detection of EML4-ALK fusion gene in Chinese non-small cell lung cancer by using a sensitive quantitative real-time reverse transcriptase PCR technique. *Diagn Mol Pathol* 2015; 23: 245–254.
72. Li T, Maus MKH, Desai SJ, *et al.* Large-scale screening and molecular characterization of EML4-ALK fusion variants in archival non-small-cell lung cancer tumor specimens using quantitative reverse transcription polymerase chain reaction assays. *J Thorac Oncol* 2014; 9: 18–25.
73. Wang R, Pan Y, Li C, *et al.* The use of quantitative real-time reverse transcriptase PCR for 5′ and 3′ portions of ALK transcripts to detect ALK rearrangements in lung cancers. *Clin Cancer Res* 2012; 18: 4725–4732.
74. International Organization for Standardization. ISO 15189:2012. Medical Laboratories – requirements for quality and competance. www.iso.org/iso/home/catalogue_ics/catalogue_detail_ics.htm?csnumber=56115. Date last accessed: May 11, 2015.
75. Thomas A, Rajan A, Lopez-Chavez A, *et al.* From targets to targeted therapies and molecular profiling in non-small cell lung carcinoma. *Ann Oncol* 2013; 24: 577–585.
76. Chung J-Y, Braunschweig T, Williams R, *et al.* Factors in tissue handling and processing that impact RNA obtained from formalin-fixed, paraffin-embedded tissue. *J Histochem Cytochem* 2008; 56: 1033–1042.
77. Bai Y, Tolles J, Cheng H, *et al.* Quantitative assessment shows loss of antigenic epitopes as a function of pre-analytic variables. *Lab Invest* 2011; 91: 1253–1261.
78. Hewitt SM, Lewis FA, Cao Y, *et al.* Tissue handling and specimen preparation in surgical pathology: issues concerning the recovery of nucleic acids from formalin-fixed, paraffin-embedded tissue. *Arch Pathol Lab Med* 2008; 132: 1929–1935.
79. Spruessel A, Steimann G, Jung M, *et al.* Tissue ischemia time affects gene and protein expression patterns within minutes following surgical tumor excision. *Biotechniques* 2004; 36: 1030–1037.
80. Medeiros F, Rigl CT, Anderson GG, *et al.* Tissue handling for genome-wide expression analysis: a review of the issues, evidence, and opportunities. *Arch Pathol Lab Med* 2007; 131: 1805–1816.
81. Hauptmann M, Stewart PA, Lubin JH, *et al.* Mortality from lymphohematopoietic malignancies and brain cancer among embalmers exposed to formaldehyde. *J Natl Cancer Inst* 2009; 101: 1696–1708.
82. Cogliano V, Grosse Y, Baan R, *et al.* Advice on formaldehyde and glycol ethers. *Lancet Oncol* 2004; 5: 528.
83. Bussolati G, Annaratone L, Medico E, *et al.* Formalin fixation at low temperature better preserves nucleic acid integrity. *PLoS One* 2011; 6: e21043.
84. Viertler C, Groelz D, Gündisch S, *et al.* A new technology for stabilization of biomolecules in tissues for combined histological and molecular analyses. *J Mol Diagn* 2012; 14: 458–466.
85. Srinivasan M, Sedmak D, Jewell S. Effect of fixatives and tissue processing on the content and integrity of nucleic acids. *Am J Pathol* 2002; 161: 1961–1971.
86. Goldstein NS, Ferkowicz M, Odish E, *et al.* Minimum formalin fixation time for consistent estrogen receptor immunohistochemical staining of invasive breast carcinoma. *Am J Clin Pathol* 2003; 120: 86–92.
87. Wolff AC, Hammond MEH, Schwartz JN, *et al.* American Society of Clinical Oncology/College of American Pathologists guideline recommendations for human epidermal growth factor receptor 2 testing in breast cancer. *J Clin Oncol* 2007; 25: 118–145.
88. Spencer DH, Sehn JK, Abel HJ, *et al.* Comparison of clinical targeted next-generation sequence data from formalin-fixed and fresh-frozen tissue specimens. *J Mol Diagn* 2013; 15: 623–633.
89. Ferrer I, Armstrong J, Capellari S, *et al.* Effects of formalin fixation, paraffin embedding, and time of storage on DNA preservation in brain tissue: a BrainNet Europe study. *Brain Pathol* 2007; 17: 297–303.
90. Zanini C, Gerbaudo E, Ercole E, *et al.* Evaluation of two commercial and three home-made fixatives for the substitution of formalin: a formaldehyde-free laboratory is possible. *Environ Health* 2012; 11: 59.
91. Lassalle S, Hofman V, Marius I, *et al.* Assessment of morphology, antigenicity, and nucleic acid integrity for diagnostic thyroid pathology using formalin substitute fixatives. *Thyroid* 2009; 19: 1239–1248.
92. Kothmaier H, Rohrer D, Stacher E, *et al.* Comparison of formalin-free tissue fixatives: a proteomic study testing their application for routine pathology and research. *Arch Pathol Lab Med* 2011; 135: 744–752.
93. Stanta G, Mucelli SP, Petrera F, *et al.* A novel fixative improves opportunities of nucleic acids and proteomic analysis in human archive's tissues. *Diagn Mol Pathol* 2006; 15: 115–123.

94. Kap M, Smedts F, Oosterhuis W, *et al.* Histological assessment of PAXgene tissue fixation and stabilization reagents. *PLoS One* 2011; 6: e27704.
95. Groelz D, Sobin L, Branton P, *et al.* Non-formalin fixative *versus* formalin-fixed tissue: a comparison of histology and RNA quality. *Exp Mol Pathol* 2013; 94: 188–194.
96. Xie R, Chung J-Y, Ylaya K, *et al.* Factors influencing the degradation of archival formalin-fixed paraffin-embedded tissue sections. *J Histochem Cytochem* 2011; 59: 356–365.
97. Naik R, Pai M, Rai S, *et al.* Microwave histoprocessing *versus* conventional histoprocessing. *Indian J Pathol Microbiol* 2008; 51: 12.
98. Amrutha N, Patil S, Rao RS. Microwaves: a revolution in histoprocessing. *J Contemp Dent Pract* 2014; 15: 149–152.
99. Bronsert P, Weißer J, Biniossek ML, *et al.* Impact of routinely employed procedures for tissue processing on the proteomic analysis of formalin-fixed paraffin-embedded tissue. *Proteomics Clin Appl* 2014; 8: 796–804.
100. Devi RB, Subashree AR, Parameaswari PJ, *et al.* Domestic microwave *versus* conventional tissue processing: a quantitative and qualitative analysis. *J Clin Diagn Res* 2013; 7: 835–839.
101. Emerson LL, Tripp SR, Baird BC, *et al.* A comparison of immunohistochemical stain quality in conventional and rapid microwave processed tissues. *Am J Clin Pathol* 2006; 125: 176–183.
102. Shruthi BS, Vinodhkumar P, Kashyap B, *et al.* Use of microwave in diagnostic pathology. *J Cancer Res Ther* 2013; 9: 351–355.
103. Pegolo E, Pandolfi M, Di Loreto C, *et al.* Implementation of a microwave-assisted tissue-processing system and an automated embedding system for breast needle core biopsy samples: morphology, immunohistochemistry, and FISH evaluation. *Appl Immunohistochem Mol Morphol* 2013; 21: 362–370.
104. Nassiri M, Ramos S, Zohourian H, *et al.* Preservation of biomolecules in breast cancer tissue by a formalin-free histology system. *BMC Clin Pathol* 2008; 8: 1.
105. Bödör C, Schmidt O, Csernus B, *et al.* DNA and RNA isolated from tissues processed by microwave-accelerated apparatus MFX-800-3 are suitable for subsequent PCR and Q-RT-PCR amplification. *Pathol Oncol Res* 2007; 13: 149–152.
106. De Marzo AM, Fedor HH, Gage WR, *et al.* Inadequate formalin fixation decreases reliability of p27 immunohistochemical staining: probing optimal fixation time using high-density tissue microarrays. *Hum Pathol* 2002; 33: 756–760.
107. Arnold MM, Srivastava S, Fredenburgh J, *et al.* Effects of fixation and tissue processing on immunohistochemical demonstration of specific antigens. *Biotech Histochem* 1996; 71: 224–230.
108. Khode R, Larsen DA, Culbreath BC, *et al.* Comparative study of epidermal growth factor receptor mutation analysis on cytology smears and surgical pathology specimens from primary and metastatic lung carcinomas. *Cancer Cytopathol* 2013; 121: 361–369.
109. Gailey MP, Stence AA, Jensen CS, *et al.* Multiplatform comparison of molecular oncology tests performed on cytology specimens and formalin-fixed, paraffin-embedded tissue. *Cancer Cytopathol* 2014; 1–10.
110. Scarpa A, Sikora K, Fassan M, *et al.* Molecular typing of lung adenocarcinoma on cytological samples using a multigene next generation sequencing panel. *PLoS One* 2013; 8: e80478.
111. Savic S, Bubendorf L. Role of fluorescence *in situ* hybridization in lung cancer cytology. *Acta Cytol* 2012; 56: 611–621.
112. Son C, Kang E-J, Roh MS. Strategic management of transthoracic needle aspirates for histological subtyping and EGFR testing in patients with peripheral lung cancer: An institutional experience. *Diagn Cytopathol* 2014; [In press DOI: 10.1002/dc.23237].
113. Huysentruyt CJR, Baldewijns MM, Rüland AM, *et al.* Modified UroVysion scoring criteria increase the urothelial carcinoma detection rate in cases of equivocal urinary cytology. *Histopathology* 2011; 58: 1048–1053.
114. Economou M, Schöni L, Hammer C, *et al.* Proper paraffin slide storage is crucial for translational research projects involving immunohistochemistry stains. *Clin Transl Med* 2014; 3: 4.
115. Smits AJJ, Kummer JA, de Bruin PC, *et al.* The estimation of tumor cell percentage for molecular testing by pathologists is not accurate. *Mod Pathol* 2014; 27: 168–174.
116. Do H, Dobrovic A. Sequence artifacts in DNA from formalin-fixed tissues: causes and strategies for minimization. *Clin Chem* 2015; 61: 64–71.

---

Disclosures: E.J.M. Speel reports receiving honoraria from Pfizer, Amgen and Roche, outside the submitted work.

Chapter 10

# Management of early stage lung cancer: a surgeon's perspective

Pascal A. Thomas

Lobectomy with lymphadenectomy is the standard of care for patients with early stage NSCLC and the use of minimally invasive approaches are associated with reduced morbidity when compared with thoracotomy. Segmentectomy with lymphadenectomy seems to provide a curative effect equivalent to that of lobectomy for stage IA tumours of ≤2 cm and for pure or predominant ground glass opacities. The combination of lung sparing resections with minimally invasive approaches results in preserved pulmonary function, improved quality of life and very low morbidity. This benefit persists in so-called high-risk patients. Among patients with clinical stage IA managed with sublobar resections, more than 25% are proved to have a more advanced pathologic stage at surgery, suggesting that alternative ablative therapies would result in an incomplete resection in a similar proportion. Moreover, resection samples tumour tissue that is adequate in quantity and quality, and provides material for "research biopsies" to consolidate tissue availability for clinical trials, translational research, and in biobanks.

Surgery, eventually followed by adjuvant platinum-based chemotherapy, is the backbone treatment for early stage NSCLC [1]. However, the idiom "early stage disease" encompasses a confusing area if characterised by the alternative wording "resectable disease", which may also cover some locally advanced T and N diseases, and even certain anecdotal oligometastatic situations. This chapter focuses on surgical perspectives in the management of clinical stage I disease, especially in the era of the implementation of individual lung cancer screening programmes. Indeed, the randomised, controlled National Lung Screening Trial (NLST) [2] recently demonstrated a reduction in lung cancer related and overall long-term mortality of 20%, when using low dose CT scanning in high-risk subjects. This finding was related to the diagnosis of lung cancer at a curable stage in the vast majority of cases, in particular stage I where it was found to be 50%. Accordingly, the detection of small lung nodules and ground-glass opacities is expected to increase substantially in the forthcoming years. Therefore, the issue of whether to perform a lobectomy or a sublobar resection, *i.e.* a segmentectomy or wedge resection, is of renewed interest within the thoracic surgeon community, as is the surgical approach of offering either open or minimally invasive surgery, to lessen the surgical insult. These controversial surgical debates now occur in a competitive context with the advent of alternative treatments, such as stereotactic body radiation therapy, radiofrequency, cryo- or microwave

Dept of Thoracic Surgery, North Hospital - APHM, Aix-Marseille University, Marseille, France.

Correspondence: Pascal A. Thomas, Dept of Thoracic Surgery, Aix-Marseille University, North Hospital, Chemin des Bourrely, 13915 Marseille, France. E-mail: pathomas@ap-hm.fr

 Print ISBN: 978-1-84984-061-3. Online ISBN: 978-1-84984-062-0. Print ISSN: 2312-508X. Online ISSN: 2312-5098.

ablation. Thus, a timely critical evaluation of outcomes should be performed, which focusses on operative risks, functional results, survival data and recurrence patterns related to modern surgical concepts concerning early stage lung cancers, in order to serve as a benchmark against which the outcomes of these ablative techniques must be compared. This is especially so in the case of the elderly and co-morbid patients in whom competitive risks of cancer-unrelated death exist.

## Sublobar resection

For decades the "good" operation to cure lung cancer was thought to be pneumonectomy [3]. In 1960, CAHAN [4] supported the so-called "radical lobectomy" with systemic mediastinal lymphadenectomy as an alternative option to achieve the balanced surgical effects of both curability and functional preservation. In line with this trend, KODAMA *et al.* [5] reported their initial experience with "radical segmentectomy" in 1992. To date, the most recently available international guidelines still recommend lobectomy over any form of sublobar resection to treat early stage NSCLC patients [1]. This recommendation is mainly based upon the results from only one randomised trial of sublobar resection *versus* lobectomy for clinical T1N0 NSCLC, which was published in 1995 [6]. In this study, the annual death rate was 30% higher in the sublobar group. In addition, the locoregional recurrence rate in the sublobar group was 300% higher than in the lobectomy group (17.2% *versus* 6.4%), with relatively worse results after wedge resection than after segmentectomy. Another large prospective, multicentre nonrandomised study showed a comparable tendency for increased local recurrence in patients undergoing sublobar resection [7]. However, in both of these studies long-term survival was not statistically different between sublobar and lobectomy resected patients. Nevertheless, since then the use of sublobar resections has been reserved for high-risk patients with small tumours who are unable to tolerate lobectomy because of significant impairment in cardiopulmonary reserve.

### Tumour type and size

The increased detection of smaller and smaller NSCLC tumours by enhanced CT screening protocols has led to the thoracic surgeon community reconsidering the appropriateness of lobectomy in all cases. A substantial body of literature, mainly from Japan, has demonstrated lower postoperative morbidity and mortality, and preserved pulmonary function, following sublobar resection (segmentectomy in particular) compared with lobectomy. Amazing long-term survival, reported historically as well by Japanese surgeons in the special setting of ground-glass opacities, helped to identify so-called indolent types of ADC for which local recurrence is infrequent. These lesions largely correspond to atypical adenomatous hyperplasia and ADC, and in particular to *in situ*, minimally invasive or invasive ADC, lepidic predominant, as emphasised by the 2011 international multidisciplinary classification of lung ADC (as defined by the International Association for the Study of Lung Cancer (IASLC)/American Thoracic Society(ATS)/European Respiratory Society (ERS)) [8]. In brief, their invasiveness correlates with the portion of solid component within the ground-glass opacities region [9]. Moreover, adherence to current international guidelines recommending the routine use of PET and brain imaging followed by selective invasive lymph node investigations, improves accuracy of clinical staging and increases the proportion of pathological early stage tumours at surgery. In addition, such precise pre-treatment work-up also carries the opportunity to disclose synchronous multifocality that emphasises the interest of lung-sparing resections.

## Resection type and margins

For decades, wedge resection and segmentectomy were, confusingly, considered as synonyms. Segmentectomy, a cancer operation initially ideated for the cure of tuberculosis, is an anatomic resection that is more likely than wedge resection to provide sufficient margins and allows access to stations 11 and 12 lymph nodes [10, 11]. A wedge resection can be easily performed for peripheral tumours located in the upper lobes, or those nodules located in the vicinity of the fissures, whereas deep lesions in the lung or those located posteriorly and inferiorly in the lower lobes are difficult to locate and/or resect with sufficient margins, unless an anatomic resection is done [11]. Wedge resection, when feasible, are an easy, quick and safe operation to undertake. The associated operative risk for a wedge resection is quite low and may be of interest in high-risk patients: a Society of Thoracic Surgery database propensity-matched analysis showed that in patients with preoperative $FEV_1$ less than 60% predicted undergoing wedge resection *versus* anatomic resection, there was a 52% reduction in perioperative mortality and incidence of a major morbidity [12]. Pure and predominant ground-glass opacities could probably be resected by wedge with excellent long-term survival, not different from that provided by anatomic resections, *i.e.* segmentectomies and lobectomies [13], especially in high-risk patients. In other cases, the increase in locoregional recurrence and possible decrease in long-term survival associated with the use of wedge resection for primary lung cancers is a matter of concern. A recent meta-analysis compared the effect of segmentectomy and lobectomy on survival in 22 observational studies published between 1994 and 2012. The hazard ratios (HR) of overall and cancer-specific survival indicated significant benefits of lobectomy for stage I, stage IA and stage IA with tumours larger than 2 cm but smaller than 3 cm at 1.20 (95% CI 1.04–1.38; p=0.011), 1.24 (95% CI 1.08–1.42; p=0.002) and 1.41 (95% CI 1.14–1.71; p=0.001), respectively. Segmentectomy provided an effect equivalent to that of lobectomy only for stage IA tumours of 2 cm or smaller (HR 1.05; 95% CI 0.89–1.24; p=0.550) [14].

Beside the tumour size, adequate resection margin is an important consideration after sublobar resection, wedge resection in particular. However, there is no clear information or consensual definition regarding what constitutes an adequate margin distance either on a fresh or a formalin-fixed shrunken lung specimen. It has been postulated that margins of 1.5 cm in a deflated lung and 2 cm in an inflated one are generally acceptable [15]. El-Sherif *et al.* [16] demonstrated that the incidence of local recurrence almost doubled (14.6% *versus* 7.5%) in case of margins less than 1 cm on deflated fresh sublobar resection specimen. A Japanese prospective multicentre study showed that cytologically positive margins, as determined by using a run-across method, by which a slide was brushed along the staple line after wedge resection, were not found when the macroscopic margin distance was greater than 20 mm and/or the maximum tumour diameter [17]. Mohiuddin *et al.* [18] recently reported on decreased local recurrence rates for a margin distance of ⩾15 mm on deflated fresh specimen, regardless of the tumour size when the tumours were ⩽2 cm, with no evidence of additional benefit with an increased margin distance beyond this value.

## Lymph node dissection

The long-term survival advantage of a segmentectomy over a wedge resection may be due to the more generous margin of resection usually obtained with anatomical segmentectomy. It also may be related to a better lymph node dissection, especially at the interlobar level.

A case-matched study on patients with peripheral cT1a N0 M0 tumours, who underwent anatomical segmentectomy or lobectomy, showed similar median number of N1 and N2 nodes following anatomical segmentectomy, when compared with standard lobectomy and equivalent 3-year survival rates [19]. In contrast, anatomical segmentectomy has been found to provide more nodes for pathology and to result in significantly better cancer-related survival than wedge resections [20]. A nonrandomised, prospective controlled study, conducted to compare lobectomy with segmental resection for the treatment of elderly clinical stage I lung cancer patients, showed that patients who underwent segmental resection with lymph node dissection experienced similar 5-year survival than those undergoing lobectomy, whereas those who underwent segmentectomy with lymph node sampling did not [21].

## Pulmonary function

The respective impact of sublobar and lobar resections on pulmonary function tests (PFT) is a problematic point. Intuitively, one may consider that the extent of the removed lung parenchyma directly affects postoperative functional loss and that segmentectomy offers significantly better functional preservation compared with lobectomy. However, few works confirmed this hypothesis following open [22–24] or VATS procedures [25]. The last study showed, for instance, a mean±SD loss of *D*LCO of 8.86%±14.03% at 12 months after lobectomy *versus* 0.80%±11.76% after sublobar resection. In fact, the effect on the postoperative PFT results depends on the emphysema status, operation side, targeted lobe, PFT indicators, and chronology. Upper lobectomies may act as a lung volume reduction surgery in COPD patients [26] and may result in better PFT than sublobar resections postoperatively. On the right side, the volume of the upper or middle lobe is relatively low compared with that of the other lobes, but the subsequent upward displacement of the right lower lobe causes an angulation of the bronchus intermedius that leads to increase airway resistance [27]. Right lower-lobe lobectomy may be associated with no difference in FEV1 when compared with that of a sublobar resection. Because the right lower lobe has a relatively large volume, the removal of it results in reductions in FVC and *D*LCO. However, as the angulation of the remaining bronchus scarcely changes after a right lower-lobe lobectomy, FEV1 could be similar to the level of sublobar resection. On the left side, the lung consists of two relatively large lobes. If one of these two lobes is removed, the remaining lobe is unlikely to appropriately compensate and thereby resulting in a reduced pulmonary function than after a sublobar resection [25]. Finally, PFT may improve dramatically between 3 and 12 months postoperatively, especially if rehabilitation is undertaken [28], after what they reach a plateau [25]. To summarise this point, sublobar resection usually saves greater pulmonary function than lobectomy. However, in right-side lobectomy, some differences may dissipate at 1 year.

## Quality of life

This outcome indicator has already been shown to be related to PFT, and especially postoperative *D*LCO values. Quality of life (QoL) is of huge relevance, particularly when caring for a high-risk patient with early stage lung cancer in whom competitive risks of death and clinical impact of the treatment are to be balanced for each treatment option. Fernando *et al.* [29] reported QoL results from a prospective multicentre study of high-risk operable patients treated with sublobar resection. Global QoL and dyspnoea did not deteriorate significantly 3 months after the operation. There were advantages, with respect to minimising postoperative dyspnoea, when VATS, rather than thoracotomy, or wedge resection, rather than segmentectomy, were used. VATS was also superior to thoracotomy with improved QoL at 3 months, lending support to the preferential use of VATS when sublobar resection is performed.

## Lymphadenectomy

The American College of Surgery Oncology Group (ACOSOG) Z0030 randomised trial concluded that, compared to systematic hilar and mediastinal lymph node sampling, systematic dissection did not improve survival in patients with early stage NSCL cancer [30]. However, a meta-analysis of the four available randomised studies, including the ACOSOG Z0030 trial, which represented 1778 patients with early stage NSCLC, demonstrated a strong trend toward a reduction in all-cause mortality with lymph node dissection relative to sampling (risk ratio 0.91, 95% CI 0.82–1.00, p=0.05, p=0.59 for heterogeneity; HR 0.86, 95% CI, 0.73–1.01, p=0.06, p=0.29 for heterogeneity) [31]. If the ACOSOG Z0030 trial was excluded, the result became statistically significant with a risk ratio of 0.87 (95% CI, 0.76–0.99, p=0.04). The three non-ACOSOG trials were all similar in that invasive staging of the mediastinum had not been done before randomisation [32–34]. In contrast, approximately 30% of the patients included in the ACOSOG Z0030 trial received preoperative mediastinoscopy. Furthermore, only patients who had intra-operatively proven negative systematic sampling with frozen sections of stations 2R, 4R, 7, and 10R, for right sided tumours, and 5, 6, 7, and 10L, for left sided tumours, were eligible for randomisation. Therefore, patients with extralobar N1 and N2 positive nodes that were discovered with sampling were excluded from the trial [30]. From these data, one may conclude that if systematic invasive hilar and mediastinal lymph node assessments are not done before or at the time of resection, then a systematic dissection should be performed as it potentially offers a better local control and a survival advantage through the detection and removal of positive nodes, thereby providing a complete resection and information for adjuvant chemotherapy. The ACOSOG Z0030 trial also suggests in early stage lung cancer patients, supposed to be N0 after invasive preoperative staging, that systematic sampling of stations 2R, 4R, 7 and 10R, for right sided tumours, and 5, 6, 7 and 10L, for left sided tumours, should be regarded as the minimal intra-operative nodal assessments.

## Minimally invasive approaches

### VATS

As for many surgical disciplines, the introduction of minimally invasive techniques has revolutionised thoracic surgical practices in recent decades (figs 1–3). In the absence of well-designed, large scale, multi-institutional randomised controlled trials, the highest level of clinical evidence that has been provided, to date, is a meta-analysis of propensity score matched patients, which compared short-term outcomes for VATS and open approaches for the treatment of NSCLC [35]. This meta-analysis reported 1817 patients who underwent VATS and 1817 propensity score-matched patients who underwent thoracotomy. It found significantly fewer overall complications after VATS. Specifically, patients who underwent VATS were significantly less likely to develop prolonged air leak, pneumonia, atrial arrhythmias and renal failure when compared with matched patients

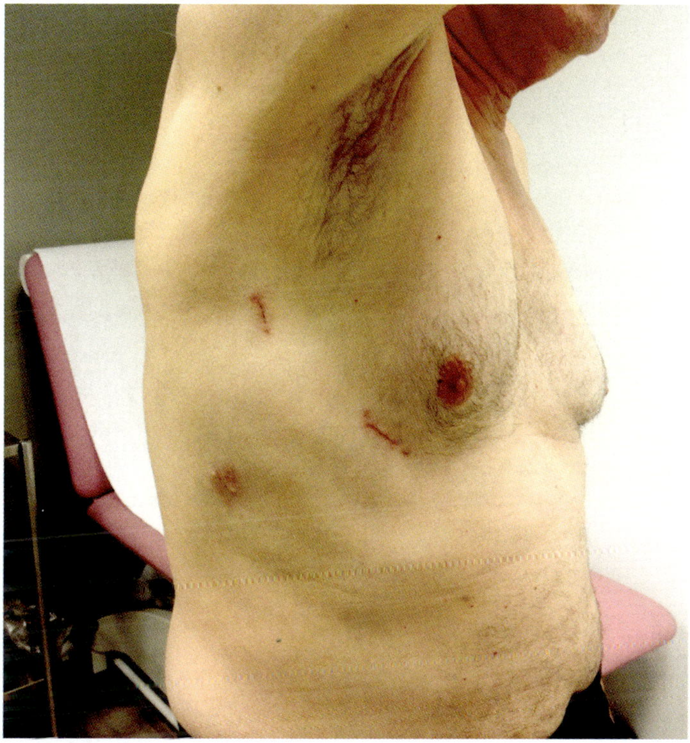

Figure 1. The surgical scars from a posterior approach with three trocar incisions: the posterior trocar placement is in the 5th intercostal space anterior to the latissimus dorsi; the anterior superior incision is located in the 5th intercostal space just below the nipple and is enlarged to 3 cm or 4 cm to remove the operative specimen; the inferior incision is located in the 8th intercostal space on the midaxillary line and is used for the thoracoscope.

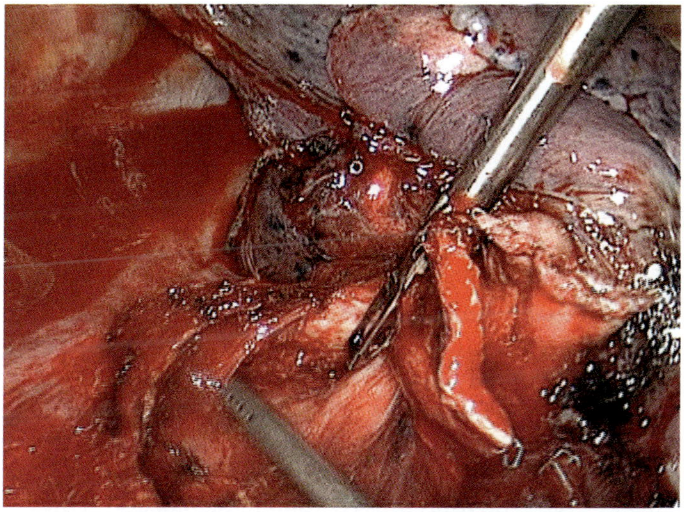

Figure 2. VATS right lower lobectomy, operative view after removal of the operative specimen and systematic lymphadenectomy at the subcarinal area (station 7).

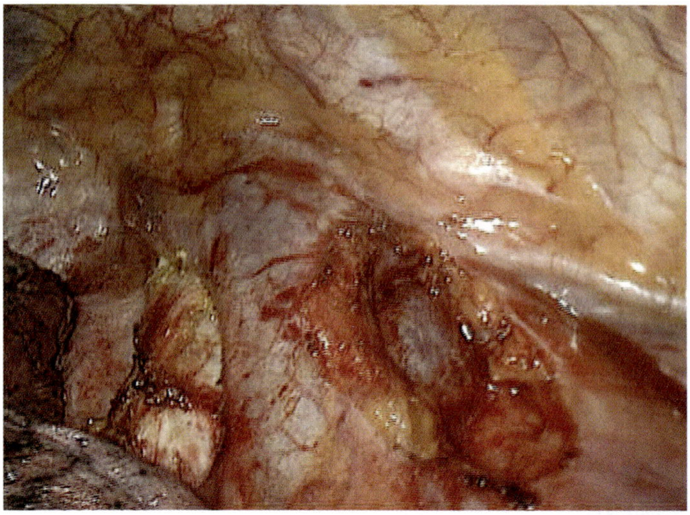

Figure 3. VATS lobectomy and systematic lymphadenectomy, upper mediastinal lymphadenectomy (stations 2R, 4R and 3A).

who underwent thoracotomy. The duration of hospitalisation was also significantly shorter after VATS, and there was a trend towards a lower perioperative mortality rate for patients in this treatment group. These results have been confirmed by the very last analysis of video-assisted approach to anatomic resection of clinical stage I lung cancer in the STS database [36]. Propensity scoring was used to match cases into 2745 well-balanced pairs. Patients undergoing VATS experienced significantly less pulmonary complications, atrial arrhythmias, and were less likely to undergo blood transfusion. Operative mortality was also lesser, but the difference did not reach statistical significance. This trend has also been confirmed in European countries in a similarly sized sample of patients. Using the European Society of Thoracic Surgeons (ESTS) database, propensity score yielded two well-matched groups of 2721 patients. Compared to the open lobectomy group, the VATS lobectomy group was associated with a lower incidence of total complications, major cardiopulmonary complications, atelectasis requiring bronchoscopy and wound infection. Finally, operative mortality was twice as low in the VATS group when compared with the open group (1% *versus* 1.9%, p=0.0201) [37].

There is now a host of institutional case series, as well as larger analyses of clinical and administrative population-based databases, that suggest a clinical benefit of VATS. However, despite the use of sophisticated matching statistical methods, the difference between VATS and thoracotomy may still be partly related to dormant unobserved confounders. The most profound ones are those changes made in perioperative care that are definitely not captured in any database. Undeniably, the advent of VATS techniques was also a timely occasion for the thoracic surgeon community to question many of the conventions of patient management after pulmonary resection as are old dogmas related to the number of chest tubes, duration of chest tubes, suction *versus* water seal, and indications for chest tube removal. More importantly, overall care paradigms have moved towards a dedicated, so-called, "fast track" care pathway based upon therapeutic education, preoperative rehabilitation, pain management that favours locoregional analgesia over systemic therapies, and standardisation of perioperative management, which all contribute to a safer postoperative course and enabling the patient to be discharged earlier. Besides other potential bias, one may presume that all these developments were not translated fully and simultaneously to the management of patients operated through a formal thoracotomy [38].

Data on long-term survival are scanty. They also carry the same methodological limitations as mentioned earlier. Nevertheless, the most recent meta-analysis of the literature, conducted on over 2000 patients in each group, suggests that long-term outcomes with VATS are at least similar, if not better, than outcomes observed with classic thoracotomy [39].

## Robot-assisted thoracic surgery (RATS)

The last development in this setting is robot-assisted thoracic surgery (RATS), which adds a computer technology-enhanced device to the interaction between the surgeon and the patient (figs 4 and 5). Robotic surgery offers some specific advantages over VATS: a 10-fold magnified three-dimensional view of the operative field; less camera manipulation is required, a more precise dissection can be undertaken, due to the suppression of any tremor; an improved hand–eye coordination; and the use of articulated instruments, which provide seven degrees of freedom. The main technical limitations of RATS are the absence of touch sensation, the relatively large size in today's already crowded operating rooms, and the ongoing need for compatible staplers and energy devices. Most of these disadvantages are likely to be remedied with time and improvements in technology. Nevertheless, whether the use of RATS translates into a clinical benefit for the patient is still controversial. When compared with open approaches, RATS should be regarded equal to a minimally invasive option, with the inherent potential advantages as listed earlier. When compared with VATS, RATS seems roughly similar to VATS in terms of early outcomes, even if it may be less painful than VATS and leads to fewer conversions [40]. Preliminary data show that long-term stage-specific survival with RATS is consistent with prior results for VATS and thoracotomy [41]. Defining the current place and future role of RATS in the management of early stage lung cancer patients is tricky. On the one hand, it seems that RATS may be an alternative option to VATS for some surgeons who do not feel comfortable with VATS. On the other hand, a better perspective may be to consider RATS as complementary to

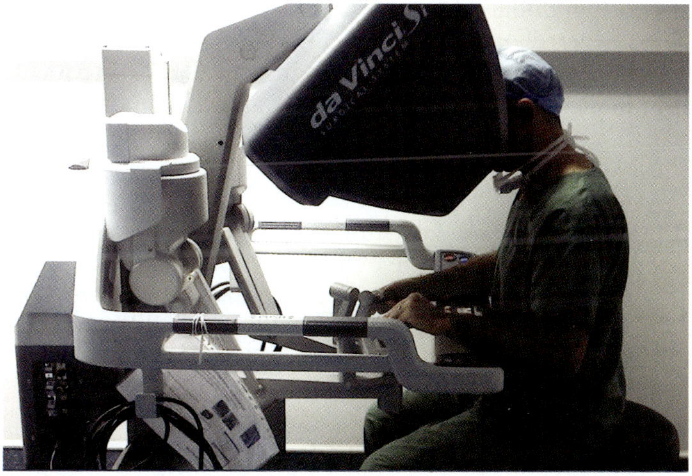


Figure 4. Robot-assisted thoracic surgery. The operating surgeon is shown seated at the console.

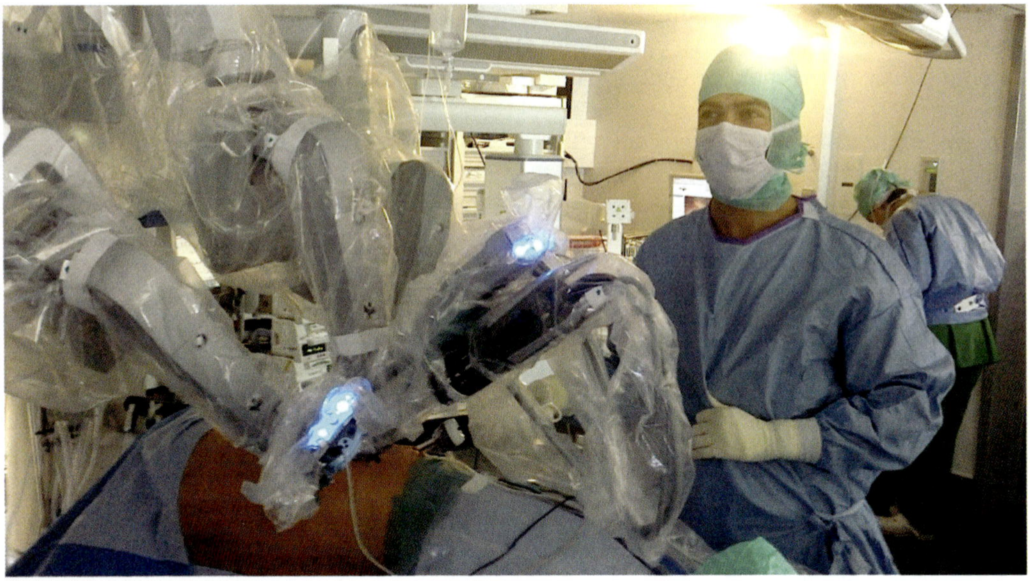

Figure 5. Robot-assisted thoracic surgery. The assistant surgeon during a three-arm and one assistant-port lobectomy procedure.

VATS for complex procedures, *i.e.* segmentectomies or bronchoplastic and angioplastic lung resections, making them easier to adopt and to perform by improving ergonomic, surgeon view and precise movements. Either way the pivotal concern is its current, nearly prohibitive, cost. If cost is not reduced for routine procedures, it is likely that robotic surgery will be restricted to high-volume referral centres and dedicated teams only.

## High-risk patients

Lung cancer resection is one of the more risky elective surgeries as patients, undergoing this operation, are usually aged >60 years and have multiple comorbidities, which are related to tobacco consumption. Therefore, a significant portion of patients with stage I lung cancer are considered inoperable or high-risk surgical candidates. Historically, sublobar resections were preferred to lobectomy in some of these patients. The advent of nonsurgical ablative therapies opened a new era that urged the thoracic surgeon community to reassess the benefit/risk ratio of surgery in these patients, as a training round before the forthcoming ultimate debate in standard risk patients.

Using a single institution, prospectively maintained database, a team from the University of Virginia, Taylor *et al.* [42], compared the outcomes of patients undergoing lobectomy with and without marginal pulmonary function tests, characterised by criteria applied in research trials (ACOSOG Z4099 and Radiation Therapy Oncology Group (RTOG) 1021) or guidelines (American College of Chest Physicians (CHEST)). According to the ACOSOG/RTOG criteria, patients with marginal PFT were defined as follows: $FEV_1 \leqslant 50\%$ or $D_{LCO} \leqslant 50\%$ or aged >75 years and $FEV_1$ 50–60% or aged >75 years and $D_{LCO}$ 50–60%. According to the CHEST criteria, patients with marginal PFT had a predictive postoperative $FEV_1$ and/or $D_{LCO}$ <40%. Despite nearly a doubled incidence of pneumonia and cardiovascular events, 30-day mortality was slightly, but not significantly, augmented in patients with marginal PFT in comparison with those with non-marginal PFT (1.5% *versus* 0.4% according to the ACOSOG/RTOG criteria and 1.3% *versus* 0.8% according to the CHEST criteria). Furthermore, in both marginal PFT categories, marginal PFT was not associated with a decrease in overall long-term survival compared with patients with non-marginal PFT.

Crabtree *et al.* [43] compared the selection criteria and short-term outcomes among three prospective clinical trials using stereotactic body radiotherapy (RTOG 0236), sublobar resection (ACOSOG Z4032), and radiofrequency ablation (ACOSOG Z4033). The overall 90-day mortality for stereotactic body radiotherapy, surgery and radiofrequency ablation was 0%, 2.4% and 2.0%, respectively. A propensity matched comparison showed no difference between stereotactic body radiotherapy and surgery for 30-day grade 3+ adverse events. Among the patients with clinical stage IA in ACOSOG Z4032, a large portion of patients (29.3%) had a more advanced pathologic stage at surgery, suggesting that alternative ablative therapies would result in an incomplete resection in almost one third of the patients.

To summarise this point, a true definition of "high-risk" remains a critical unmet need in patient care in early stage lung cancer [44].

## The surgeon's role in the biomolecular era

Despite adequate treatment, including adjuvant platinum-based chemotherapy in some cases, 20–50% of patients with so-called stage I–II NSCLC will recur, with distant metastases in two out of three of the cases. Obtaining tissue specimens from recurrent or metastatic diseases is not always possible, due to altered general condition of the patient or various technical and anatomical reasons. This practical information supports the pivotal role of tumour resection, as it highlights the need for a precise initial pathology diagnosis and the appropriate handling of tissue samples for genomic profiling, when needed. Indeed, the identification of specific genetic and molecular abnormalities followed by the administration of a specific inhibitor to the target, are the basis of personalised lung cancer treatment of advanced stages. For instance, testing for EGFR mutations and ALK gene rearrangements has become an essential component of daily clinical practice, in order to select advanced NSCLC patients who are most likely to benefit from TKI. A similar paradigm is under investigation in early stage NSCLC to identify patients who could derive benefit from targeted adjuvant therapy [45]. This approach now also includes immunotherapy. In fact, the development of a new therapeutic class of drugs, which inhibit immune checkpoints such as antibodies targeting CTLA4, programmed cell death 1 and programmed cell death ligand 1, has recently emerged as a potent strategy in oncology. In this new paradigm, the role of the surgeon is crucial. Resection definitely offers the best sampling of tumour tissue that is representative and is adequate in quantity and quality, but also provides material for "research biopsies" to consolidate tissue availability for clinical trials, translational research and in biobanks [46].

## References

1. Vansteenkiste J, Crinò L, Dooms C, *et al.* 2nd ESMO Consensus Conference on Lung Cancer: early-stage non-small-cell lung cancer consensus on diagnosis, treatment and follow-up. *Ann Oncol* 2014; 25: 1462–1474.
2. National Lung Screening Trial Research Team. Reduced lung-cancer mortality with low-dose computed tomographic screening. *N Engl J Med* 2011; 365: 395–409.

3. Churchill ED, Sweet RH, Scoutter L, *et al.* The surgical management of carcinoma of the lung; a study of the cases treated at the Massachusetts General Hospital from 1930–1950. *J Thorac Surg* 1950; 20: 349–365.
4. Cahan WG. Radical lobectomy. *J Thorac Cardiovasc Surg* 1960; 39: 555–572.
5. Kodama K, Doi O, Yasuda T, *et al.* Radical laser segmentectomy for T1 N0 lung cancer. *Ann Thorac Surg* 1992; 54: 1193–1195.
6. Ginsberg RJ, Rubinstein LV. Randomized trial of lobectomy *versus* limited resection for T1 N0 non-small cell lung cancer. *Ann Thorac Surg* 1995; 60: 615–622.
7. Landreneau RJ, Sugarbaker DJ, Mack MJ, *et al.* Wedge resection *versus* lobectomy for stage 1 (T1N0M0) non-small cell lung cancer. *J Thorac Cardiovasc Surg* 1997; 113: 698–700.
8. Travis WD, Brambilla E, Noguchi M, *et al.* International Association for the Study of Lung Cancer/American Thoracic Society/European Respiratory Society international multidisciplinary classification of lung adenocarcinoma. *J Thorac Oncol* 2011; 6: 244–285.
9. Van Schil PE, Asamura H, Rusch VW, *et al.* Surgical implications of the new IASLC/ATS/ERS adenocarcinoma classification. *Eur Respir J* 2012; 39: 478–486.
10. Kent M, Landreneau R, Mandrekar S, *et al.* Segmentectomy *versus* wedge resection for non-small cell lung cancer in high-risk operable patients. *Ann Thorac Surg* 2013; 96: 1747–1755.
11. Sienel W, Stremmel C, Kirschbaum A, *et al.* Frequency of local recurrence following segmentectomy of stage IA non-small cell lung cancer is influenced by segment localisation and width of resection margins—implications for patient selection for segmentectomy. *Eur J Cardiothorac Surg* 2007; 31: 522–527.
12. Linden PA, D'Amico TA, Perry Y, *et al.* Quantifying the safety benefits of wedge resection: a Society of Thoracic Surgery database propensity-matched analysis. *Ann Thorac Surg* 2014; 98: 1705–1712.
13. Tsutani Y, Miyata Y, Nakayama H, *et al.* Appropriate sublobar resection choice for ground glass opacity-dominant clinical stage IA lung adenocarcinoma: wedge resection or segmentectomy. *Chest* 2004; 97: 1701–1707.
14. Bao F, Ye P, Yang Y, *et al.* Segmentectomy or lobectomy for early stage lung cancer: a meta-analysis. *Eur J Cardiothorac Surg* 2014; 46: 1–7.
15. Fell SC, Kirby TJ. Limited pulmonary resection. *In*: Dienemann HD and Hoffmann H eds. Thoracic Surgery. 2nd Edn. New York, Churchill Livingstone, 2002; 36: 1002–1004.
16. El-Sherif A, Fernando HC, Santos R, *et al.* Margin and local recurrence after sublobar resection of non-small cell lung cancer. *Ann Surg Oncol* 2007; 14: 2400–2405.
17. Sawabata N, Ohta M, Matsumura A, *et al.* Optimal distance of malignant negative margin in excision of nonsmall cell lung cancer: a multicenter prospective study. *Ann Thorac Surg* 2004; 77: 415–420.
18. Mohiuddin K, Haneuse S, Sofer T, *et al.* Relationship between margin distance and local recurrence among patients undergoing wedge resection for small (⩽2 cm) non-small cell lung cancer. *J Thorac Cardiovasc Surg* 2014; 147: 1169–1175.
19. Mattioli S, Ruffato A, Puma F, *et al.* Does anatomical segmentectomy allow an adequate lymph node staging for cT1a non-small cell lung cancer? *J Thorac Oncol* 2011; 6: 1537–1541.
20. Sienel W, Dango S, Kirschbaum A, *et al.* Sublobar resections in stage IA non-small cell lung cancer: segmentectomies result in significantly better cancer-related survival than wedge resections. *Eur J Cardiothorac Surg* 2008; 33: 728–734.
21. Cheng YD, Duan CJ, Dong S, *et al.* Clinical controlled comparison between lobectomy and segmental resection for patients over 70 years of age with clinical stage I non-small cell lung cancer. *Eur J Surg Oncol* 2012; 38: 1149–1155.
22. Keenan RJ, Landreneau RJ, Maley RH Jr, *et al.* Segmental resection spares pulmonary function in patients with stage I lung cancer. *Ann Thorac Surg* 2004; 78: 228–233.
23. Harada H, Okada M, Sakamoto T, *et al.* Functional advantage after radical segmentectomy *versus* lobectomy for lung cancer. *Ann Thorac Surg* 2005; 80: 2041–2045.
24. Yoshikawa K, Tsubota N, Kodama K, *et al.* Prospective study of extended segmentectomy for small lung tumors: the final report. *Ann Thorac Surg* 2002; 73: 1055–1059.
25. Kim SJ, Lee YJ, Park JS, *et al.* Changes in pulmonary function in lung cancer patients after video-assisted thoracic surgery. *Ann Thorac Surg* 2015; 99: 210–217.
26. Kushibe K, Takahama M, Tojo T, *et al.* Assessment of pulmonary function after lobectomy for lung cancer-upper lobectomy might have the same effect as lung volume reduction surgery. *Eur J Cardiothorac Surg* 2006; 29: 886–890.
27. Seok Y, Cho S, Lee JY, *et al.* The effect of postoperative change in bronchial angle on postoperative pulmonary function after upper lobectomy in lung cancer patients. *Interact Cardiovasc Thorac Surg* 2014; 18: 183–188.
28. Edvardsen E, Skjønsberg OH, Holme I, *et al.* High-intensity training following lung cancer surgery: a randomised controlled trial. *Thorax* 2015; 70: 244–250.
29. Fernando HC, Landreneau RJ, Mandrekar SJ, *et al.* Analysis of longitudinal quality of life data in high-risk operable patients with lung cancer: results from ACOSOG Z4032 (Alliance) a multicenter randomized trial. *J Thorac Cardiovasc Surg* 2015; 149: 718–726.

30. Darling GE, Allen MS, Decker PA, *et al.* Randomized trial of mediastinal lymph node sampling *versus* complete lymphadenectomy during pulmonary resection in the patient with N0 or N1 (less than hilar) non-small cell carcinoma: results of the American College of Surgery Oncology Group Z0030 trial. *J Thorac Cardiovasc Surg* 2011; 141: 662–670.
31. Takagi H, Matsui M, Umemoto T. Alice in wonderland of mediastinal lymph nodes. *J Thorac Cardiovasc Surg* 2011; 142: 477–478.
32. Sugi K, Nawata K, Fujita N, *et al.* Systematic lymph node dissection for clinically diagnosed peripheral non-small cell lung cancer less than 2 cm in diameter. *World J Surg* 1998; 22: 290–294.
33. Izbicki JR, Passlick B, Pantel K, *et al.* Effectiveness of radical systematic mediastinal lymphadenectomy in patients with resectable non–small cell lung cancer: results of a prospective randomized trial. *Ann Surg* 1998; 227: 138–144.
34. Wu YI, Huang ZF, Wang SY, *et al.* A randomized trial of systematic nodal dissection in resectable non-small cell lung cancer. *Lung Cancer* 2002; 36: 1–6.
35. Cao C, Manganas C, Ang SC, *et al.* Video-assisted thoracic surgery *versus* open thoracotomy for non-small cell lung cancer: a meta-analysis of propensity score-matched patients. *Interact Cardiovasc Thorac Surg* 2013; 16: 244–249.
36. Boffa DJ, Dhamija A, Kosinski AS, *et al.* Fewer complications result from a video-assisted approach to anatomic resection of clinical stage I lung cancer. *J Thorac Cardiovasc Surg* 2014; 148: 637–643.
37. Falcoz PE, Puyraveau M, Thomas PA, *et al.* Thoracoscopic *versus* open lobectomy for primary non-small cell lung cancer: a propensity-matched analysis of outcome from the ESTS database. *Eur J Cardiothorac Surg* 2015; [In press DOI: 10.1093/ejcts/ezv167].
38. Wood DE. What is most important in improving outcomes after pulmonary lobectomy: the surgeon or the approach? *Eur J Cardiothorac Surg* 2013; 43: 817–819.
39. Taioli E, Lee DS, Lesser M, *et al.* Long-term survival in video-assisted thoracoscopic lobectomy *vs* open lobectomy in lung-cancer patients: a meta-analysis. *Eur J Cardiothorac Surg* 2013; 44: 591–597.
40. Farivar AS, Cerfolio RJ, Vallières E, *et al.* Comparing robotic lung resection with thoracotomy and video-assisted thoracoscopic surgery cases entered into the Society of Thoracic Surgeons database. *Innovations (Phila)* 2014; 9: 10–15.
41. Park BJ, Melfi F, Mussi A, *et al.* Robotic lobectomy for non-small cell lung cancer (NSCLC): long-term oncologic results. *J Thorac Cardiovasc Surg* 2012; 143: 383–389.
42. Taylor MD, LaPar DJ, Isbell JM, *et al.* Marginal pulmonary function should not preclude lobectomy in selected patients with non-small cell lung cancer. *J Thorac Cardiovasc Surg* 2014; 147: 738–744.
43. Crabtree T, Puri V, Timmerman R, *et al.* Treatment of stage I lung cancer in high-risk and inoperable patients: comparison of prospective clinical trials using stereotactic body radiotherapy (RTOG 0236), sublobar resection (ACOSOG Z4032), and radiofrequency ablation (ACOSOG Z4033). *J Thorac Cardiovasc Surg* 2013; 145: 692–699.
44. Puri V, Crabtree TD, Bell JM, *et al.* National cooperative group trials of "high-risk" patients with lung cancer: are they truly "high-risk"? *Ann Thorac Surg* 2014; 97: 1678–1683.
45. Wislez M, Barlesi F, Mazières J, *et al.* Customized adjuvant phase II trial in patients with non-small cell lung cancer: IFCT-0801 TASTE. *J Clin Oncol* 2014; 32: 1256–1261.
46. Opitz I, D'Amico TA, Rocco G. The biomolecular era for thoracic surgeons: the example of the ESTS Biology Club. *J Thorac Dis* 2014; 6: Suppl. 2, S265–S271.

---

Disclosure: P.A. Thomas reports personal fees from Ethicon Endosurgery and Covidien.

Chapter 11

# Management of early stage lung cancer: a radiation oncologist's perspective

Esther G.C. Troost[1], Krista C.J. Wink[1], Jaap D. Zindler[1] and Dirk De Ruysscher[2,3]

Stereotactic body radiation therapy (SBRT) and stereotactic ablative body radiotherapy (SABR) are increasingly being delivered to medically inoperable patients with peripheral stage I NSCLC or to patients refusing surgery. The outcome and toxicity profiles of SBRT and SABR are favourable when compared to surgery. Even though retrospective reports of SABR/SBRT for central tumours report comparably safe and effective results, prospective clinical studies should be performed in order to gain solid evidence. Imaging during follow-up of operable patients and resectable tumours should primarily consist of CT, with the addition of PET when recurrence is suspected. With the lack of direct comparison of SABR/SBRT *versus* surgery in randomised, prospective clinical trials, patients should be offered shared-decision making.

Even though most patients present with distant metastases, increasingly, patients are diagnosed with early stage disease on chest imaging that was performed for other indications. Guidelines usually regard primary surgery with lobectomy and mediastinal lymph node dissection as the preferred treatment [1, 2]. Surgical resection of early stage NSCLC leads to a 5-year overall survival rate of 50–77%, whereas for untreated patients, the 5-year overall survival is only 6–14% [3–6]. Obviously, these series are not directly comparable because of their divergent case mix.

However, one in three patients presenting with lung cancer is aged 75 years or older and/or suffers from significant comorbidity [7]. Due to an ageing of the general population, the number of elderly patients with lung cancer is increasing even though the incidence of lung cancer per age group is falling [7, 8]. Elderly patients are more prone not to receive curative treatment options because of the aforementioned comorbidity, higher (peri)operative risk, low performance index, personal choice or a perceived lack of treatment benefit [9–11].

[1]Dept of Radiation Oncology (MAASTRO), GROW School for Oncology and Developmental Biology, Maastricht University Medical Centre, Maastricht, The Netherlands. [2]Dept of Oncology, Experimental Radiation Oncology, Leuven, KU Leuven - University of Leuven, Belgium. [3]Dept of Radiation Oncology, University Hospitals Leuven, Leuven, Belgium.

Correspondence: Esther G.C. Troost, Helmholtz-Zentrum Dresden-Rossendorf, OncoRay – National Center for Radiation Research in Oncology, University Hospital and Medical Faculty Carl Gustav Carus of Technische Universität Dresden, Department of Radiation Oncology, Fetscherstraße 74, 01307 Dresden, Germany. E-mail: esther.troost@uniklinikum-dresden.de

 Print ISBN: 978-1-84984-061-3. Online ISBN: 978-1-84984-062-0. Print ISSN: 2312-508X. Online ISSN: 2312-5098.

For inoperable patients and patients unwilling to undergo surgery, alternative treatment options have been explored. External beam radiotherapy with conventional fractionation schedules demonstrated only a marginal improvement in overall survival when compared with no treatment [6, 12]. Notably, at that time, the radiation fields were based on bony anatomy on X-ray imaging and, consequently, large when compared with today's techniques. Advances in patient positioning, image acquisition (breathing-related CT), radiation treatment planning (three-dimensional (3D) and four-dimensional radiotherapy) and radiotherapy delivery techniques (intensity-modulated radiation therapy) have paved the way for stereotactic body radiotherapy (SBRT) or stereotactic ablative body radiotherapy (SABR) as the treatment of choice for medically inoperable stage I NSCLC patients (fig. 1) [13–17].

Both SABR and SBRT are stereotactic techniques in which high doses of radiotherapy are very precisely delivered with steep dose gradients and in a short overall treatment. This achieves a very high biological dose [18]. Although SABR and SBRT are frequently used as synonyms, they may indeed not be exchangeable. SABR refers to so-called ablative doses, such as three fractions of 18 Gy, which are able to eradicate any living cell in the high-dose volume. SBRT may include these high ablative doses but also contain more "gentle" fractionation schedules such as eight fractions of 7.5 Gy, 10 fractions of 5 Gy or lower. The latter also achieves high local control rates, but possibly to a lesser degree than ablative doses. It is important to distinguish ablative from nonablative doses because mixing them

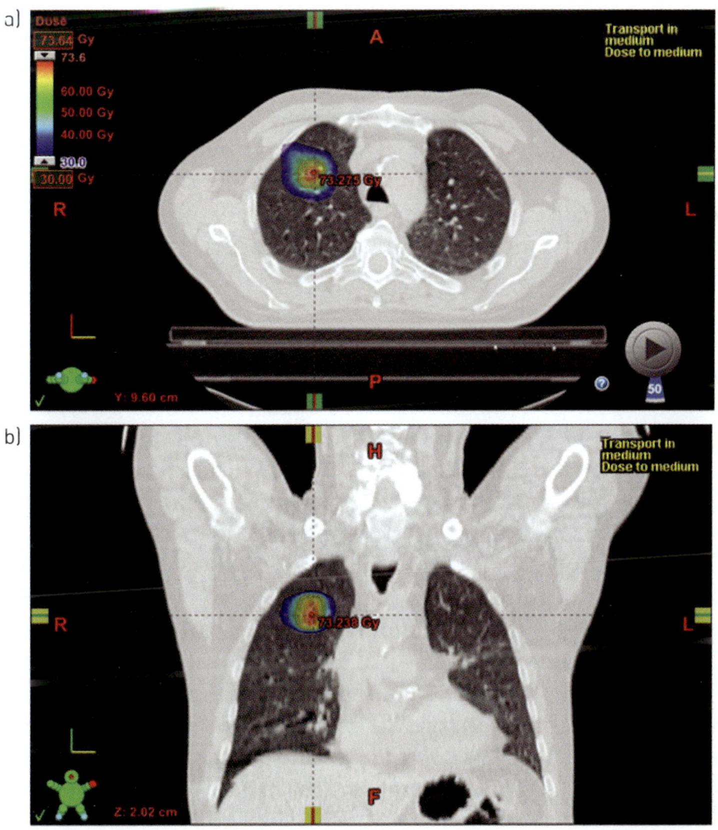


Figure 1. Stereotactic radiotherapy plan of a patient with a cT1aN0M0 NSCLC of the right upper lobe in a) transverse and b) frontal view. The colours indicate the radiation dose ranging from 30 Gy (blue) to 74 Gy (red) for a prescribed tumour dose of 60 Gy in eight fractions.

leads to confusion over what is considered to be "safe" [19]. With an increasing number of radiation oncology departments being equipped with linear accelerators facilitating image-guided radiation delivery, SBRT/SABR are rapidly gaining ground for the entire cohort of medically inoperable stage I NSCLC patients. A recent systematic review of SBRT/SABR for stage I NSCLC patients found it to be equivalent to surgery regardless of the patients' comorbidity [20].

## Outcome

45 studies of stereotactic radiotherapy in early stage NSCLC have been reported [20]. 13 studies, including 996 patients, were prospective and 32 reports with, in total, 2645 patients were retrospective.

When all 45 studies on SBRT/SABR, with in total 3641 patients, are taken into account, the 2-year overall survival was 70% (95% CI 67–92%) and the average local tumour control after 2 years was 91% (95% CI 90–93%) [20]. Even though the patient selection will have been different between the reports and older reports used obviously more outdated techniques, neither the 2-year overall survival nor the 2-year local control differed significantly [20]. The 2-year local control was 91% (95% CI 89–93%) for linear accelerated-based techniques, 88% (95% CI 78–94%) for Cyberknife (Accuray Inc., Sunnyvale, CA, USA) and 80% (95% CI 68–91%) for other technologies. The 2-year overall survival was 69% (95% CI 66–71%), 73% (95% CI 61–83%) and 75% (95% CI 65–83%), respectively. These figures remain stable for at least 5 years [20]. After 5 years, the locoregional recurrences rates were about 15%, with approximately 20% of the patients developing distant metastases [20]. Taking into account the reproducibility of these findings over many reports across the world, it is reasonable to claim that SBRT/SABR outcomes are similar to lobectomy and lymph node dissection [21, 22]. Indeed, in the International Association for the Study of Lung Cancer database, which consists of large, relatively nonselected groups of patients, the 2-year overall survival was 68% (95% CI 66–70%) [20].

Table 1 summarises the data of numerous prospective and retrospective studies of treatment outcome following SABR for medically inoperable stage I NSCLC. Importantly, even in a cohort of 193 stage I NSCLC patients aged 75 years or older, a reasonable 3-year overall survival rate of 45.1% was reported for SABR [34]. Senthi *et al.* [42] recently reviewed the available literature on SABR for centrally located tumours and summarised 20 eligible studies. Cause-specific survival at 2–3 years was reported to be greater than 80%, with high local control rates [29, 30, 38]. Regional and distant control rates specifically for stage I NSCLC have scarcely been published, and it is known that outcome for peripheral and central tumours was reported to be identical (3-year rates were 86% and 75% *versus* 91% and 73%, respectively) [34]. Care should be taken to limit waiting time between the diagnostic $^{18}$F-fluordeoxyglucose (FDG)-PET/CT scan and initiation of SABR to avoid progression in tumour size, metabolic tumour activity, and regional and distant disease [43]. Importantly, the patterns of failure for stage I NSCLC patients following surgery (*i.e.* lobectomy/pneumonectomy) or SABR were found to be comparable and this variable should, therefore, not be taken into account in the decision-making process [44].

Palma *et al.* [45] found evidence for the increasing number of stage I NSCLC patients being treated when SBRT/SABR was available as therapeutic option. They assessed the Amsterdam Cancer Registry in three eras (1999–2001 (pre-SABR), 2002–2004 (some

Table 1. Overview of local control and overall survival (OS) following stereotactic ablative body radiotherapy/stereotactic body radiation therapy for stage I NSCLC

| First author [ref.] | Patients n | Fractionation schedule Gy | Follow-up time months median (range) | Local control rate % (at time years) | OS months median | 1-year OS % | 3-year OS % |
|---|---|---|---|---|---|---|---|
| **Baumann [23]** | 60 | 3×15 | 23 (3–42) | 96 (2.2) | NA | NA | NA |
| **Chang [24]** | 27 | 4×10, 4×12.5 | 17 (6–40) | 100$^{\#}$ | NA | NA | NA |
| **Fakiris [25]** | 70 | 3×20, 3×22 | 50.2 (1.4–64.8) | 88.1 (3) | 32.4 | NA | 42.7 |
| **Kopek [26]** | 88 | 3×15, 3×22.5 | 44 (1.6–96.5) | 89 (4) | 21.8 | 67 | 36 |
| **Milano [27]** | 53 | 30–63×2.5–5 | | 73 (2) | NA | 72 (2 years) | NA |
| **Stephans [28]** | 92 | 3×20, 5×10, 10×5 | 18.4 (1.7–48) | 98 (NA) | 18 | NA | NA |
| **Baba [29]** | 124 | 4×11, 4×12, 4×13 | NA | 80 (3) | NA | NA | 71 |
| **Bradley [30]** | 91 | 3×18, 5×9 | 18 (6–42) | 86 (2) | NA | NA | NA |
| **Ricardi [31]** | 62 | 3×15 | 28 (9–60.7) | 87.8 (3) | NA | NA | 57.1 |
| **Timmerman [22]** | 59 | 3×18 | 34.4 (4.8–49.9) | 97.6 (3) | 48.1 | NA | 55.8 |
| **Andratschke [32]** | 92 | 3–5×7–15 | NA | 64 (3) | 29 | 79 | 17 |
| **Bral [33]** | 40 | 3×20 | 16 (5–33) | 97 (1) | NA | 52 (2 years) | NA |
| **Haasbeek [34]** | 63 | 8×7.5 | 35 | 92.6 (3) | 47 | NA | 64.3 |
| **Olsen [35]** | 130 | 5×9, 5×10, 3×18 | 11, 16, 13 | 75, 100, 99 (1) | 14, NR, 34 | NA | NA |
| **Chang [36]** | 130 | 4×12.5 | 26 (6–78) | 98.5 (2) | 60 | 93.0 | 65.3 |
| **Janssen [37]** | 65 | 3×12.5, 8×6 | 13.8 (1–41) | 93 (1) | NA | 79 | NA |
| **Nuyttens [38]** | 56 | 6×8, 5×9, 5×10, 5×12 | 23 | 91 (1) | NA | 53 (2 years) | NA |
| **Duncker-Rohr [39]** | 39 | 5×7, 3×12.5 | NA | 95 (1) | NA | 65.4 | NA |
| **Lee [40]** | 58 (40 primary, 18 recurrent) | 30–60 in median 5 fractions | 23.8 (1.5–77.2) | 95.3 (1)$^{¶}$, 77.9 (3)$^{+}$ | NA | 55.6 (2 years) | NA |
| **Videtic [41]** | 80 | 1×30, 1×34 | 18.7 (1.8–43.0), 17.8 (0.1–39.4) | 98 (1), 86.2 (1) | NA | 75.0, 64.0 | NA |

NA: not available; NR: not reached. $^{\#}$: for 50-Gy cohort; $^{¶}$: at 1 year; $^{+}$: at 3 years.

availability of SABR) and 2005–2007 (full access to SABR)), and compared treatment patterns and overall survival in three treatment groups (surgery, radiotherapy or no therapy). In total, 875 patients diagnosed with stage I NSCLC met the inclusion criteria. Primary treatment was surgery in 299 (34%) patients, SBRT/SABR in 299 (34%) patients and neither in 277 (32%) patients. Over time, the proportion of patients undergoing radiotherapy increased significantly (26% in the era 1999–2001 to 42% in the timespan 2005–2007), with correspondingly fewer patients receiving no treatment at all (38% to 26%, respectively). The 30-day mortality calculated from the date of treatment was 7.4% for the surgical cohort as compared with 1.0% for radiotherapy. Estimated overall survival rates for the surgically treated patients were 34, 30 and 36 months, respectively, for the three consecutive eras, as compared with 20, 18 and 26 months for the radiotherapy cohort. For patients not receiving treatment, median overall survival was 6 months with 21% dying within 30 days of diagnosis. In summary, the introduction of SBRT/SABR was associated with a significant increase in radiotherapy usage, a decline in the proportion of untreated elderly patients, and an improved overall survival rate.

Apart from the effectiveness of SBRT/SABR, and the favourable outcome both in clinical practice and when compared to best supportive care, the radiation dose delivered to the stage I NSCLC patients may be of importance. Van Baardwijk *et al.* [46], therefore, analysed the freedom from local progression in patients treated with SBRT/SABR or accelerated high-dose conventional radiotherapy. The delivered dose was converted to a dose in 2-Gy fractions calculated from the periphery of the planning target volume (PTV). The authors concluded that fractionated and accelerated schedules with equivalent biological doses achieved the same tumour control rates as SBRT/SABR. Thus, lower, but more uniform, doses than the entire PTV may be sufficient to achieve similar control rates, and adapted fractionation schedules in proximity of radiation-sensitive structures may be safely applied.

## Toxicity

The toxicity of SBRT/SABR is favourable: approximately 3% of the patients experience significant side-effects (Common Terminology Criteria for Adverse Events grade ⩾3), which makes this treatment modality also suitable for elderly and/or frail patients [22, 47].

### Pulmonary toxicity

When embarking on SABR for pulmonary lesions, radiation treatment was generally delivered in 2-Gy fractions and traditional dose constraints predicting normal tissue complication probability rates based thereupon were potentially unreliable. Most patients referred for SABR were medically inoperable due to pulmonary comorbidity and compromised lung function (measured by FEV1 and *D*LCO). Despite this, pulmonary toxicity following SABR has been found to be remarkably low. In 88 stage I lung cancer patients treated with SABR reported on by Kopek *et al.* [26], four patients deteriorated in performance status by ⩾3 grade points and one patient had a 3-grade-point worsening of dyspnoea. In 130 patients with stage I NSCLC undergoing SABR (50 Gy in four fractions), 15 patients developed radiation pneumonitis (12 patients grade 2 and three patients grade 3) with a median time to onset of 4 months (range 1–11 months) [36]. In-depth analysis showed that dosimetric variables (lung volumes receiving a dose between 5 and 40 Gy as well as the mean lung doses) were associated with the incidence of grade 2 to 3 radiation pneumonitis, whereas other patient characteristics (FEV1, tumour location, performance status and gross tumour volume) were not. Interestingly, Henderson *et al.* [48] found pulmonary toxicity grade 2 or greater not to depend on the baseline *D*LCO or baseline FEV1. Pulmonary function (FEV1 and *D*LCO) does not deteriorate after SABR, even in individuals with a bad baseline lung function [49]. SABR is therefore not contraindicated in patients with severe COPD.

## Oesophageal toxicity

Stephans *et al.* [50] assessed risk factors for grade ⩾3 late oesophageal toxicity after SABR to lesions in the lung or liver. This retrospective analysis included 52 patients treated with a median dose of 50 Gy in five fractions (range 37.5–60 Gy in three to 10 fractions) and the median maximum dose to 1 $cm^3$ of the oesophagus (oesophageal 1-$cm^3$ dose) was 24.0 Gy (range 7.8–50.9 Gy). The risk of fistula for oesophageal 1-$cm^3$ doses exceeding 40, 45 and 50 Gy was 25% (two out of nine subjects), 50% (two out of four subjects) and 50% (two out of four subjects), respectively. Noteworthy, the two patients with fistula received adjuvant antiangiogenic agents (VEGF) within 2 months of completing SABR.

## Toxicity to bone and skin

In tumours located in proximity of the chest wall, complications of the skin, subcutaneous tissue, bone and peripheral nervous system may arise. Kopek *et al.* [26] reported on seven cases of rib fracture, all of which occurred between 9 and 24 months of treatment. Chang *et al.* [36] reported 12 patients to have developed chest wall pain (11 grade 2 and one grade 3) with a median onset time after SABR of 8 months (range 0–27 months). Furthermore, eight patients in the cohort had grade 2 or 3 dermatitis (median onset time 2 months, range 0–10 months). The VU University Medical Center group (Amsterdam, the Netherlands) [51] published the incidence of chest wall pain and rib fractures in a cohort of 500 patients (with 530 tumours) treated with risk-adapted SABR: 3×20 Gy for T1 tumours not adjacent to the chest wall, 5×12 Gy for T1 lesions in broad contact with the chest wall and for T2 tumours, and 8×7.5 Gy for central lesions. Chest wall pain was reported in 57 (11.4%) patients and scored as grade 3 in 10 (20%) patients. Most patients (6.4%) developed their complaints within 3 months of the start of SABR. Rib fractures developed in eight patients at a median time of 24 months of the start of SABR (range 6–27 months). Factors univariately predicting chest wall pain were smaller tumour-to-chest-wall distance, larger tumour diameters and larger treatment volumes. The first factor also predicted rib fractures. The fractionation schedule was not a significant risk factor for chest-wall toxicity.

## Toxicity of mediastinal structures

More serious complications, such as bronchial stenosis, airway necrosis, fatal haemoptysis, pericardial effusion have been reported after SABR of centrally located tumours [33, 52–54]. Although it has been suggested that centrally located tumours can be treated with SABR, extreme hypofractionation schedules such as 54 Gy delivered in three fractions have not been delivered in these series. Most authors used a more fractionated schedule, such as 60 Gy in eight to 10 fractions, and even then it is unclear what is meant by a "central" tumour. No detailed evaluation of the dose–volume relationship of critical organs has been published and many institutions allow a lower dose in the PTV when it overlaps with critical central structures such as the pulmonary artery. As a consequence, the PTV dose homogeneity may have been compromised. This may not necessarily compromise local tumour control but this should not be interpreted as an argument that some central structures may tolerate ablative radiation doses. On top of that, all series are retrospective. Therefore, the European Organisation for Research and Treatment of Cancer initiated the international, multicentre phase II study of SABR/SBRT in inoperable, centrally located NSCLC treated to a dose of 60 Gy in eight fractions (LungTech, www.clinicaltrials.gov identifier number NCT01795521). The primary end-point of this study, which aims to include 150 stage I NSCLC patients, is freedom from local progression at 3 years, and the secondary end-points include acute and late toxicity, patterns of recurrence, overall survival, and cause of death. After completion of SABR, patients will be followed-up by clinical examination and FDG-PET/CT imaging. A subsequent phase III clinical study is aimed for.

Even though the summarised data underline the importance of SABR/SBRT as a therapeutic option in stage I NSCLC patients, we want to express a note of caution. The data on toxicity presented here have been acquired both in a few prospective and numerous retrospective analyses. It is well-known that the latter analyses tend to be based on nonstandardised data obtained from incomplete medical records, and may thus be an underestimation of the incidence and severity of toxicity.

## SABR as an alternative to surgery (lobectomy and sublobar resection)

Even though outcome data for SABR are favourable, no prospective study directly comparing surgery with SABR in stage I NSCLC has successfully been completed (NCT00840749 and NCT00687986). Therefore, a population-based, matched-pair comparison of SABR with lobectomy, the gold standard surgical procedure in stage I NSCLC patients, has been performed [55]. A total of 120 elderly stage I NSCLC patients treated in the Dutch provinces of North Holland and Flevoland between 2005 and 2007 were matched regarding age, stage, sex and treatment year. Details on comorbidity were lacking. Of the 61 deaths, 26 occurred in the surgery group and 35 in the SABR cohort. The 30-day mortality calculated from the start date of treatment was 8.3% for surgery and 1.7% for SABR. Dividing the 30-day mortality by age (below 80 years *versus* 80 years or older), it was 2.6% for the first and 18.2% for the latter in the surgically treated patients, as opposed to 0% and 4.4% in the patients undergoing SABR. Overall survival at 1 and 3 years was 75% and 60% after surgery and 87% and 42% after SABR, respectively. In the absence of comorbidity data, the authors hypothesised that there may have been a bias against SABR, since the SABR patients generally have more comorbidity, making them unideal candidates for surgery.

Recently, sublobar resections have gained acceptance as lung-sparing surgery in selected patients. Randomised trials comparing lobectomy to sublobar resections are ongoing. Crabtree *et al.* [56] compared short-term outcomes among three prospective clinical trials: SABR (Radiation Therapy Oncology Group 0236), sublobar resection (American College of Surgeons Oncology Group (ACOSOG) trial Z4032) and radiofrequency ablation (ACOSOG trial 4033). The 90-day mortality for SABR, surgery and radiofrequency ablation was 0%, 2.4% (five out of 211 patients) and 2.0% (one out of 51), respectively. Unadjusted 30-day adverse events of grade 3 or higher were significantly more common in the patients undergoing surgery than those treated with SABR (28% *versus* 9.1%).

Both groups, Palma *et al.* [55] and Crabtree *et al.* [56], stress the importance of performing a randomised clinical trial to define the relative survival benefit for each treatment modality and to help tailor treatment for the individual patient.

## Imaging for follow-up

Huang *et al.* [57] systematically reviewed the literature and identified high-risk CT changes (*e.g.* bulging margin, air bronchogram disappearance and increasing opacity after 12 months) as signs of disease progression after SABR. Besides, it is known that a focal increase of the maximum standardised uptake value measured by FDG-PET or FDG-PET/CT is a warning sign suggestive of disease progression after SABR [58, 59]. When surgery can be considered salvage therapy, follow-up of patients treated with SABR using serial CT scans is advised, which ought to be complemented by FDG-PET/CT in the case of suspected disease recurrence [57]. Alternative (functional) imaging modalities, such as magnetic resonance imaging, dynamic contrast-enhanced CT or dual-energy CT, may offer additional information but are thus far unexplored.

Because of the excellent local tumour control, the most important reason to follow up these patients is the occurrence of second primary lung cancer at a rate of 2–4% per year, without evidence of decreasing frequency beyond 5 and even 10 years [2].

## Shared decision-making

In the light of lacking level 1 evidence for choosing between the treatment modalities, taking into account the treatments' varying reported mortality and morbidity rates, and the patient population currently referred, it is of utmost importance to involve the patient through a shared decision-making (SDM) process. SDM is increasingly incorporated in routine clinical practice, especially in situations where treatments are equivalent or differ only marginally. Regarding treatment of stage I NSCLC patients, surgery and SABR are equally effective therapeutic options, but differ regarding risk of morbidity and 30-day mortality. Therefore, a dedicated patient decision aid providing in depth information about options, benefits, harms, and uncertainties of both treatment options should be developed. Decision aids are increasingly being used in the clinic (*e.g.* for patients with early stage prostate cancer) and are reasonably easy to design (www.eLearning4health.com). These aids may form the basis for the dialogue between the physician and patient and possibly result in less patient-experienced regret when experiencing side-effects [60–62].

## Recommendations

1) The interval between diagnostic FDG-PET/CT and initiation of SABR should be kept short, preferably less than 4 weeks to avoid disease progression (local, regional or distant).

2) SABR (*i.e.* high-dose fractionated or single high-dose treatment) is advised for peripheral tumours irrespective of the lung function. For patients with central tumours, the LungTech trial (delivering SBRT in eight fractions of 7.5 Gy) will start accrual shortly.

3) Follow-up imaging in patients with resectable disease should be performed with CT scans. FDG-PET is mandatory only in case of suspected recurrent disease.

4) Due to similar overall survival but differing toxicity patterns, patients should be offered a choice (*e.g.* by SDM).

## References


1. Oncoline. Richtlijnen oncologische zorg [Oncological care guidelines]. www.oncoline.nl Date last updated: February 17, 2015.
2. Vansteenkiste J, De Ruysscher D, Eberhardt WE, *et al.* Early and locally advanced non-small-cell lung cancer (NSCLC): ESMO Clinical Practice Guidelines for diagnosis, treatment and follow-up. *Ann Oncol* 2013; 24: Suppl. 6, vi89–vi98.
3. Martini N, Bains MS, Burt ME, *et al.* Incidence of local recurrence and second primary tumors in resected stage I lung cancer. *J Thorac Cardiovasc Surg* 1995; 109: 120–129.
4. Rami-Porta R, Ball D, Crowley J, *et al.* The IASLC Lung Cancer Staging Project: proposals for the revision of the T descriptors in the forthcoming (seventh) edition of the TNM classification for lung cancer. *J Thorac Oncol* 2007; 2: 593–602.
5. Raz DJ, Zell JA, Ou SH, *et al.* Natural history of stage I non-small cell lung cancer: implications for early detection. *Chest* 2007; 132: 193–199.
6. Wisnivesky JP, Bonomi M, Henschke C, *et al.* Radiation therapy for the treatment of unresected stage I–II non-small cell lung cancer. *Chest* 2005; 128: 1461–1467.
7. Edwards BK, Howe HL, Ries LA, *et al.* Annual report to the nation on the status of cancer, 1973–1999, featuring implications of age and aging on U.S. cancer burden. *Cancer* 2002; 94: 2766–2792.
8. Palma DA, Tyldesley S, Sheehan F, *et al.* Stage I non-small cell lung cancer (NSCLC) in patients aged 75 years and older: does age determine survival after radical treatment? *J Thorac Oncol* 2010; 5: 818–824.
9. Sigel K, Bonomi M, Packer S, *et al.* Effect of age on survival of clinical stage I non-small-cell lung cancer. *Ann Surg Oncol* 2009; 16: 1912–1917.
10. Owonikoko TK, Ragin CC, Belani CP, *et al.* Lung cancer in elderly patients: an analysis of the surveillance, epidemiology, and end results database. *J Clin Oncol* 2007; 25: 5570–5577.
11. Janssen-Heijnen ML, Schipper RM, Razenberg PP, *et al.* Prevalence of co-morbidity in lung cancer patients and its relationship with treatment: a population-based study. *Lung Cancer* 1998; 21: 105–113.
12. Rowell NP, Williams CJ. Radical radiotherapy for stage I/II non-small cell lung cancer in patients not sufficiently fit for or declining surgery (medically inoperable). *Cochrane Database Syst Rev* 2001; CD002935.
13. Ong CL, Verbakel WF, Cuijpers JP, *et al.* Stereotactic radiotherapy for peripheral lung tumors: a comparison of volumetric modulated arc therapy with 3 other delivery techniques. *Radiother Oncol* 2010; 97: 437–442.
14. Ong CL, Palma D, Verbakel WF, *et al.* Treatment of large stage I–II lung tumors using stereotactic body radiotherapy (SBRT): planning considerations and early toxicity. *Radiother Oncol* 2010; 97: 431–436.
15. Chi A, Liao Z, Nguyen NP, *et al.* Systemic review of the patterns of failure following stereotactic body radiation therapy in early stage non-small-cell lung cancer: clinical implications. *Radiother Oncol* 2010; 94: 1–11.
16. Cuijpers JP, Verbakel WF, Slotman BJ, *et al.* A novel simple approach for incorporation of respiratory motion in stereotactic treatments of lung tumors. *Radiother Oncol* 2010; 97: 443–448.
17. Han K, Cheung P, Basran PS, *et al.* A comparison of two immobilization systems for stereotactic body radiation therapy of lung tumors. *Radiother Oncol* 2010; 95: 103–108.
18. De Ruysscher D, Nakagawa K, Asamura H. Surgical and nonsurgical approaches to small-size nonsmall cell lung cancer. *Eur Respir J* 2014; 44: 483–494.
19. Nestle U, Faivre-Finn C, DeRuysscher D, *et al.* Stereotactic body radiotherapy (SBRT) in central non-small cell lung cancer (NSCLC): solid evidence or "no-go"? *Radiother Oncol* 2013; 109: 178–179.
20. Solda F, Lodge M, Ashley S, *et al.* Stereotactic radiotherapy (SABR) for the treatment of primary non-small cell lung cancer; systematic review and comparison with a surgical cohort. *Radiother Oncol* 2013; 109: 1–7.
21. Taremi M, Hope A, Dahele M, *et al.* Stereotactic body radiotherapy for medically inoperable lung cancer: prospective, single-center study of 108 consecutive patients. *Int J Radiat Oncol Biol Phys* 2012; 82: 967–973.
22. Timmerman R, Paulus R, Galvin J, *et al.* Stereotactic body radiation therapy for inoperable early stage lung cancer. *JAMA* 2010; 303: 1070–1076.
23. Baumann P, Nyman J, Hoyer M, *et al.* Stereotactic body radiotherapy for medically inoperable patients with stage I non-small cell lung cancer – a first report of toxicity related to COPD/CVD in a non-randomized prospective phase II study. *Radiother Oncol* 2008; 88: 359–367.
24. Chang JY, Balter PA, Dong L, *et al.* Stereotactic body radiation therapy in centrally and superiorly located stage I or isolated recurrent non-small-cell lung cancer. *Int J Radiat Oncol Biol Phys* 2008; 72: 967–971.
25. Fakiris AJ, McGarry RC, Yiannoutsos CT, *et al.* Stereotactic body radiation therapy for early stage non-small-cell lung carcinoma: four-year results of a prospective phase II study. *Int J Radiat Oncol Biol Phys* 2009; 75: 677–682.
26. Kopek N, Paludan M, Petersen J, *et al.* Co-morbidity index predicts for mortality after stereotactic body radiotherapy for medically inoperable early stage non-small cell lung cancer. *Radiother Oncol* 2009; 93: 402–407.
27. Milano MT, Chen Y, Katz AW, *et al.* Central thoracic lesions treated with hypofractionated stereotactic body radiotherapy. *Radiother Oncol* 2009; 91: 301–306.

28. Stephans KL, Djemil T, Reddy CA, *et al.* A comparison of two stereotactic body radiation fractionation schedules for medically inoperable stage I non-small cell lung cancer: the Cleveland Clinic experience. *J Thorac Oncol* 2009; 4: 976–982.
29. Baba F, Shibamoto Y, Ogino H, *et al.* Clinical outcomes of stereotactic body radiotherapy for stage I non-small cell lung cancer using different doses depending on tumor size. *Radiat Oncol* 2010; 5: 81.
30. Bradley JD, El Naqa I, Drzymala RE, *et al.* Stereotactic body radiation therapy for early stage non-small-cell lung cancer: the pattern of failure is distant. *Int J Radiat Oncol Biol Phys* 2010; 77: 1146–1150.
31. Ricardi U, Filippi AR, Guarneri A, *et al.* Stereotactic body radiation therapy for early stage non-small cell lung cancer: results of a prospective trial. *Lung Cancer* 2010; 68: 72–77.
32. Andratschke N, Zimmermann F, Boehm E, *et al.* Stereotactic radiotherapy of histologically proven inoperable stage I non-small cell lung cancer: patterns of failure. *Radiother Oncol* 2011; 101: 245–249.
33. Bral S, Gevaert T, Linthout N, *et al.* Prospective, risk-adapted strategy of stereotactic body radiotherapy for early stage non-small-cell lung cancer: results of a Phase II trial. *Int J Radiat Oncol Biol Phys* 2011; 80: 1343–1349.
34. Haasbeek CJ, Lagerwaard FJ, Slotman BJ, *et al.* Outcomes of stereotactic ablative radiotherapy for centrally located early stage lung cancer. *J Thorac Oncol* 2011; 6: 2036–2043.
35. Olsen JR, Robinson CG, El Naqa I, *et al.* Dose-response for stereotactic body radiotherapy in early stage non-small-cell lung cancer. *Int J Radiat Oncol Biol Phys* 2011; 81: e299–e303.
36. Chang JY, Liu H, Balter P, *et al.* Clinical outcome and predictors of survival and pneumonitis after stereotactic ablative radiotherapy for stage I non-small cell lung cancer. *Radiat Oncol* 2012; 7: 152.
37. Janssen S, Dickgreber NJ, Koenig C, *et al.* Image-guided hypofractionated small volume radiotherapy of non-small cell lung cancer – feasibility and clinical outcome. *Onkologie* 2012; 35: 408–412.
38. Nuyttens JJ, van der Voort van Zyp NC, Praag J, *et al.* Outcome of four-dimensional stereotactic radiotherapy for centrally located lung tumors. *Radiother Oncol* 2012; 102: 383–387.
39. Duncker-Rohr V, Nestle U, Momm F, *et al.* Stereotactic ablative radiotherapy for small lung tumors with a moderate dose. Favorable results and low toxicity *Strahlenther Onkol* 2013; 189: 33–40.
40. Lee DS, Kim YS, Yoo Ie R, *et al.* Long term clinical experience of high-dose ablative lung radiotherapy: high pre-treatment [18F]fluorodeoxyglucose-positron emission tomography maximal standardized uptake value of the primary tumor adversely affects treatment outcome. *Lung Cancer* 2013; 80: 172–178.
41. Videtic GM, Stephans KL, Woody NM, *et al.* 30 Gy or 34 Gy? Comparing 2 single-fraction SBRT dose schedules for stage I medically inoperable non-small cell lung cancer. *Int J Radiat Oncol Biol Phys* 2014; 90: 203–208.
42. Senthi S, Haasbeek CJ, Slotman BJ, *et al.* Outcomes of stereotactic ablative radiotherapy for central lung tumours: a systematic review. *Radiother Oncol* 2013; 106: 276–282.
43. Murai T, Shibamoto Y, Baba F, *et al.* Progression of non-small-cell lung cancer during the interval before stereotactic body radiotherapy. *Int J Radiat Oncol Biol Phys* 2012; 82: 463–467.
44. Robinson CG, DeWees TA, El Naqa IM, *et al.* Patterns of failure after stereotactic body radiation therapy or lobar resection for clinical stage I non-small-cell lung cancer. *J Thorac Oncol* 2013; 8: 192–201.
45. Palma D, Visser O, Lagerwaard FJ, *et al.* Impact of introducing stereotactic lung radiotherapy for elderly patients with stage I non-small-cell lung cancer: a population-based time-trend analysis. *J Clin Oncol* 2010; 28: 5153–5159.
46. van Baardwijk A, Tome WA, van Elmpt W, *et al.* Is high-dose stereotactic body radiotherapy (SBRT) for stage I non-small cell lung cancer (NSCLC) overkill? A systematic review. *Radiother Oncol* 2012; 105: 145–149.
47. Shibamoto Y, Hashizume C, Baba F, *et al.* Stereotactic body radiotherapy using a radiobiology-based regimen for stage I nonsmall cell lung cancer: a multicenter study. *Cancer* 2012; 118: 2078–2084.
48. Henderson M, McGarry R, Yiannoutsos C, *et al.* Baseline pulmonary function as a predictor for survival and decline in pulmonary function over time in patients undergoing stereotactic body radiotherapy for the treatment of stage I non-small-cell lung cancer. *Int J Radiat Oncol Biol Phys* 2008; 72: 404–449.
49. Widder J, Postmus D, Ubbels JF, *et al.* Survival and quality of life after stereotactic or 3D-conformal radiotherapy for inoperable early stage lung cancer. *Int J Radiat Oncol Biol Phys* 2011; 81: e291–e297.
50. Stephans KL, Djemil T, Diaconu C, *et al.* Esophageal dose tolerance to hypofractionated stereotactic body radiation therapy: risk factors for late toxicity. *Int J Radiat Oncol Biol Phys* 2014; 90: 197–202.
51. Bongers EM, Haasbeek CJ, Lagerwaard FJ, *et al.* Incidence and risk factors for chest wall toxicity after risk-adapted stereotactic radiotherapy for early stage lung cancer. *J Thorac Oncol* 2011; 6: 2052–2057.
52. Song SY, Choi W, Shin SS, *et al.* Fractionated stereotactic body radiation therapy for medically inoperable stage I lung cancer adjacent to central large bronchus. *Lung Cancer* 2009; 66: 89–93.
53. Timmerman R, McGarry R, Yiannoutsos C, *et al.* Excessive toxicity when treating central tumors in a phase II study of stereotactic body radiation therapy for medically inoperable early stage lung cancer. *J Clin Oncol* 2006; 24: 4833–4839.
54. Corradetti MN, Haas AR, Rengan R. Central-airway necrosis after stereotactic body-radiation therapy. *N Engl J Med* 2012; 366: 2327–2329.
55. Palma D, Visser O, Lagerwaard FJ, *et al.* Treatment of stage I NSCLC in elderly patients: a population-based matched-pair comparison of stereotactic radiotherapy *versus* surgery. *Radiother Oncol* 2011; 101: 240–244.

56. Crabtree T, Puri V, Timmerman R, *et al.* Treatment of stage I lung cancer in high-risk and inoperable patients: comparison of prospective clinical trials using stereotactic body radiotherapy (RTOG 0236), sublobar resection (ACOSOG Z4032), and radiofrequency ablation (ACOSOG Z4033). *J Thorac Cardiovasc Surg* 2013; 145: 692–699.
57. Huang K, Dahele M, Senan S, *et al.* Radiographic changes after lung stereotactic ablative radiotherapy (SABR) – can we distinguish recurrence from fibrosis? A systematic review of the literature. *Radiother Oncol* 2012; 102: 335–342.
58. Hicks RJ. Role of $^{18}$F-FDG PET in assessment of response in non-small cell lung cancer. *J Nucl Med* 2009; 50: Suppl. 1, 31S–42S.
59. Takeda A, Kunieda E, Fujii H, *et al.* Evaluation for local failure by $^{18}$F-FDG PET/CT in comparison with CT findings after stereotactic body radiotherapy (SBRT) for localized non-small-cell lung cancer. *Lung Cancer* 2013; 79: 248–253.
60. van Tol-Geerdink JJ, Stalmeier PF, van Lin EN, *et al.* Do patients with localized prostate cancer treatment really want more aggressive treatment? *J Clin Oncol* 2006; 24: 4581–4586.
61. Schrijvers J, Vanderhaegen J, Van Poppel H, *et al.* How do patients between the age of 65 and 75 use a web-based decision aid for treatment choice in localized prostate cancer? *J Evid Base Med* 2013; 6: 167–172.
62. Isebaert S, Van Audenhove C, Haustermans K, *et al.* Evaluating a decision aid for patients with localized prostate cancer in clinical practice. *Urol Int* 2008; 81: 383–388.

---

Disclosures: None declared.

Chapter 12

# Mediastinal staging

Christophe Dooms[1], Herbert Decaluwe[2] and Paul De Leyn[2]

In the absence of distant metastasis, accurate mediastinal nodal staging is the most important prognostic factor for lung cancer. Contrast enhanced CT is an imperfect means of staging the mediastinum, but it provides information on lymph node size and anatomical borders of the nodal stations. An integrated PET-CT, guides clinicians in the next step, *i.e.* either tissue verification of mediastinal nodes or direct to surgery.

Linear endosonography has become the preferred invasive procedure to perform mediastinal nodal staging of lung cancer. A combined EBUS and oesophageal EUS approach enables systematic mediastinal nodal sampling of at least nodal stations 4R, 4L and 7.

A low threshold for considering a confirmatory video-assisted mediastinoscopy (VAM) should be maintained after a negative combined endosonography. The role of VAM has been redefined: it lowers the post-test probability after a negative endosonography to approximately 5%, and allows bimanual nodal dissection of stations 2L and 4L, which are rarely dissected at the time of lung resection.

Clinical tumour, node, metastasis (TNM) staging of lung cancer is important for each patient in order to determine the anatomic extent of the disease, define the best treatment strategy for the patient and to assess the prognosis, based on the applied stage group. In the absence of distant metastasis, accurate nodal staging guides treatment and becomes the most important prognostic factor. Each individual patient requires a probability assessment to be made on the presence of metastases in the regional lymph nodes. This probability assessment is based on imaging characteristics (contrast enhanced spiral CT scan of the chest and integrated PET-CT scans) and endoscopic and/or surgical techniques (EBUS transbronchial needle aspiration (TBNA), EUS-FNA, EUS- bronchoscopic (B) FNA, cervical mediastinoscopy, VATS). The aim of mediastinal staging is to exclude with the highest certainty and the lowest morbidity patients with mediastinal nodal disease, since these patients will not benefit from upfront surgery. The concepts of decision analysis and Bayes' theorem form the basis for a mediastinal staging strategy. The post-test probability of malignancy can be calculated based on the pre-test probability and the specific test's sensitivity and specificity. The goal of the clinical staging strategy is to lower the post-test probability sufficiently so that it falls below the testing threshold. Ideally the goal is to select a staging strategy with a post-test probability of 5% or less, which ascertains the clinician that the result is accurate. The European Society of Thoracic Surgery (ESTS) working group

[1]Dept of Respiratory Diseases, University Hospitals KU Leuven, Leuven, Belgium. [2]Dept of Thoracic Surgery, University Hospitals KU Leuven, Leuven, Belgium

Correspondence: Christophe Dooms, Dept of Respiratory Diseases, University Hospitals KU Leuven, Leuven, Belgium.
E-mail: christophe.dooms@uzleuven.be

 Print ISBN: 978-1-84984-061-3. Online ISBN: 978-1-84984-062-0. Print ISSN: 2312-508X. Online ISSN: 2312-5098.

considers a rate of unforeseen mediastinal nodal disease less than 10%, at the time of anatomic resection with lymph node dissection, as acceptable [1].

## Chest CT scan

CT scanning is an imperfect means of staging the mediastinum. Based on combined studies with 7368 patients and a mediastinal nodal disease prevalence of 30%, the median sensitivity and positive predictive value for identifying mediastinal nodal involvement were 55% and 58%, respectively, while the negative predictive value was 83% [2]. However, a contrast-enhanced multidetector CT scan has an excellent spatial resolution. As such it remains important for lung cancer staging, providing information on lymph node size and nodal station. A lymph node is pathologically enlarged when it is 10 mm or larger, in short axis. The anatomical borders of the lymph node stations are clearly defined from a CT scan, which did result in an internationally accepted nodal map [3]. It is important to realise that the oncological mediastinal midline is located at the left paratracheal margin. A CT scan may help select the appropriate procedure for tissue sampling, due to the anatomical images it provides.

## Integrated PET-CT scan

A noninvasive assessment of mediastinal lymph nodes by PET with F18-fluorodeoxyglucose (FDG) is more accurate than a CT scan alone [4]. A Cochrane review evaluated the integrated PET-CT for assessing mediastinal lymph node involvement in resectable NSCLC [5]. The summary sensitivity and specificity for studies applying a visual interpretation with FDG activity more than background of mediastinal blood pool as positivity criterion (n=2823; prevalence of mediastinal nodal disease 29%) were 77% (95% CI 65–86%) and 90% (95% CI 85–94%), respectively. The summary for the sensitivity and specificity for the studies applying a standardised uptake value (SUV) measurement, with $SUV_{max} \geqslant 2.5$ as positivity criterion (n=1656, prevalence of mediastinal nodal disease 28%), were 81% (95% CI 70–89%) and 79% (95% CI 70–87%), respectively [5]. These results varied, greatly, between the studies in each analysis. The review showed that the accuracy of PET-CT scanning is insufficient to allow management using a PET-CT scan alone; however, PET-CT can be used to guide clinicians in the next step (either a biopsy or direct to surgery). The suboptimal specificity of mediastinal lymph nodes found positive on PET-CT scan, require tissue confirmation. There are additional conditions where invasive staging is also mandatory, despite a normal mediastinum on PET-CT, as the prevalence of N2/N3 disease remains significant. These conditions include a primary tumour >3 cm, any central primary tumour, PET/CT hilar N1 disease, and low FDG uptake in the primary tumour [6]. A recent meta-analysis has shown that the negative predictive value of PET-CT scans for tumours ⩽3 cm was 94% (n=649), compared to 89% for tumours >3 cm (n=130) staged as T2 (6th Edition of TNM Atlas [7]) [8]. This finding was confirmed in a recent prospective study from Spain [9]. For peripheral tumours ⩽3 cm the negative predictive value of PET-CT was 92% while it was 85% for tumours>3 cm [9]. Lee *et al.* [10] examined the prevalence of pathologic N2 disease in patients with clinical stage I NSCLC [7], with negative mediastinum on PET and CT images. N2 disease was found in 2.9% of peripheral tumours (the outer third of the lung), while the prevalence of N2 disease was 21.6% in central tumours. Based on these studies, further mediastinal staging can be omitted for peripheral tumours ⩽3 cm without enlarged (hilar and/or mediastinal) lymph nodes on CT images and with PET-negative nodes. In a study from Japan, 30% of 143 patients with N1 disease found after a CT-scan (lymph node short axis >1 cm) were found to have pathologic N2–N3 [11]. Similarly, a recent prospective study on clinical N1 lung cancer (mainly PET positive hilar nodes) found a microscopic N2/3 rate of 24% [12].

## Cervical mediastinoscopy

A conventional cervical mediastinoscopy through a pre-tracheal suprasternal incision was introduced in 1959 and for decades considered the gold standard for invasive mediastinal nodal staging of patients with potentially operable lung cancer. Recently, a very large (n=721, prevalence of mediastinal nodal disease 47%) retrospective single centre study reported on safety and efficacy of cervical mediastinoscopy performed by general thoracic surgeons [13]. There was no mortality, a low perioperative complication rate at 1.3%, and an unexpected hospital (re)admission rate of 0.46%. The sensitivity, negative predictive value and post-test probability were 0.90 (95% CI 0.87–0.92), 0.92 (95% CI 0.90–0.94), and 0.09 (95% CI 0.07–0.11), respectively. It is performed under general anaesthesia and allows a full mapping of the ipsilateral and contralateral superior mediastinal lymph nodes. Many patients stay one night in the hospital, although it can be safely done as an outpatient procedure [14]. Since 1995, the use of video techniques has been introduced leading to video-assisted mediastinoscopy (VAM) clearly improving visualisation and teaching [15]. In addition, VAM allows bimanual dissection with possibilities to perform nodal dissection and removal rather than sampling or biopsy. This is especially important as stations 2L and 4L are rarely dissected at the time of lung resection (*i.e.* VATS or open thoracotomy), whether the primary tumour is on the right or left side. The ESTS working group recommends performing VAM [1]. A best evidence topic (108 papers published between 1989 and 2011) has been published on the safety and accuracy of VAM compared to conventional mediastinoscopy [16]. Both procedures are safe, without mortality and with low morbidity (0.83–2.9% for VAM and 0–5.3% for conventional mediastinoscopy). The negative predictive value and test accuracy were identical, although more lymph node stations are sampled by VAM.

## Left-sided VATS

Left-sided VATS is a surgical technique that enables the extraction of large tissue samples from the para-aortic lymph nodes in station 6 and subaortic lymph nodes in station 5. This is indicated when suspected (enlarged or PET-positive) lymph nodes are visualised on scans in stations 5 or 6, as these nodal stations cannot be biopsied by routine cervical mediastinoscopy or endosonography. An alternative to VATS is the left anterior mediastinotomy or an extended cervical mediastinoscopy. The latter is performed in some experienced centres with negative predictive values ranging from 0.89 to 0.97 [17].

## EUS and EBUS

In the last decade, the predominant role of cervical mediastinoscopy has been challenged by EUS and EBUS using a convex probe. This convex ultrasound transducer is located at the tip of a flexible scope and allows linear scanning parallel to the insertion direction of the flexible scope in order to assess structures around the oesophagus or central airways. A dedicated working channel allows the introduction of a needle for aspiration under real-time guidance. It is possible to visualise and sample lymph nodes with a short axis of ⩾5 mm and the optimal number of aspirations per station for nodal staging has been reported to be three [18]. Even if some ultrasound features might be predictive of lymph node malignancy, *e.g.* round shape, distinct margin or heterogeneous echogenicity, no single echogenic aspect of a visualised lymph node can exclude tissue sampling [19, 20].

When mediastinal nodal staging is required, systematic nodal sampling seems feasible but some primary choices have to be made. At least mediastinal nodal stations 4R, 4L and 7 should be sought. All FDG-positive node(s) or the largest node measuring ⩾5 mm in each nodal station should be biopsied. To avoid contamination, the order of sampling should begin at the level of N3 stations followed by N2 stations before N1. There is no evidence to suggest that sampling of all visible nodes in each nodal station is superior to a systematic nodal sampling of the largest or PET-positive node in each station. EBUS allows the exploration of the same lymph node stations as a cervical mediastinoscopy (table 1). It must be stressed that EBUS cannot access the pre-vascular nodes (station 3a), the subaortic and para-aortic nodes (stations 5 and 6) as well as the paraoesophageal and pulmonary ligament nodes (stations 8 and 9). However, some of these nodes (stations 8 and 9) can be reached using EUS-FNA, illustrating that EUS is complementary to EBUS (table 1). Several authors have, therefore, extended the use of the EBUS scope to an oesophageal exploration with EUS-bronchoscopic (B) sampling of stations 4L, 7, 8 and 9 [22, 23]. A recent randomised controlled trial (RCT) compared tolerance of EBUS-TBNA and EUS-FNA. The study concluded that EUS-FNA was associated with a shorter procedural duration ($p<0.001$), lower doses of intravenous midazolam ($p=0.02$) and higher operator satisfaction

Table 1. Accessibility to nodal stations with different sampling techniques

| | Mediastinoscopy | EBUS-TBNA | EUS-FNA |
|---|---|---|---|
| **Supraclavicular zone** | | | |
| 1 | +/– | – | – |
| **Superior mediastinal nodes** | | | |
| 2R | + | + | – |
| 2L | + | + | + |
| 4R | + | + | – |
| 4L | + | + | + |
| 3a | – | – | – |
| 3p | – | +/– | +/– |
| **Aortic nodes** | | | |
| 5 | – | – | –# |
| 6 | – | – | –# |
| **Inferior mediastinal nodes** | | | |
| 7 | + | + | + |
| 8 | – | – | + |
| 9 | – | – | + |
| **N1 nodes** | | | |
| 10 hilar | +/– | + | +/– |
| 11 interlobar | – | + | – |
| 12 lobar | – | + | – |

TBNA: transbronchial needle aspiration; FNA: fine-needle aspiration. +: accessible; –: inaccessible; +/–: may be accessible. #: casuistic reports that it is feasible. Reproduced and modified from [21] with permission from the publisher.

($p<0.001$), while no significant difference was observed in patient tolerance [24]. In terms of safety, EBUS (within a recent prospective registry) and EUS (within a recent systematic review) have a low complication or serious adverse event rate of 1.4 and 0.3%, respectively [25, 26].

The two staging strategies proposed in the 2007 ESTS guidelines, surgical staging alone on the one hand and combined EUS/EBUS followed by surgical staging, whenever endosonography was negative, on the other hand, were compared in a pivotal RCT [27, 28]. It was concluded that invasive mediastinal nodal staging should start with combined linear endosonography, as the trial showed that a staging strategy starting with combined linear endosonography (EUS+EBUS) detected significantly ($p=0.02$) more mediastinal nodal N2/N3 disease compared to cervical mediastinoscopy alone, resulting in a significantly higher sensitivity of 0.94 (95% CI 0.85–0.98) compared to 0.79 (95% CI 0.66–0.88), respectively [28]. Another RCT did compare two strategies of combined (both the oesophageal and airway route were performed using an EBUS-scope) linear endosonography by randomising towards either an EUS-B centred approach (commencing with the oesophageal route) or an EBUS centred approach (commencing with the airway route) [29]. There was no significant difference in overall diagnostic accuracy between both arms [29]. The EBUS-centred approach did not result in a statistical significant increase in sensitivity when an EUS-B procedure was added, but a nodal stage shift was observed in 7% of patients based on the second (EUS-B) procedure. The EUS-centred approach resulted in a significant increase in sensitivity when an EBUS procedure was added, responsible for a nodal stage shift in 48% of patients. This study suggested that EBUS-TBNA is the preferred primary procedure in combined linear endosonography for mediastinal nodal staging of resectable stage I–III lung cancer [29]. There is no RCT comparing combined EBUS-EUS(-B) to EBUS-TBNA alone for mediastinal nodal staging, but a meta-analysis suggested that the combined EBUS-EUS is more sensitive than EBUS-TBNA alone to detect mediastinal nodal disease [30]. The absolute increase in sensitivity of the combined approach compared to EBUS-TBNA alone depends on the quality of the EBUS-TBNA procedure, but published studies suggest an increase in sensitivity up to 10% [22, 23, 29, 31]. An unsolved issue is how the combined EBUS-EUS procedure should be applied in the staging process of patients with lung cancer. Should invasive mediastinal nodal staging using EUS or EUS-B be considered as "selected complementary to EBUS" for mediastinal station(s), which inaccessible or difficult to access by EBUS, or should EUS or EUS-B be "systematically combined with EBUS" in all patients and in all accessible nodal stations. There is no RCT comparing these strategies and as such no definite answer can be given.

A meta-analysis on combined linear endosonography, which included studies until 2011, reported a post-test probability of 0.15 (95% CI 0.09–0.25). This implied that the probability of having mediastinal nodal involvement for the individual patient with a negative combined linear endosonography result is not low enough to directly proceed to an anatomical surgical resection [30]. Several prospective cohort studies on combined EBUS+EUS(-B) linear endosonography have been reported since 2011, confirming that endosonography is the standard test for initial complete invasive mediastinal nodal staging with a post-test probability of around 0.10 (table 2). Overall, a confirmatory VAM is still warranted as this further lowers the post-test probability to 0.05. This has been clearly shown within the ASTER trial (Assessment of Surgical sTaging *vs* Endoscopic Ultrasound in Lung Cancer: a Randomized Clinical Trial) for patients with a radiographical abnormal mediastinum on either a CT and/or a PET scan image (clinical stage III lung cancer, prevalence of mediastinal nodal disease 63%), as the post-test probability of a negative linear combined endosonography

Table 2. Prospective studies[#] on combined endosonography for mediastinal nodal staging and with surgical lymph node dissection at resection as gold standard

| First author [ref.] | Endosonography combined modality | Clinical stage lung cancer on imaging | Prevalence N2/3 % | Patients n | | Sensitivity (95% CI) | NPV (95% CI) | Post-test probability (95% CI) |
|---|---|---|---|---|---|---|---|---|
| | | | | Included | Analysed | | | |
| Wallace [32] | EBUS+EUS | I–III | 30 | 138 | 134 | 0.93 (0.79–0.98) | 0.97 (0.90–0.99) | 0.03 (0.01–0.10) |
| Szlubowski [33] | EUS+EBUS | I–II | 23 | 120 | 120 | 0.68 (0.48–0.83) | 0.91 (0.83–0.95) | 0.10 (0.05–0.19) |
| Herth [22] | EBUS+EUS-B | II–III | 51 | 150 | 139 | 0.96 (0.87–0.99) | 0.96 (0.87–0.99) | 0.04 (0.01–0.13) |
| Annema [28] | EUS+EBUS | I–III | 54 | 123 | 123 | 0.85 (0.74–0.92) | 0.85 (0.75–0.92) | 0.15 (0.10–0.25) |
| Hwangbo [23] | EBUS+EUS-B | I–III | 31 | 150 | 143 | 0.91 (0.78–0.97) | 0.96 (0.90–0.99) | 0.04 (0.02–0.11) |
| Ohnishi [31] | EBUS+EUS | I–III | 28 | 115 | 110 | 0.84 (0.66–0.94) | 0.94 (0.86–0.98) | 0.06 (0.03–0.15) |
| Kang [29] | EBUS+EUS-B | I–III | 40 | 160 | 148 | 0.88 (0.76–0.95) | 0.93 (0.85–0.97) | 0.08 (0.04–0.16) |
| Oki [34] | EBUS+EUS-B | I–III | 23 | 150 | 150 | 0.69 (0.51–0.83) | 0.91 (0.85–0.95) | 0.10 (0.05–0.17) |
| Liberman [35] | EBUS+EUS | I–IV[¶] | 32 | 166 | 166 | 0.89 (0.76–0.95) | 0.95 (0.89–0.98) | 0.05 (0.02–0.12) |
| Dooms [12] | EBUS+/-EUS(-B) | II | 24 | 100 | 100 | 0.38 (0.18–0.57) | 0.81 (0.71–0.91) | 0.19 (0.13–0.27) |

NPV: negative predictive value; B: bronchoscopic. [#]: studies contained >50 patients; [¶]: 8% of patients included had stage IV based on PET-CT.

of 20% could be lowered to 5% by adding a cervical mediastinoscopy [36]. The situation was less clear for patients who had a normal mediastinum on a CT and PET scan image, due to a low number of patients within ASTER and a lack of other prospective clinical data. One prospective study on clinical stage I–II (n=120, prevalence of mediastinal nodal disease 23%) found a post-test probability of a negative combined endosonography of 10% [33]. However, in this study a negative endosonography was directly followed by a nodal dissection (instead of mediastinoscopy), what was striking was that the endosonography gave a false positive in two patients in the subcarinal nodal station, demonstrating that extreme care needs to be taken not to overstage a centrally located primary tumour. Another, more recent, prospective cohort study on clinical stage II lung cancer, based on the presence of clinical N1 disease on imaging (n=100, prevalence of mediastinal nodal disease 24%), showed that the post-test probability of a negative endosonography was 19%, which could be lowered to 9% by adding a cervical mediastinoscopy [12]. In addition, a confirmatory VAM could be considered part of the mediastinal nodal dissection process when surgical resection is performed.

In conclusion, combined EBUS-EUS(-B) linear endosonography is the standard for initial baseline mediastinal nodal staging and clearly reduces the need for invasive surgical mediastinal nodal staging in patients with stage I–III lung cancer. A preoperative surgical mediastinal staging procedure is still recommended in the routine clinical practice after a negative (or incomplete) combined linear endosonography.

## References

1. De Leyn P, Dooms C, Kuzdzal J, *et al.* Revised ESTS guidelines for preoperative mediastinal lymph node staging for non-small-cell lung cancer. *Eur J Cardiothorac Surg* 2014; 45: 787–798.
2. Silvestri GA, Gonzalez AV, Jantz MA, *et al.* Methods for staging non-small cell lung cancer: diagnosis and management of lung cancer, 3rd Edn: American College of Chest Physicians evidence-based clinical practice guidelines. *Chest* 2013; 143; Suppl. 5, e211s–e250s.
3. Rusch VW, Asamura H, Watanabe H, *et al.* The IASLC lung cancer staging project: a proposal for a new international lymph node map in the forthcoming seventh edition of the TNM classification for lung cancer. *J Thorac Oncol* 2009; 4: 568–577.
4. Gould MK, Kuschner WG, Rydzak CE, *et al.* Test performance of positron emission tomography and computed tomography for mediastinal staging in patients with non-small-cell lung cancer: a meta-analysis. *Ann Intern Med* 2003; 139: 879–892.
5. Schmidt-Hansen M, Baldwin DR, Hasler E, *et al.* PET-CT for assessing mediastinal lymph node involvement in patients with suspected resectable non-small cell lung cancer. *Cochrane Database Syst Rev* 2014; 11: CD009519.
6. De Leyn P, Lardinois D, Van Schil PE, *et al.* ESTS guidelines for preoperative lymph node staging for non-small cell lung cancer. *Eur J Cardiothorac Surg* 2007; 32: 1–8.
7. Wittekind C, Asamura H, Sobin LH. TNM Atlas. 6th Edn. Chichester, Wiley-Blackwell, 2014.
8. Wang J, Welch K, Wang L, *et al.* Negative predictive value of positron emission tomography for stage T1–2N0 non-small-cell lung cancer: a meta-analysis. *Clin Lung Cancer* 2012; 13: 81–89.
9. Gómez-Caro A, Boada M, Cabañas M, *et al.* False-negative rate after positron emission tomography/computer tomography scan for mediastinal staging in cI stage non-small-cell lung cancer. *Eur J Cardiothorac Surg* 2012; 42: 93–100.
10. Lee P, Port J, Korst R, *et al.* Risk factors for occult mediastinal metastases in clinical stage I non-small cell lung cancer. *Ann Thorac Surg* 2007; 84: 177–181.
11. Hishida T, Yoshida J, Nishimura M, *et al.* Problems in the current diagnostic standards of clinical N1 non-small cell lung cancer. *Thorax* 2008; 63: 526–531.
12. Dooms C, Tournoy KG, Schuurbiers O, *et al.* Endosonography for mediastinal nodal staging of clinical N1 non-small cell lung cancer: a prospective multicenter study. *Chest* 2015: 147; 209–215.
13. Wei B, Bryant A, Minnich D, *et al.* The safety and efficacy of mediastinoscopy when performed by general thoracic surgeons. *Ann Thorac Surg* 2014; 97: 1878–1884.
14. Luke WP, Pearson FG, Todd TR, *et al.* Prospective evaluation of mediastinoscopy for assessment of carcinoma of the lung. *J Thorac Cardiovasc Surg* 1986; 91: 53–56.

15. Martin-Ucar AE, Chetty GK, Vaughan R, *et al.* A prospective audit evaluating the role of video-assisted cervical mediastinoscopy (VAM) as a training tool. *Eur J Cardiothorac Surg* 2001; 26: 393–395.
16. Zakkar M, Tan C, Hunt I. Is video mediastinoscopy a safer and more effective procedure than conventional mediastinoscopy? *Interact Cardiovasc Thorac Surg* 2012; 14: 81–84.
17. Rami-Porta R, Call S. Invasive staging of mediastinal lymph nodes: mediastinoscopy and remediastinoscopy. *Thorac Surg Clin* 2012; 22: 177–189.
18. Lee HS, Lee GK, Lee HS, *et al.* Real-time endobronchial ultrasound-guided transbronchial needle aspiration in mediastinal staging of non-small cell lung cancer: how many aspirations per target lymph node station? *Chest* 2008; 134: 368–374.
19. Fujiwara T, Yasufuku K, Nakajima T, *et al.* The utility of sonographic features during endobronchial ultrasound-guided transbronchial needle aspiration for lymph node staging in patients with lung cancer: a standard endobronchial ultrasound image. *Chest* 2010; 138: 641–647.
20. Memoli JS, El-Bayoumi E, Pastis NJ, *et al.* Using endobronchial ultrasound features to predict lymph node metastasis in patients with lung cancer. *Chest* 2011; 140: 1550–1556.
21. Dooms C, Muylle I, Yserbyt J, *et al.* Endobronchial ultrasound in the management of nonsmall cell lung cancer. *Eur Respir Rev* 2013; 22: 169–177.
22. Herth FJF, Krasnik M, Kahn N, *et al.* Combined endoscopic endobronchial ultrasound-guided fine-needle aspiration of mediastinal lymph nodes through a single bronchoscope in 150 patients with suspected lung cancer. *Chest* 2010; 138: 790–794.
23. Hwangbo B, Lee GK, Lee HS, *et al.* Transbronchial and transesophageal fine-needle aspiration using an ultrasound bronchoscope in mediastinal staging of potentially operable lung cancer. *Chest* 2010; 138: 795–802.
24. Oki M, Saka H, Ando M, *et al.* Transbronchial *versus* transesophageal needle aspiration using an ultrasound bronchoscope for the diagnosis of mediastinal lesions: a randomized study. *Chest* 2014 [In press DOI: 10.1378/chest.14-1283].
25. Eapen G, Shah A, Lei X, *et al.* Complications, consequences, and practice patterns of endobronchial ultrasound-guided transbronchial needle aspiration: results of the AQuIRE registry. *Chest* 2013; 143: 1044–1053.
26. von Bartheld MB, van Breda A, Annema JT, *et al.* Complication rate of endosonography (endobronchial and endoscopic ultrasound): a systematic review. *Respiration* 2014; 87: 343–351.
27. De Leyn P, Lardinois D, Van Schil PE, *et al.* ESTS guidelines for preoperative lymph node staging for non-small cell lung cancer. *Eur J Cardiothorac Surg* 2007; 32: 1–8.
28. Annema JT, van Meerbeeck JP, Rintoul RC, *et al.* Mediastinoscopy *vs* endosonography for mediastinal nodal staging of lung cancer: a randomized trial. *JAMA* 2010; 304: 2245–2252.
29. Kang H, Hwangbo B, Lee GK, *et al.* EBUS-centered *versus* EUS-centered mediastinal staging in lung cancer: a randomised controlled trial. *Thorax* 2014; 69: 261–268.
30. Zhang R, Ying K, Shi L *et al.* Combined endobronchial and endoscopic ultrasound-guided fine needle aspiration for mediastinal lymph node staging of lung cancer: a meta-analysis. *Eur J Cancer* 2013; 49: 1860–1867.
31. Ohnishi R, Yasuda I, Kato T, *et al.* Combined endobronchial and endoscopic ultrasound-guided fine needle aspiration for mediastinal nodal staging of lung cancer. *Endoscopy* 2011; 43: 1082–1089.
32. Wallace MB, Pascual JM, Raimondo M, *et al.* Minimally invasive endoscopic staging of suspected lung cancer. *JAMA* 2008; 299: 540–546.
33. Szlubowski A, Zieliński M, Soja J, *et al.* A combined approach of endobronchial and endoscopic ultrasound-guided needle aspiration in the radiologically normal mediastinum in non-small-cell lung cancer staging: a prospective trial. *Eur J Cardiothorac Surg* 2010; 37: 1175–1179.
34. Oki M, Saka H, Ando M, *et al.* Endoscopic ultrasound-guided fine needle aspiration and endobronchial ultrasound-guided transbronchial nedle aspiration: are two better than one in mediastinal staging of non-small cell lung cancer? *J Thorac Cardiovasc Surg* 2014; 148: 1169–1177.
35. Liberman M, Sampalis J, Duranceau A, *et al.* Endosonographic mediastinal lymph node staging of lung cancer. *Chest* 2014; 146: 389–397.
36. Tournoy KG, Keller SM, Annema JT. Mediastinal staging of lung cancer: novel concepts. *Lancet Oncol* 2012; 13: e221–e229.

---

Discolsures: None declared.

# Chapter 13

# Approaches in patients with locally advanced NSCLC: a surgeon's perspective

Paul E. Van Schil, Michèle De Waele, Jeroen M. Hendriks and Patrick R. Lauwers

Locally advanced NSCLC represents a heterogeneous group of different disease entities, ranging from initially resectable to potentially resectable after induction therapy, and finally to nonresectable tumours.

In restaging after induction therapy, repeat mediastinoscopy provides pathological evidence of response after induction therapy but is less accurate than a first procedure. When N2 disease is discovered during thoracotomy after negative, careful preoperative staging, a resection should be performed if it is possible for it to be complete. In discrete N2 involvement, surgical resection may be recommended in patients with proven mediastinal downstaging after induction therapy who can preferentially be treated by lobectomy. Infiltrative, bulky N2 disease is mostly treated with combined chemoradiation. In stage IIIB NSCLC, surgical resection is only indicated in carefully selected cases. Complete resection remains the most important prognostic factor.

Every patient with locally advanced lung cancer should be discussed within a multidisciplinary tumour board. As surgical resection might be challenging in these cases, treatment in an experienced centre is recommended.

Stage III NSCLC represents locally advanced disease and consists of a heterogeneous spectrum of quite different entities regarding T and N involvement. These include upfront resectable disease, tumours that may become resectable after induction therapy and nonresectable cancers [1]. Most patients will be treated using combined modality therapy, which in many cases consists of concurrent or sequential chemoradiation. The role of surgery remains controversial in both the evaluation of the extent of these tumours and in their specific management. In a recent analysis of 83 913 patients with clinical stage IIIA-N2 disease, biopsies of lymph nodes were obtained in only 23% of patients who were treated without surgery [2]. In surgical patients, clinical N2 stage was pathologically confirmed in only 56% of treatment-naive patients. Clearly, there is room for improvement. Every patient should be discussed within a multidisciplinary team in order to determine

Dept of Thoracic and Vascular Surgery, Antwerp University Hospital, Edegem, Belgium.

Correspondence: Paul E. Van Schil, Dept of Thoracic and Vascular Surgery, Antwerp University Hospital, Wilrijkstraat 10, B-2650 Edegem, Belgium. E-mail: paul.van.schil@uza.be

 Print ISBN: 978-1-84984-061-3. Online ISBN: 978-1-84984-062-0. Print ISSN: 2312-508X. Online ISSN: 2312-5098.

the optimal diagnostic and therapeutic strategy. Technically challenging procedures should be performed in centres with considerable experience in difficult thoracic surgical procedures. The ultimate aim is still to obtain a complete resection as this is the most important prognostic factor.

In this chapter, we will discuss the precise definition of complete resection, the different indications for surgery in locally advanced disease, the current role of invasive restaging in NSCLC, and surgical treatment of stages IIIA and IIIB NSCLC. Finally, recently published guidelines on the management of locally advanced NSCLC will be discussed.

## Locally advanced NSCLC: complete resection and indications for surgery

When discussing surgical treatment for early stage or locally advanced NSCLC, the ultimate goal is to accomplish a complete resection. Although this seems rather straightforward, specific criteria remain difficult to determine. For this reason, the International Association for the Study of Lung Cancer (IASLC) created a specific subcommittee to define generally accepted criteria for complete, incomplete and so-called uncertain resections when not all criteria are fulfilled [3]. In the context of this chapter, the definition of complete or R0 resection is particularly important. It implies that macroscopically the tumour has been completely removed; on a microscopic level, all section margins are free of disease, as well the bronchial, vascular and any peripheral margins. A precise lymph node dissection is also required. The surgeon should perform a systematic lymph node dissection or at least a lobe-specific nodal dissection, removing a minimum of six lymph node stations, of which three should be in the mediastinum. Subcarinal lymph node station number 7 should always be included. Moreover, there should be no extracapsular extension in nodes removed separately or in those at the margin of the lung specimen. The highest mediastinal node must be negative. These are rather strict criteria but they constitute a complete resection of the primary tumour and draining of the lymph nodes.

Indications for surgical treatment can be subdivided into accepted, investigational and exceptional, depending on the extent of the primary tumour and lymph node involvement [4]. An overview is provided in table 1.

## Restaging after induction therapy: is there a role for invasive techniques?

The rationale for induction therapy in patients with locally advanced lung cancer consists of downstaging the disease process to increase the chances of a subsequent complete resection and to eradicate systemic micrometastases. The aims are to increase resectability, to conserve functional lung parenchyma and to prolong disease-free and overall survival. The disadvantages include potentially increased morbidity and mortality due to chemotherapy, chemoradiation or a subsequent surgical procedure. The latter is often more technically challenging due to an intense fibrotic reaction that occurs around the pulmonary vessels. Several series show that patient compliance is better for induction therapy than for adjuvant therapy [5]. Better patient selection may also occur as patients with progressive disease after induction therapy present locoregionally aggressive disease, which is unlikely to be cured by surgical resection.

Table 1. Indications for surgery in clinical stage III NSCLC

**Accepted indications, c stage IIIA**
T3N1M0 in all functionally operable patients
T4N0-1M0 in selected patients
T1-3N2M0 in occult or "surprise" N2
**Investigational, c stage IIIA**
T1-3N2M0 in discrete N2
T4N0-1M0 in certain subgroups
**Exceptional, c stages IIIA–IIIB**
T1-3N2M0 in infiltrative, bulky N2
T4N2M0 in all subgroups
T1-4N3M0 in all subgroups

Induction therapy is mostly applied in patients with N2 or N3 involvement and in those with T4 tumours considered initially nonresectable. In patients with nodal disease, there is still ongoing discussion regarding how accurate restaging procedures should be performed. As mediastinal downstaging has been shown to be an important prognostic factor, this issue deserves special attention [6–8]. A summary of available techniques and their results is provided in tables 2 and 3. Noninvasive staging techniques, such as CT, PET or combined CT-PET, are not accurate enough for precious restaging. Minimally invasive techniques have recently been introduced that represent promising staging modalities. They include transbronchial needle aspiration (TBNA), EBUS and EUS, which are increasingly used for lung cancer staging as well as restaging. However, false-negative rates of 20–30% have been reported for restaging procedures [12, 19, 20].

More invasive methods include repeat mediastinoscopy (or remediastinoscopy) and exploration *via* VATS or thoracoscopy, which are part of the armamentarium of the thoracic surgeon.

Remediastinoscopy is technically more difficult than a first procedure and has lower accuracy; however, it provides pathological proof of response after induction therapy [21]. Survival depends on the findings of remediastinoscopy. As can be expected, patients with a positive remediastinoscopy result have a poor prognosis compared to those with a negative repeat

Table 2. Restaging with PET-CT, EUS and EBUS after induction therapy

| First author [ref.] | Year | Technique | Subjects n | Sensitivity | Specificity | Accuracy |
|---|---|---|---|---|---|---|
| De Leyn [9] | 2006 | PET-CT | 30 | 77 | 92 | 83 |
| Cerfolio [10] | 2006 | PET-CT | 93 | 62 | 88 | 79 |
| Krasnik [11] | 2006 | EBUS | 83 | 70 | 100 | 75 |
| Herth [12] | 2008 | EBUS | 124 | 76[#] | 100 | 77 |
| Stigt [13] | 2009 | EUS | 25 | 92 | 100 | 92 |
| | | PET-CT | | 83 | 31 | 56 |
| von Bartheld [14] | 2011 | EUS | 58 | 44; false-negative rate 58 | NR | 60 |

Data are presented as %, unless otherwise stated. NR: not reported. #: negative predictive value was only 20%.

Table 3. Results of remediastinoscopy after induction therapy since 2005

| First author [ref.] | Year | Subjects n | Induction therapy | Morbidity | Mortality | Sensitivity | NPV | Accuracy |
|---|---|---|---|---|---|---|---|---|
| Stamatis [15] | 2005 | 165 | Chemo-radio | 2.5 | 0 | 74 | 86 | 93 |
| De Waele [8] | 2006 | 32 | Chemo (n=26), Chemo-radio (n=6) | 3.1 | 0 | 71 | 75 | 84 |
| De Leyn [9] | 2006 | 30 | Chemo | 0 | 0 | 29 | 52 | 60 |
| De Waele [16]# | 2008 | 104 | Chemo (n=79), Chemo-radio (n=25) | 3.9 | 1 | 70 | 73 | 84 |
| Marra [17]¶ | 2008 | 104 | Chemo-radio | 1.9 | 0 | 61 | 85 | 88 |
| Call [18]+ | 2011 | 84 | Chemo (n=49) Chemo-radio (n=35) | 4.0 | 1 | 74 | 79 | 87 |

Data are presented as %, unless otherwise stated. NPV: negative predictive value; chemo: chemotherapy; chemo-radio: chemoradiotherapy. #: combined, updated series; ¶: subset of patients of Stamatis *et al.* [15]; +: results of restaging after induction therapy.

procedure [8]. In a series of 104 patients at two thoracic centres in Barcelona (Spain) and Antwerp (Belgium), nodal status was found to be the only significant factor for survival in multivariate analysis [16]. The largest series of repeat mediastinoscopies was reported in 2005 and described a total of 279 repeat mediastinoscopies [15]. Results were similar in a subset of 104 patients who underwent remediastinoscopy after induction chemoradiotherapy for stage IIIA-IIIB NSCLC [17]. So, even combined chemoradiation does not give rise to increased difficulties or a lower accuracy of remediastinoscopy compared with chemotherapy alone.

Although VATS has been used for restaging, experience is limited. In a phase II study of the Cancer and Leukaemia group B (CALGB 39803), 70 patients with stage IIIA-N2 NSCLC underwent restaging using VATS [22]. A positive result was defined as pathological proof of persisting N2 disease, demonstration of pleural metastases or pleural carcinomatosis. A negative result was defined as a negative lymph node biopsy of at least three lymph node stations. Sensitivity in this series was 75%, specificity was 100% and negative predictive value was 76%. Although useful, a VATS approach is limited to one hemithorax only, requires double-lumen intubation and does not offer a higher level of accuracy than repeat mediastinoscopy.

For thoracic surgeons with no experience of remediastinoscopy, an alternative approach would be the initial use of minimally invasive staging procedures such as TBNA, EBUS or EUS to obtain cytological proof of mediastinal nodal involvement [21]. After induction therapy, patients are subsequently restaged using mediastinoscopy. In this way, technically more demanding remediastinoscopy can be avoided but prospective validation is necessary [23]. Figure 1 presents the restaging algorithm currently used at our institute, the Antwerp University Hospital (Edegem, Belgium).

## Stage IIIA NSCLC

Stage IIIA NSCLC consists of a heterogeneous spectrum of locally advanced disease. The different subgroups are listed in table 1.

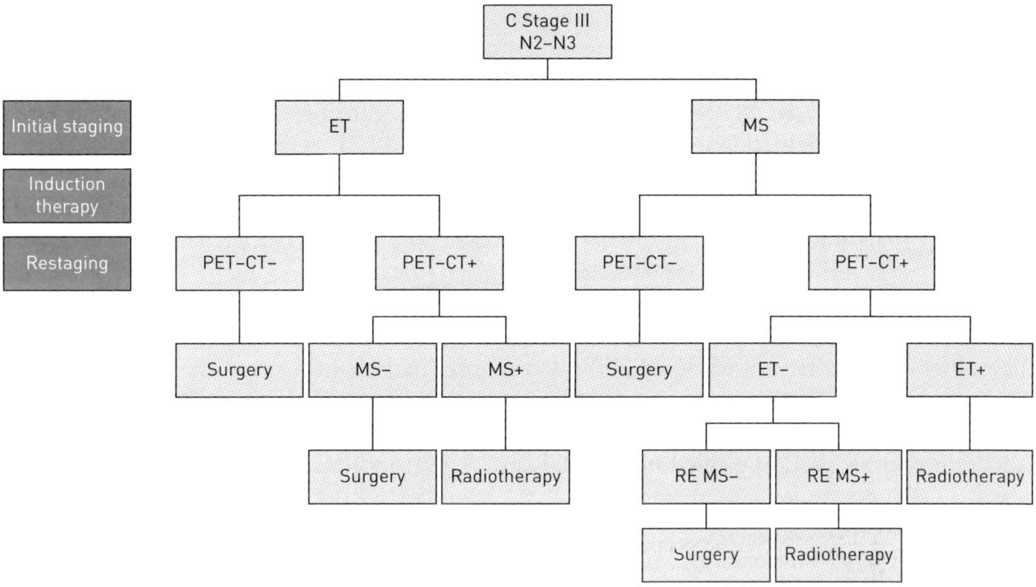


Figure 1. Restaging algorithm currently used at the Antwerp University Hospital (Edegem, Belgium) depending on whether initial proof of N2 disease was obtained using an endosonographic technique (ET) (such as EBUS or EUS) or mediastinoscopy (MS). RE MS: repeat MS. +: positive; –: negative.

T3N1 disease is usually an incidental finding during resection of a clinical T3 tumour and is a rather uncommon event. The surgeon should proceed with the intervention when a complete resection can be obtained. Adjuvant chemotherapy is indicated due to N1 involvement [24, 25].

N2 disease implies ipsilateral mediastinal or subcarinal lymph node involvement (stage IIIA-N2 disease). It is subdivided into: occult, unexpected or non-imaged N2 discovered at thoracotomy; discrete N2 proven at preoperative staging, which is potentially resectable; and nonresectable, infiltrative N2 [25].

When N2 disease is discovered during thoracotomy after negative preoperative staging, so-called occult or "surprise" N2 involvement, a resection should be performed if it is possible for this to be complete according to the definition previously outlined. Careful preoperative staging is necessary and during thoracotomy, a systematic nodal dissection should be performed to obtain precise pathological staging [26]. Adjuvant chemotherapy increases survival and is currently recommended in these cases [25]. The addition of postoperative radiotherapy remains controversial. The specific question as to whether adjuvant radiotherapy has an impact on survival is addressed in the Lung ART trial, which is currently open for inclusion (NCT00410683; https://clinicaltrials.gov/).

Most patients with discrete, pathologically proven N2 disease detected during preoperative work-up will be treated using induction therapy. It is clear from the recent literature that whilst surgery is feasible after induction therapy for locally advanced NSCLC, it is often more complex and may carry a higher risk, mainly due to a higher incidence of empyema and bronchopleural fistula. In initial series, mainly from North America, mortality of pneumonectomy was shown to be high, particularly in right pneumonectomy after induction chemoradiation, which had a reported mortality of 23.9% compared with 11.3% for lobectomies and pneumonectomies combined [27]. Lower mortality is reported in other series, although the incidence of bronchopleural fistula remains elevated [28–33]. In one series from two high-volume centres, the 90-day mortality rate was shown to be only 3% [32]. A meta-analysis of the mortality of pneumonectomy after induction therapy demonstrated that right pneumonectomy is associated with a significantly higher mortality compared with left pneumonectomy [34]. For 90-day mortality, the cumulative mortalities were 20% and 9% for right and left pneumonectomies, respectively. The alternative interventions to pneumonectomy are bronchoplastic procedures, which can also be safely performed after induction therapy [35, 36].

Prognostic factors after induction therapy include complete tumour resection and chemotherapy activity consisting of clinical response, pathological response and mediastinal downstaging [37]. Improving on chemotherapy as induction therapy usually means adding radiotherapy, but a recent meta-analysis demonstrated that for stage IIIA-N2 NSCLC, induction chemoradiation yielded no clear advantage over induction chemotherapy alone [38].

For locally advanced stage IIIA-N2 lung cancer, the major question remains whether better local control and survival are obtained using induction therapy followed by surgery, compared with standard chemoradiotherapy. This specific question was addressed in two large randomised trials (table 4).

In the Intergroup 0139 trial, patients with pathologically proven stage IIIA-N2 NSCLC were randomised between a full course of chemoradiation and induction chemoradiation followed by surgery [39]. There was no significant difference in overall survival between both arms. However, there was a difference in PFS, favouring the surgical arm. Patients downstaged to

Table 4. Comparison of European Organisation for Research and Treatment of Cancer (EORTC) 08941 [28, 40] with the Intergroup (INT) 0139 trial [39]

| | EORTC 08941 | INT 0139 |
|---|---|---|
| **Induction regimen** | Chemotherapy | Chemoradiation |
| **Complete resection# %** | 50.0 | 71.0 |
| **Exploratory thoracotomy %** | 13.6 | 4.5 |
| **Rate of pneumonectomy %** | 46.8 | 32.9 |
| **ypN factor %** | N0-1: 41.4; N2: 55.8 | N0: 46; N1-N3: 54 |
| **ypT0N0 %** | 5.2 | 14.4 |
| **30-day mortality %** | | |
| Overall | 3.9 | 5 |
| Lobectomy | 0 | 1 |
| Pneumonectomy | 6.9; R: 5.3; L: 9.1 | 26; R simple: 29; R complex: 50; L simple: 0; L complex: 16 |
| **Median survival months** | | |
| Overall | Radio: 17.5; surgery: 16.4 | Radio: 22.2; surgery: 23.6 |
| Progression-free | Radio: 11.3; surgery: 9.0 | Radio: 10.5; surgery: 12.8 |
| **Local recurrence %** | Radio: 55; surgery: 32 (p=0.001) | Radio: 22; surgery: 10 (p=0.002) |
| **5-year survival %** | | |
| Lobectomy | 27 | 36 |
| Pneumonectomy | 12 (p=0.009) | 22 |
| ypN factor | N0-1: 29; N2-3: 7 (p=0.0009) | N0: 41; N1-3: 24 (p<0.0001) |

R: right; L: left; radio: radiotherapy. #: definition was different in the two trials.

N0 disease had the best prognosis, and the rate of locoregional recurrence was significantly lower in the surgical arm. In a subsequent exploratory analysis, patients undergoing lobectomy were matched to a similar group treated with chemoradiation. There was a significant survival advantage for the surgical group. However, no difference was found for a matched group undergoing pneumonectomy.

In the European Organisation for Research and Treatment of Cancer (EORTC) 08941 phase III trial, patients with histologically proven stage IIIA-N2 disease were randomised between surgery and radiotherapy after responding to induction chemotherapy [28, 40]. Patients with a minor response were also included. There was no difference in overall survival and PFS between both arms. In an exploratory analysis, patients downstaged to N0 or N1 disease had a significantly better prognosis than those with persisting N2 disease. The rate of locoregional recurrence was also significantly less in the surgical arm. Patients treated with lobectomy had a significantly better survival than those who had a pneumonectomy. A comparison between both trials is provided in table 4. Although not clearly proven, surgical resection could provide a survival benefit in downstaged patients when a pneumonectomy can be avoided, as the latter intervention entails a significantly higher mortality and morbidity rate compared to lobectomy, especially after combined induction chemoradiation [41].

In order to determine the optimal local treatment, a study that evaluates the role of surgery *versus* radiotherapy after induction treatment in patients achieving mediastinal downstaging would be of interest [42]. Another attractive research strategy would be to improve the induction therapy.

The majority of patients with infiltrative, bulky N2 disease are treated with combination platinum-based chemotherapy and radiotherapy. Concurrent chemoradiotherapy is preferable to sequential application for improved performance status and minimal weight loss [24, 25]. However, the optimal treatment schedule remains a matter of investigation.

## Stage IIIB NSCLC

Generally, patients with stage IIIB NSCLC (T4-N3 disease) have a poor overall prognosis. However, in carefully selected cases, long-term survival may be achieved after surgical resection in experienced centres, sometimes in combination with chemotherapy or radiotherapy. Most important prognostic parameters include a complete surgical resection, excellent performance status and no involvement of mediastinal lymph nodes [43]. In selected subgroups of T4N0 disease, a 5-year survival of 30% has been reported. This is particularly true of tumours invading the main carina or distal trachea, left atrium, superior vena cava and vertebral bodies. An extended resection is often necessary, sometimes followed by a technically demanding and challenging reconstruction, which should be performed in an experienced centre by a specialised, multidisciplinary team. Induction therapy may improve resectability but no randomised studies are available. As a result of this relatively good prognosis, T4N0-1 lung cancer was reclassified as stage IIIA disease in the seventh edition of the TNM classification [44]. Good prognosis in selected patients was also seen in Spanish phase II study, which included 136 patients with stage IIIA and IIIB disease who were treated with induction chemotherapy using a cisplatin-based triplet followed by surgical resection [45]. In patients with T4N0-1 disease in whom a complete resection was obtained, the 5-year survival rate was 53%, which is a remarkably good result.

Additional malignant nodules in the primary lobe represent a particular entity. Several series have shown that they represent a rather favourable subgroup, which was confirmed by survival analysis of the large IASLC database [44]. Additional malignant nodules in the primary lobe are currently classified as T3 disease, and additional malignant nodules in an ipsilateral, non-primary lobe are currently classified as T4 disease.

In general, patients with stage IIIB-N3 disease are treated using combined chemoradiotherapy as they are not good candidates for surgical resection [46]. In the Southwest Oncology Group (SWOG) 8805 trial, selected patients with stage IIIA-N2 and stage IIIB-T4,N3 underwent induction chemoradiation followed by surgical resection when there was no progressive disease shown on the chest CT scan [47]. There was no survival difference between stages IIIA and IIIB. The strongest predictor of long-term survival was absence of tumour in the mediastinal nodes. So, in case of N3 disease, an intervention can only be considered when mediastinal downstaging is pathologically proven by minimally invasive or invasive techniques, which represents an exceptional situation.

Pancoast or superior sulcus tumours with clinical T4 characteristics, such as Horner's syndrome, invasion of the brachial plexus or vertebral bodies, are very challenging. Significant downstaging can be achieved with induction chemoradiotherapy, which facilitates subsequent resection. Even patients with stable disease should undergo thoracotomy, as pathological downstaging can be observed without any clinical response on the chest CT scan due to the development of necrosis inside these tumours. In a series of 110 patients presenting with T3-4N0-1 superior sulcus tumours (SWOG 9416 trial), induction chemoradiation consisted of two cycles of cisplatin and etoposide given concurrently with 45 Gy of radiotherapy, followed by surgical resection where clinical response was seen or in stable disease [48]. Postoperatively, two more cycles of chemotherapy were administered. The 5-year survival rate for all patients was 44%, and 54% for those patients who had a complete resection, with no significant difference between T3 and T4 tumours.

## Current guidelines for locally advanced NSCLC

The controversial nature of stage III disease is reflected in recent guidelines published by the American College of Chest Physicians (ACCP) and the European Society for Medical Oncology (ESMO) [24, 25, 46].

Infiltrative, bulky N2 is the most easy to deal with. The ACCP and ESMO guidelines recommend a combination of platinum-based doublet chemotherapy and radiotherapy (60–66 Gy), preferentially in a concurrent scheme.

For discrete N2 involvement detected by preoperative staging, the ACCP recommends that a treatment plan should be made by a multidisciplinary team that at least includes a thoracic surgeon, a medical oncologist and a radiation oncologist. Definitive chemoradiation or induction therapy followed by surgery is recommended over either surgery or radiation alone. ESMO guidelines state that treatment in these cases remains a matter of debate. Both definitive chemoradiation and induction therapy followed by surgery are considered valid options. Surgery is preferably considered in those patients in whom a complete resection by lobectomy is anticipated.

For incidental, unexpected, occult or surprise N2 disease after thorough preoperative staging, the ACCP recommends that a planned resection is performed in association with a systematic nodal dissection, provided that a complete resection can be obtained. Adjuvant chemotherapy is recommended. Sequential adjuvant radiotherapy should be considered when there is a high likelihood of local recurrence. The same treatment schedule is proposed by ESMO.

Concurrent induction chemoradiotherapy is recommended by the ACCP for potentially resectable superior sulcus or Pancoast tumours. As for other lung cancers, every effort should be made to achieve a complete resection.

For cT4N0-1M0, the ACCP recommends that in patients who are considered for curative resection, the surgical procedure should only be performed in dedicated thoracic surgical units.

## Conclusion

Stage III NSCLC comprises quite different subgroups of patients with locally advanced disease due to extrapulmonary extension of the primary tumour or nodal involvement beyond the pulmonary hilum into the mediastinum. Guidelines for diagnosis and management were recently updated but many grey and controversial areas remain. For this reason, each patient should be discussed within a dedicated multidisciplinary team. Technically challenging procedures should be performed in an experienced thoracic surgery department, not only to deal with challenging aspects of the intervention but also to take care of the postoperative complications that are frequently observed in this patient population. Cooperative efforts are required to better define the indications for surgical resection within a multimodality setting and to determine the significant factors related to overall and disease-free survival.

## References

1. Van Schil PE, De Waele M, Hendriks JM, *et al.* Surgical treatment of stage III non-small cell lung cancer. *Eur J Cancer* 2009; 45: Suppl. 1, 106–112.
2. Hancock J, Rosen J, Moreno A, *et al.* Management of clinical stage IIIA primary lung cancers in the National Cancer Database. *Ann Thorac Surg* 2014; 98: 424–432.
3. Rami-Porta R, Wittekind C, Goldstraw P. Complete resection in lung cancer surgery: proposed definition. *Lung Cancer* 2005; 49: 25–33.
4. Van Schil PE, Hendriks JM, Hertoghs M, *et al.* Current surgical treatment of non-small-cell lung cancer. *Expert Rev Anticancer Ther* 2011; 11: 1577–1585.
5. Lim E, Harris G, Patel A, *et al.* Preoperative *versus* postoperative chemotherapy in patients with resectable non-small cell lung cancer: systematic review and indirect comparison meta-analysis of randomized trials. *J Thorac Oncol* 2009; 4: 1380–1388.
6. Betticher DC, Hsu Schmitz SF, Totsch M, *et al.* Mediastinal lymph node clearance after docetaxel-cisplatin neoadjuvant chemotherapy is prognostic of survival in patients with stage IIIA pN2 non-small-cell lung cancer: a multicenter phase II trial. *J Clin Oncol* 2003; 21: 1752–1759.
7. Kim ES, Bosquee L. The importance of accurate lymph node staging in early and locally advanced non-small cell lung cancer: an update on available techniques. *J Thorac Oncol* 2007; 2: Suppl. 2, S59–S67.
8. De Waele M, Hendriks J, Lauwers P, *et al.* Nodal status at repeat mediastinoscopy determines survival in non-small cell lung cancer with mediastinal nodal involvement, treated by induction therapy. *Eur J Cardiothorac Surg* 2006; 29: 240–243.
9. De Leyn P, Stroobants S, De Wever W, *et al.* Prospective comparative study of integrated positron emission tomography-computed tomography scan compared with remediastinoscopy in the assessment of residual mediastinal lymph node disease after induction chemotherapy for mediastinoscopy-proven stage IIIA-N2 non-small-cell lung cancer: a Leuven Lung Cancer Group Study. *J Clin Oncol* 2006; 24: 3333–3339.
10. Cerfolio RJ, Bryant AS, Ojha B. Restaging patients with N2 (stage IIIa) non-small cell lung cancer after neoadjuvant chemoradiotherapy: a prospective study. *J Thorac Cardiovasc Surg* 2006; 131: 1229–1235.

11. Krasnik M, Vilmann P, Herth F. EUS-FNA and EBUS-TBNA; the pulmonologist's and surgeon's perspective. *Endoscopy* 2006; 38: Suppl. 1, S105–S109.
12. Herth FJ, Annema JT, Eberhardt R, *et al.* Endobronchial ultrasound with transbronchial needle aspiration for restaging the mediastinum in lung cancer. *J Clin Oncol* 2008; 26: 3346–3350.
13. Stigt JA, Oostdijk AH, Timmer PR, *et al.* Comparison of EUS-guided fine needle aspiration and integrated PET-CT in restaging after treatment for locally advanced non-small cell lung cancer. *Lung Cancer* 2009; 66: 198–204.
14. von Bartheld MB, Versteegh MI, Braun J, *et al.* Transesophageal ultrasound-guided fine-needle aspiration for the mediastinal restaging of non-small cell lung cancer. *J Thorac Oncol* 2011; 6: 1510–1515.
15. Stamatis G, Fechner S, Hillejan L, *et al.* Repeat mediastinoscopy as a restaging procedure. *Pneumologie* 2005; 59: 862–866.
16. De Waele M, Serra-Mitjans M, Hendriks J, *et al.* Accuracy and survival of repeat mediastinoscopy after induction therapy for non-small cell lung cancer in a combined series of 104 patients. *Eur J Cardiothorac Surg* 2008; 33: 824–828.
17. Marra A, Hillejan L, Fechner S, *et al.* Remediastinoscopy in restaging of lung cancer after induction therapy. *J Thorac Cardiovasc Surg* 2008; 135: 843–849.
18. Call S, Rami-Porta R, Obiols C, *et al.* Repeat mediastinoscopy in all its indications: experience with 96 patients and 101 procedures. *Eur J Cardiothorac Surg* 2011; 39: 1022–1027.
19. Annema JT, Veselic M, Versteegh MI, *et al.* Mediastinal restaging: EUS-FNA offers a new perspective. *Lung Cancer* 2003; 42: 311–318.
20. de Cabanyes Candela S, Detterbeck FC. A systematic review of restaging after induction therapy for stage IIIa lung cancer: prediction of pathologic stage. *J Thorac Oncol* 2010; 5: 389–398.
21. Van Schil P, De Waele M, Hendriks J, *et al.* Remediastinoscopy. *J Thorac Oncol* 2007; 2: 365–366.
22. Jaklitsch MT, Gu L, Demmy T, *et al.* Prospective phase II trial of preresection thoracoscopic mediastinal restaging after neoadjuvant therapy for IIIA (N2) non-small cell lung cancer: results of CALGB protocol 39803. *J Thorac Cardiovasc Surg* 2013; 146: 9–16.
23. De Leyn P, Dooms C, Kuzdzal J, *et al.* Revised ESTS guidelines for preoperative mediastinal lymph node staging for non-small-cell lung cancer. *Eur J Cardiothorac Surg* 2014; 45: 787–798.
24. Vansteenkiste J, De Ruysscher D, Eberhardt WE, *et al.* Early and locally advanced non-small-cell lung cancer (NSCLC): ESMO Clinical Practice Guidelines for diagnosis, treatment and follow-up. *Ann Oncol* 2013; 24: Suppl. 6, vi89–vi98.
25. Ramnath N, Dilling TJ, Harris LJ, *et al.* Treatment of stage III non-small cell lung cancer: diagnosis and management of lung cancer, 3rd ed: American College of Chest Physicians evidence-based clinical practice guidelines. *Chest* 2013; 143: Suppl. 5, e314S–e340S.
26. Detterbeck F. What to do with "Surprise" N2?: intraoperative management of patients with non-small cell lung cancer. *J Thorac Oncol* 2008; 3: 289–302.
27. Martin J, Ginsberg RJ, Abolhoda A, *et al.* Morbidity and mortality after neoadjuvant therapy for lung cancer: the risks of right pneumonectomy. *Ann Thorac Surg* 2001; 72: 1149–1154.
28. Van Schil P, Van Meerbeeck J, Kramer G, *et al.* Morbidity and mortality in the surgery arm of EORTC 08941 trial. *Eur Respir J* 2005; 26: 192–197.
29. Mansour Z, Kochetkova EA, Ducrocq X, *et al.* Induction chemotherapy does not increase the operative risk of pneumonectomy! *Eur J Cardiothorac Surg* 2007; 31: 181–185.
30. Alifano M, Boudaya MS, Salvi M, *et al.* Pneumonectomy after chemotherapy: morbidity, mortality, and long-term outcome. *Ann Thorac Surg* 2008; 85: 1866–1873.
31. Gudbjartsson T, Gyllstedt E, Pikwer A, *et al.* Early surgical results after pneumonectomy for non-small cell lung cancer are not affected by preoperative radiotherapy and chemotherapy. *Ann Thorac Surg* 2008; 86: 376–382.
32. Weder W, Collaud S, Eberhardt WE, *et al.* Pneumonectomy is a valuable treatment option after neoadjuvant therapy for stage III non-small-cell lung cancer. *J Thorac Cardiovasc Surg* 2010; 139: 1424–1430.
33. Alan S, Jan S, Tomas H, *et al.* Does chemotherapy increase morbidity and mortality after pneumonectomy? *J Surg Oncol* 2009; 99: 38–41.
34. Kim AW, Boffa DJ, Wang Z, *et al.* An analysis, systematic review, and meta-analysis of the perioperative mortality after neoadjuvant therapy and pneumonectomy for non-small cell lung cancer. *J Thorac Cardiovasc Surg* 2012; 143: 55–63.
35. Veronesi G, Solli PG, Leo F, *et al.* Low morbidity of bronchoplastic procedures after chemotherapy for lung cancer. *Lung Cancer* 2002; 36: 91–97.
36. Gomez-Caro A, Boada M, Reguart N, *et al.* Sleeve lobectomy after induction chemoradiotherapy. *Eur J Cardiothorac Surg* 2012; 41: 1052–1058.
37. Betticher DC, Hsu Schmitz SF, Totsch M, *et al.* Prognostic factors affecting long-term outcomes in patients with resected stage IIIA pN2 non-small-cell lung cancer: 5-year follow-up of a phase II study. *Br J Canc* 2006; 94: 1099–1106.

38. Shah AA, Berry MF, Tzao C, *et al.* Induction chemoradiation is not superior to induction chemotherapy alone in stage IIIA lung cancer. *Ann Thorac Surg* 2012; 93: 1807–1812.
39. Albain KS, Swann RS, Rusch VW, *et al.* Radiotherapy plus chemotherapy with or without surgical resection for stage III non-small-cell lung cancer: a phase III randomised controlled trial. *Lancet* 2009; 374: 379–386.
40. van Meerbeeck JP, Kramer GW, Van Schil PE, *et al.* Randomized controlled trial of resection *versus* radiotherapy after induction chemotherapy in stage IIIA-N2 non-small-cell lung cancer. *J Natl Cancer Inst* 2007; 99: 442–450.
41. Van Schil PE. Mortality associated with pneumonectomy after induction chemoradiation *versus* chemotherapy alone in stage IIIA-N2 non-small cell lung cancer. *J Thorac Cardiovasc Surg* 2008; 135: 718.
42. McCloskey P, Balduyck B, Van Schil PE, *et al.* Radical treatment of non-small cell lung cancer during the last 5 years. *Eur J Cancer* 2013; 49: 1555–1564.
43. Rice TW, Blackstone EH. Radical resections for T4 lung cancer. *Surg Clin North Am* 2002; 82: 573–587.
44. Rami-Porta R, Ball D, Crowley J, *et al.* The IASLC Lung Cancer Staging Project: proposals for the revision of the T descriptors in the forthcoming (seventh) edition of the TNM classification for lung cancer. *J Thorac Oncol* 2007; 2: 593–602.
45. Garrido P, Gonzalez-Larriba JL, Insa A, *et al.* Long-term survival associated with complete resection after induction chemotherapy in stage IIIA (N2) and IIIB (T4N0–1) non small-cell lung cancer patients: the Spanish Lung Cancer Group Trial 9901. *J Clin Oncol* 2007; 25: 4736–4742.
46. Kozower BD, Larner JM, Detterbeck FC, *et al.* Special treatment issues in non-small cell lung cancer: diagnosis and management of lung cancer, 3rd ed: American College of Chest Physicians evidence-based clinical practice guidelines. *Chest* 2013; 143, : Suppl. 5, e369S–e399S.
47. Albain KS, Rusch VW, Crowley JJ, *et al.* Concurrent cisplatin/etoposide plus chest radiotherapy followed by surgery for stages IIIA (N2) and IIIB non-small-cell lung cancer: mature results of Southwest Oncology Group phase II study 8805. *J Clin Oncol* 1995; 13: 1880–1892.
48. Rusch VW, Giroux DJ, Kraut MJ, *et al.* Induction chemoradiation and surgical resection for superior sulcus non-small-cell lung carcinomas: long-term results of Southwest Oncology Group Trial 9416 (Intergroup Trial 0160). *J Clin Oncol* 2007; 25: 313–318.

Disclosures: None declared.

Chapter 14

# Approaches in patients with locally advanced NSCLC: a radiation oncologist's perspective

Dirk De Ruysscher[1,2], Stéphanie Peeters[1,2] and Esther G.C. Troost[3]

The backbone of treatment for locally advanced NSCLC should be chemotherapy in all suitable patients.

In fit patients with resectable disease, concurrent chemotherapy and radiotherapy, intensive chemotherapy followed by resection, chemotherapy followed by intensive (*i.e.* accelerated) radiotherapy or concurrent chemoradiotherapy followed by resection are all viable options with none proven to be superior over the other. Across all trials, tri-modality therapy was shown to be the best way to achieve local tumour control; however, no randomised trial has been large enough to show a possible overall survival benefit. Bi-modality therapy thus remains the standard, except in situations where local tumour control is a prerequisite, *e.g.* in exemplary cases with Pancoast tumours.

In nonresectable locally advanced NSCLC, concurrent chemoradiotherapy is the standard of care with doses of 60–66 Gy in 2 Gy fractions. In patients who are unsuitable for concurrent schedules, induction chemotherapy followed by accelerated radiotherapy is an alternative treatment with curative intent.

It is clear that locally advanced NSCLC is a heterogeneous disease. In addition to its different histological entities, such as ADC and SCC and their heterogeneous genetic characteristics, its anatomical presentation and volume varies widely in individual patients [1]. Locally advanced NSCLC is therefore a basket containing several entities, which may also explain the variety of opinions regarding the treatment of this disease. To add to the complexity of treatment decisions, patients with NSCLC are often old and have many smoking-related diseases that should be taken into consideration in the treatment decision [2, 3].

For the sake of clarity, in this chapter, locally advanced NSCLC is defined as patients with N2 or N3 disease and/or with a cT4 tumour [1]. Issues regarding radiotherapy techniques, integration with imaging and quality assurance will not be discussed, as these are covered elsewhere in previously published literature ([4], for example).

[1]Dept of Oncology, Experimental Radiation Oncology, KU Leuven - University of Leuven, Leuven, Belgium. [2]Dept of Radiation Oncology, University Hospitals Leuven, Leuven, Belgium. [3]Dept of Radiation Oncology (MAASTRO), GROW School for Oncology and Developmental Biology, Maastricht University Medical Centre, Maastricht, the Netherlands.

Correspondence: Dirk De Ruysscher, Dept of Radiation Oncology, University Hospital Leuven, Herestraat 49, 3000 Leuven, Belgium.
E-mail: dirk.deruysscher@uzleuven.be

 Print ISBN: 978-1-84984-061-3. Online ISBN: 978-1-84984-062-0. Print ISSN: 2312-508X. Online ISSN: 2312-5098.

## Chemotherapy

Chemotherapy is an integral part of the treatment of locally advanced NSCLC as it improves survival in all subgroups of patients, whether treated with surgery or radiotherapy; this has been demonstrated in meta-analyses based on individual patient data [5–7]. The hazard ratio (HR) for overall survival when adding chemotherapy after primary surgery, quite a rare situation in locally advanced NSCLC, is 0.83 [7]. Preoperative chemotherapy also improves 5-year survival rates by ~5%, with a HR of 0.87, an effect that was independent of the chemotherapy regimen or schedule, and of the possible addition of postoperative radiotherapy (PORT) [8]. The administration of chemotherapy before radiotherapy increases 2-year overall survival, with a HR of 0.70 [6].

The optimisation of systemic treatment in relation to local therapy is discussed further in another chapter of this *Monograph* [9].

## Radiotherapy in resectable locally advanced NSCLC

Patients are defined as having resectable disease when a complete resection (R0) is deemed possible at diagnosis. A nonresectable cancer at diagnosis will thus not be converted to an oncological resectable disease after any type of induction therapy. In the following section, we will assume that the patient is fit enough to undergo an aggressive local treatment, surgery, radiotherapy or a combination of all three [3].

As many of the questions have not been addressed by the randomised trials that were designed for this purpose, answering them is not straightforward. Moreover, patient selection, staging procedures and other factors may contribute to differences in outcome between studies. In all studies, improved local tumour control only translated into better overall survival with follow-up times of >2 years; short-term survival is dominated by distant metastases that were present but undetected at the time of diagnosis [10, 11]. However, general conclusions may still be drawn.

### Is neoadjuvant chemotherapy combined with radiotherapy before surgery better than preoperative chemotherapy alone?

Although induction chemotherapy followed by resection has been practiced in many centres, randomised studies are very scarce. Moreover, many studies do not report on an intention-to-treat basis but only describe those patients who eventually underwent surgery, *i.e.* patients were eligible for surgery as they had resectable disease and their favourable response to induction chemotherapy meant they were considered fit enough. It is clear that these are major selection criteria. The general condition of a significant proportion of patients will deteriorate as chemotherapy will make them unfit for surgery. As an example, in an intention-to-treat analysis, only 75 (57%) of 131 patients who started induction chemotherapy eventually underwent surgery [12]. The 5-year survival of the whole group was 21%, with 28% of patients experiencing a local failure as the first site of recurrence; in contrast, the 5-year survival of patients who underwent tumour resection was 35%. These findings have been reproduced elsewhere in literature [13].

To the best of our knowledge, only one randomised trial addresses this topic, and was presented at the 2014 annual meeting of the European Society for Medical Oncology

Table 1. Summary of selected phase III studies of radiotherapy with surgery in resectable locally advanced NSCLC

| Trial [ref.] | Subjects n | Study design | 5-year overall survival | Local relapse# | 30-day mortality¶ |
|---|---|---|---|---|---|
| **SAKK 16/00 [11]** | 232 | Intensive C→R (44 Gy)→S | 40% | 24% | 3% |
| | | Intensive C→S | 34% (NS) | 35% | 0% |
| **INT 0139 [12]** | 429 | C/R (45 Gy)→S→C | 27% | 10% | 8% |
| | | C/R (61 Gy)→C | 20% (NS) | 22% | 2% |
| **ESPATÜ [13]** | 246 | C→C/R (45 Gy)→S | 44% | NR | 6% |
| | | C→C/R (65 Gy) | 40% (NS) | NR | 2% |

Further details of intensive study design are provided in the main text. SAKK: Swiss Group for Clinical Cancer Research; INT: North American Intergroup Trial; ESPATÜ: ESen PAris TÜbingen; C: chemotherapy; R: radiotherapy; S: surgery; NS: not significantly different; NR: not reported. #: first site of recurrence is local or loco-regional; ¶: mortality up to 30 days post-treatment.

(ESMO): the Swiss Group for Clinical Cancer Research (SAKK) 16/00 phase III trial (table 1) [14]. 232 patients with cN2 NSCLC were randomised to: chemotherapy that was more intensive than that generally administered (cisplatin 100 mg·m$^{-2}$ and docetaxel 85 mg·m$^{-2}$ every 3 weeks for three cycles plus granulocyte colony-stimulating factor) followed by resection; the same chemotherapy followed by accelerated radiotherapy (44 Gy in 22 fractions in 3 weeks) and surgery. Patients were staged with a whole-body $^{18}$F-fluoro-2-deoxy-D-glucose PET ($^{18}$FDG-PET)-CT scan and appropriate brain imaging. The event-free survival and overall survival were similar for the two arms of the study, with estimated 5-year survival rates of ~35%; only 55 patients were at risk 4 years post-randomisation. The first site of recurrence was local only in 35% of the patients randomised to the chemotherapy–surgery arm and 24% in the chemotherapy–radiotherapy–surgery group. The proportion of R0 resections was 91% in the triple-therapy group and 78% in the chemotherapy–surgery arm. This trial was only powered for event-free survival and detailed statistics are not yet available. At the time of writing these results were unpublished and should therefore be interpreted with caution; however, they indicate that the addition of preoperative radiotherapy to intensive chemotherapy reduces local recurrences by 31%, increasing complete resection rates, but does not improve overall survival. As toxicity was hardly increased, it is tempting to speculate that a possible gain in overall survival may have remained undetected because of the lack of power of this study. Tri-modality treatment may achieve the best local control rates.

### Is induction chemotherapy and radiotherapy before surgery better than concurrent chemotherapy and radiotherapy?

In the Lung Intergroup Trial 0139 (INT 0139) (table 1), 429 patients with resectable cN2 disease (75% had single nodal station cN2 disease) were randomised to: concurrent radiotherapy to a dose of 45 Gy and cisplatin – etoposide followed by surgery; or definitive concurrent chemoradiation to a dose of 61 Gy [15]. No staging $^{18}$FDG-PET-CT scan was performed. No statistically significant survival differences were observed. The 5-year overall survival was 20% in the concurrent chemoradiotherapy-only arm and 27% in the concurrent chemoradiotherapy and surgery group. PFS favoured the surgically treated patients. In an exploratory unplanned, matched subgroup analysis, patients being treated with a lobectomy after induction concurrent chemoradiotherapy had a better survival than those treated nonsurgically or with a pneumonectomy. The first site of relapse was local in 22% of the nonsurgical group and in 10% of patients randomised to receive surgery.

This study has been interpreted in many ways. A gain in overall survival may have remained nonsignificant because of the excess mortality in the group of patients undergoing pneumonectomy and because of the lack of statistical power. However, the study also found that tri-modality treatment achieved the best local control.

At the American Society of Clinical Oncology (ASCO) meeting in 2014, the results of the German ESPATÜ (ESen PAris TÜbingen) study were presented [16]. At the time of writing, no full length article was available. 246 patients were randomised to: three cycles of cisplatin-paclitaxel followed by concurrent cisplatin-vinorelbine and radiotherapy (45 Gy) and then surgery; or the same regimen but instead of surgery a radiotherapy boost to a total dose of 65 Gy. The 5-year survival was similar in both groups: 44% for the surgery group *versus* 40% for the no surgery group. However, in this study too, the number of patients eventually having received surgery (n=81) or a radiotherapy boost (n=80) may be too low to achieve sufficient statistical power for detecting a survival difference. Data on the patterns of recurrence are as yet unavailable.

These two randomised trials do not show a survival benefit for concurrent chemoradiotherapy over concurrent chemoradiotherapy followed by surgery. However, in both studies, there was a trend towards a numerical survival benefit of tri-modality treatment at 5 years: 7% in INT 0139 and 4% in ESPATÜ. It would take more patients to have enough statistical power to show whether these differences are real.

### Postoperative or preoperative radiotherapy?

The German Lung Cancer Cooperative Group randomised 558 resectable stage III patients to: arm 1, chemotherapy followed by surgery and postoperative radiotherapy; and arm 2, chemotherapy followed by concurrent chemoradiotherapy (45 Gy) and surgery [17]. A risk-adapted schedule of PORT was given; briefly, this was 54 Gy in 28 fractions for a R0 resection or 68.4 Gy in 38 fractions for an incomplete resection or nonresectable disease. The majority of the patients received PORT. Although not often referred this way and somewhat simplified, this trial indirectly thus compared induction chemotherapy followed by resection and PORT to induction concurrent chemoradiotherapy and surgery. The 5-year overall survival rates were similar: 21% in arm 1 and 18% in arm 2. Local failure as the first site of recurrence was observed in 40% of the patients in arm 1 and in 34% of the patients in arm 2.

The conclusion of this study was that preoperative concurrent chemotherapy and low-dose (45 Gy) radiotherapy are equivalent to induction chemotherapy followed by PORT (also after R0 resections) to a higher dose.

In all trials, toxicity of tri-modality treatments was higher than that of bi-modality, but never to such an extent that this was deemed unfeasible. An exception might be right-sided pneumonectomy [15, 17].

## Radiotherapy in nonresectable locally advanced NSCLC

### Surgery or radiotherapy after induction chemotherapy?

In the European Organisation for Research and Treatment of Cancer (EORTC) 08941 trial, 579 patients with nonresectable cN2 disease who showed at least a minimal tumour response after three cycles of induction chemotherapy were randomised between radiotherapy (60 Gy in 30 fractions in 6 weeks) and surgery [18]. No survival differences were observed, with 5-year survival rates of 16% and 14% for surgery and radiotherapy, respectively. Local recurrence as the first site of failure was seen in 58% of patients treated with radiotherapy and in 32% of surgical patients.

### Sequential or concurrent chemotherapy and radiotherapy?

In a meta-analysis based on individual data from 1205 patients and a median follow-up of 6 years, concurrent chemotherapy and radiotherapy (mostly delivered to a dose of 60–66 Gy in 2 Gy daily fractions) lead to a significantly higher 5-year survival than sequential chemoradiotherapy [10]. The HR for survival was 0.84, representing an absolute benefit at 5 years of 4.5%. Concurrent chemoradiotherapy did not affect the rate of distant metastases but did decrease loco-regional progression (HR 0.77), with an absolute benefit of 6%. No increase in late toxicity was observed. Importantly, an increased survival benefit due to better loco-regional control rates was only observed after 1.5 years of follow-up, pointing to the importance of adequate follow-up time before drawing conclusions.

### Optimal radiotherapy after induction chemotherapy?

In a meta-analysis based on individual patient data from phase III trials, including 2000 individuals, accelerated radiotherapy schedules (*i.e.* delivered in short overall treatment times) lead to higher 5-year overall survival rates at the expense of transient acute oesophagitis in patients treated with non-concurrent schedules [11]. The HR for survival was 0.88, representing an absolute benefit of 2.5% at 5 years. No increased late toxicity was observed. Accelerated radiotherapy can be delivered in once-daily fractionation and is then less costly than conventional 2 Gy per day fractionation [1].

Accelerated radiotherapy has therefore been recommended in many guidelines [1].

## Experimental strategies to improve radiotherapy

Although the survival of patients with locally advanced NSCLC has improved in the last few decades, the best recent series with concurrent chemoradiotherapy still leaves room for improvement, reporting median survivals of ~24 months and 5-year survival rates of 20–25%. At least 30% of the patients developed a local recurrence [18]. As a consequence, radiotherapy dose intensification continues to be regarded as a logical policy for improving outcome in lung cancer. Dose intensification can be achieved by dose escalation or acceleration.

RTOG 0617 was a randomised study with a 2×2 factorial design. Patients were primarily randomised to either 60 Gy in 6 weeks or 74 Gy in 7.5 weeks, and secondarily were randomised to the addition of cetuximab or not. Radiotherapy was delivered concurrently with carboplatin and paclitaxel. Following the radiotherapy regimen, patients in all study arms received two additional cycles of consolidation chemotherapy with or without cetuximab. The overall survival of the 74 Gy arm was shown to be worse than the 60 Gy arm, possibly due to increased cardiac toxicity [18]. Local recurrences were similar, supporting pre-existing knowledge that extending the overall treatment time beyond 6 weeks in concurrent chemoradiotherapy schedules counteracts the cancer cell kill of higher doses.

Clearly, adding 2 Gy fractions delivered once daily to the currently used radiotherapy schedules does not seem to be the way to go.

Several clinical trials have investigated whether intensified radiotherapy, delivered concurrently with chemotherapy, will improve local tumour control and survival. Many of them also include innovative radiotherapy techniques and concepts. The common factor in these clinical trials is an individualised dose prescription based on the radiation dose to the organs at risk, and a decreased overall treatment time of radiotherapy.

INDividualised Accelerated isotoxic Radiotherapy (INDAR), based on organ-at-risk constraints, is the backbone of the experimental arms of the IDEAL-CRT (Isotoxic Dose Escalation and Acceleration in Lung Cancer ChemoRadiotherapy) [20], the I-START (ISoToxic Accelerated Radiotherapy for Non-small cell lung cancer; ongoing trial www.clinicaltrials.gov), the Isotoxic IMRT (Isotoxic Intensity-Modulated RadioTherapy) [19, 20], the CHART-ED (Continuous Hyper fractionated Accelerated Radiotherapy - Escalated Dose Study; ongoing trial www.clinicaltrials.gov) and the BIG Lung Trial (consisting of the CARSoN and ASCaN trials) in the UK [21, 22]. The European PET-Boost trial investigates the possible beneficial effect of radiation dose redistribution within the tumour based on FDG uptake on PET scans using an INDAR schedule [23]. The PET-plan trial in Germany randomises nonaccelerated dose escalation based on the omission of elective nodal irradiation on FDG-PET scan to CT-based planning [24]. In the USA, RTOG 1106/ACRIN 6697 (ongoing trial) is a randomised trial studying individualised dose escalation based on FDG-PET response within the experimental arm to doses of up to 85.5 Gy given in 30 daily fractions in 6 weeks, compared to the same control arm as RTOG 0617 of 60 Gy in 6 weeks with concurrent carboplatin-paclitaxel.

Finally, radiotherapy may be used to induce immunogenic cell death, leading to regression of distant metastases when combined with immune modulatory agents such as anti-CTLA4 and anti-PD1 [25].

## Conclusion

As long as they are fit enough to undergo treatment with radical intent, patients with locally advanced NSCLC can be treated with different approaches, all of which may be suited for an individual patient. The backbone of the treatment should be chemotherapy in all suitable patients.

In patients with resectable disease, concurrent chemotherapy and radiotherapy, intensive chemotherapy followed by resection, chemotherapy followed by intensive (*i.e.* accelerated) radiotherapy or concurrent chemoradiotherapy followed by resection are all viable options, with none proven to be superior over the other. Tri-modality therapy (chemotherapy, surgery and radiotherapy) may be the best way to achieve local tumour control. However, numerically, a large difference in local recurrence can be seen between the studies. The

5-year overall survival may increase by 4–5%. None of the randomised trials was large enough to show the possible overall survival benefit of tri-modality over bi-modality therapy. As such, the superiority of tri- over bi-modality therapy remains a hypothesis, except in situations where local tumour control is a prerequisite, such as in exemplary cases with Pancoast tumours [26].

In nonresectable locally advanced NSCLC, concurrent chemoradiotherapy is the standard of care to doses of 60–66 Gy in 2 Gy fractions. In patients who are unsuitable for concurrent schedules, induction chemotherapy followed by accelerated radiotherapy is a curative intent alternative.

Real novel approaches are needed to improve the survival of these patients significantly.

## References

1. Vansteenkiste J, De Ruysscher D, Eberhardt WE, *et al.* Early and locally advanced non-small-cell lung cancer (NSCLC): ESMO Clinical Practice Guidelines for diagnosis, treatment and follow-up. *Ann Oncol* 2013; 24: Suppl. 6, vi89–vi98.
2. De Ruysscher D, Botterweck A, Dirx M, *et al.* Eligibility for concurrent chemotherapy and radiotherapy of locally advanced lung cancer patients: a prospective, population-based study. *Ann Oncol* 2009; 20: 98–102.
3. Brunelli A, Charloux A, Bolliger CT, *et al.* ERS/ESTS clinical guidelines on fitness for radical therapy in lung cancer patients (surgery and chemo-radiotherapy). *Eur Respir J* 2009; 34: 17–41.
4. De Ruysscher D, Faivre-Finn C, Nestle U, *et al.* European Organisation for Research and Treatment of Cancer recommendations for planning and delivery of high-dose, high-precision radiotherapy for lung cancer. *J Clin Oncol* 2010; 28: 5301–5310.
5. NSCLC Meta-analyses Collaborative Group, Arriagada R, Auperin A, *et al.* Adjuvant chemotherapy, with or without postoperative radiotherapy, in operable non-small-cell lung cancer: two meta-analyses of individual patient data. *Lancet* 2010; 375: 1267–1277.
6. Pignon JP, Stewart LA. Randomized trials of radiotherapy alone *versus* combined chemotherapy and radiotherapy in stages IIIa and IIIb non-small cell lung cancer: a meta-analysis. *Cancer* 1996; 77: 2413–2414.
7. Pignon JP, Tribodet H, Scagliotti GV, *et al.* Lung adjuvant cisplatin evaluation: a pooled analysis by the LACE Collaborative Group. *J Clin Oncol* 2008; 26: 3552–3559.
8. NSCLC Meta-analysis Collaborative Group. Preoperative chemotherapy for non-small-cell lung cancer: a systematic review and meta-analysis of individual participant data. *Lancet* 2014; 383: 1561–1571.
9. Januszewski A, Popat S. Chemotherapy. *In* Dingemans A-MC, Reck M, Westeel V, eds. Lung Cancer. *ERS Monogr* 2015; 68: 186–201.
10. Aupérin A, Le Péchoux C, Rolland E, *et al.* Meta-analysis of concomitant *versus* sequential radiochemotherapy in locally advanced non-small-cell lung cancer. *J Clin Oncol* 2010; 28: 2181–2190.
11. Mauguen A, Le Péchoux C, Saunders MI, *et al.* Hyperfractionated or accelerated radiotherapy in lung cancer: an individual patient data meta-analysis. *J Clin Oncol* 2012; 30: 2788–2797.
12. Lorent N, De Leyn P, Lievens Y, *et al.* Long-term survival of surgically staged IIIA-N2 non-small-cell lung cancer treated with surgical combined modality approach: analysis of a 7-year prospective experience. *Ann Oncol* 2004; 15: 1645–1653.
13. Billiet C, Decaluwé H, Peeters S, *et al.* Modern post-operative radiotherapy for stage III non-small cell lung cancer may improve local control and survival: a meta-analysis. *Radiother Oncol* 2014; 110: 3–8.
14. Pless M, Stupp R, Ris H, *et al.* Final results of the SAKK 16/00 trial: a randomized phase III trial comparing neoadjuvant chemoradiation to chemotherapy alone in stage IIIA/N2 non-small cell lung cancer. *Ann Oncol* 2014; 25: Suppl. 4, iv417–iv425.
15. Albain KS, Swann RS, Rusch VW, *et al.* Radiotherapy plus chemotherapy with or without surgical resection for stage III non-small-cell lung cancer: a phase III randomised controlled trial. *Lancet* 2009; 374: 379–386.
16. Eberhardt WEE, Gauler TC, Pöttgen C, *et al.* Phase III study of surgery (S) *versus* definitive concurrent chemoradiotherapy boost (def ccCRTx-BOx) in patients (pts) with operable (OP+) stage IIIA(N2)/selected IIIb (sel IIIb) non-small cell lung cancer (NSCLC) following induction (IND) chemotherapy (CTx) and concurrent CRTx (ESPATUE). *J Clin Oncol* 2014; 32: Suppl. 15, 7510.
17. Thomas M, Rübe C, Hoffknecht P, *et al.* Effect of preoperative chemoradiation in addition to preoperative chemotherapy: a randomised trial in stage III non-small-cell lung cancer. *Lancet Oncol* 2008; 9: 636–648.

18. van Meerbeeck JP, Kramer GW, Van Schil PE, *et al.* Randomized controlled trial of resection *versus* radiotherapy after induction chemotherapy in stage IIIA-N2 non-small-cell lung cancer. *J Natl Cancer Inst* 2007; 99: 442–450.
19. Bradley JD, Paulus R, Komaki R, *et al.* Standard-dose *versus* high-dose conformal radiotherapy with concurrent and consolidation carboplatin plus paclitaxel with or without cetuximab for patients with stage IIIA or IIIB non-small-cell lung cancer (RTOG 0617): a randomised, two-by-two factorial phase 3 study. *Lancet Oncol* 2015; 16: 187–199.
20. Warren S, Panettieri V, Panakis N, *et al.* Optimizing collimator margins for isotoxically dose-escalated conformal radiation therapy of non-small cell lung cancer. *Int J Radiat Oncol Biol Phys* 2014; 88: 1148–1153.
21. van Baardwijk A, Wanders S, Boersma L, *et al.* Mature results of an individualized radiation dose prescription study based on normal tissue constraints in stages I to III non-small-cell lung cancer. *J Clin Oncol* 2010; 28: 1380–1386.
22. van Baardwijk A, Reymen B, Wanders S, *et al.* Mature results of a phase II trial on individualized accelerated radiotherapy (INDAR) based on normal tissue constraints in concurrent chemo-radiation for stage III non-small cell lung cancer (NSCLC). *Eur J Cancer* 2012; 48: 2339–2346.
23. van Elmpt W, De Ruysscher D, van der Salm A, *et al.* The PET-boost randomised phase II dose-escalation trial in non-small cell lung cancer. *Radiother Oncol* 2012; 104: 67–71.
24. Fleckenstein J, Hellwig D, Kremp S, *et al.* F-18-FDG-PET confined radiotherapy of locally advanced NSCLC with concomitant chemotherapy: results of the PET-PLAN pilot trial. *Int J Radiat Oncol Biol Phys* 2011; 81: e283–e289.
25. Pilones KA, Vanpouille-Box C, Demaria S. Combination of radiotherapy and immune checkpoint inhibitors. *Semin Radiat Oncol* 2015; 25: 28–33.
26. Rusch VW. Management of Pancoast tumours. *Lancet Oncol* 2006; 7: 997–1005.

Disclosures: None declared

Chapter 15

# Chemotherapy

Adam Januszewski and Sanjay Popat

Chemotherapy continues to be the cornerstone of lung cancer therapeutics in patients without known actionable mutations, despite advances in molecular therapeutics. In NSCLC, a therapeutic plateau had been reached with platinum-doublet chemotherapy. However, the development of pemetrexed and its differential activity by histology has heralded a new era in lung cancer diagnostics such that NSCLC subtypes are now critical to decision-making. Nevertheless, several questions still remain, including the optimal treatment cycle number, to use cisplatin or carboplatin, the role of maintenance therapy, and optimal management of performance status 2 patients. For SCLC, chemotherapy has been the cornerstone of therapy for the last 30 years. A therapeutic plateau has been reached for first-line therapy where despite trials of newer schedules, doses, supportive care and drugs, platinum–etoposide remains a standard. Chemotherapy plays a minor but important role for relapsed SCLC and an important challenge is the identification of patients most likely to benefit from systemic therapy.

Over the years, chemotherapy has become the cornerstone for the treatment of lung cancer: both SCLC and NSCLC. Multiple studies have established a survival and symptom control benefit for chemotherapy. In this chapter, we review data that underpin standard clinical practice and highlight areas of controversy.

## NSCLC

Early studies enrolled all patients with lung cancer and did not consider treatment stratification by histological variant [1–3]. The activity of alkylating agents such as nitrogen mustard were first demonstrated in 1969 and the discovery that striking variation in response was dependent upon histological subtype became the forerunner of stratified treatments in lung cancer [4]. Polychemotherapy regimens, such as methotrexate, cyclophosphamide, procarbazine and vincristine, were subsequently developed aiming to increase response rates and overall survival, this particular combination demonstrating superior remissions when administered simultaneously [5]. In 1977, cisplatin started to be used to treat NSCLC and was shown to increase overall survival compared with dianhydrogalactitol, paving the way to platinum-based combination chemotherapy [6]. While platinum-based chemotherapy developed quickly in SCLC due to excellent response rates, outcomes for NSCLC were controversial in the context of small trials with heterogeneous patient populations [7–12].

One of the first large randomised phase 3 trials to confirm a survival advantage for chemotherapy for NSCLC was a National Cancer Institute of Canada trial of vindesine–cisplatin or cyclophosphamide–doxorubicin–cisplatin *versus* best supportive care (BSC).

Royal Marsden Hospital, London, UK.

Correspondence: Sanjay Popat, Royal Marsden Hospital, Fulham Road, London SW3 6JJ, UK. E-mail: sanjay.popat@rmh.nhs.uk

 Print ISBN: 978-1-84984-061-3. Online ISBN: 978-1-84984-062-0. Print ISSN: 2312-508X. Online ISSN: 2312-5098.

Here, overall survival was 32.6 (p=0.01), 24.7 (p=0.05) and 17 weeks, respectively, with responses also favouring vindesine-cisplatin [7]. Similarly, Woods *et al.* [13] confirmed a similar overall survival advantage for vindesine–cisplatin, although toxicities remained significant and, therefore, cytotoxic use in NSCLC remained questionable. The high emetogenicity of cisplatin considerably limited its early use. However, with the later introduction of serotonin antagonists in the early 1990s, concomitant improvements in clinical outcomes were also observed [14, 15].

It was not until an individual-patient meta-analysis in 1995 of chemotherapy *versus* BSC that chemotherapy became more widely used in advanced NSCLC [16]. Here, 1190 patients were included across 11 trials and patients who received chemotherapy had a significant overall survival advantage (hazard ratio (HR) 0.73, p<0.0001) with a 10% improvement in absolute survival at 1 year (from 5% to 15%). This analysis did not, however, discriminate between individual schedules.

### Platinum-based chemotherapy

Over the subsequent years, a plethora of studies using various schedules were trialled in advanced NSCLC. Two meta-analyses published in 2005 and 2006 concluded that platinum-based schedules were superior to nonplatinum ones [17, 18]. D'Addario *et al.* [17] analysed 37 trials and demonstrated a 62% relative significant response rate favouring platinum-based treatment (OR 1.62, 95% CI 1.46–1.8; p<0.001). Similarly, in a meta-analysis of 14 phase 3 trials, Pujol *et al.* [18] confirmed an improved overall survival at 1 year (OR 0.88, 95% CI 0.78–0.99; p=0.044) for platinum-based regimes. However, an increased risk of grade 3/4 gastrointestinal and haematological toxicities was observed.

These meta-analyses did not identify the optimal platinum partner. During the early part of this century, third-generation cytotoxics, including gemcitabine, vinorelbine and paclitaxel, were developed and compared (as doublets). In a seminal trial in 2002, the Eastern Cooperative Oncology Group compared cisplatin–paclitaxel with three comparators (cisplatin–gemcitabine, cisplatin–docetaxel and carboplatin–paclitaxel) in 1207 patients [19]. No significant response rate or overall survival differences were observed. These findings were replicated in another large randomised phase 3 trial, with no overall survival or response rate benefit between third-generation cytotoxic doublets (gemcitabine, paclitaxel and vinorelbine) [20] and suggesting a therapeutic plateau.

An individual-patient data meta-analysis in 2008 (including third-generation cytotoxics) demonstrated a significant and meaningful overall survival improvement with chemotherapy compared with BSC (HR 0.77, 95% CI 0.71–0.83; p<0.0001) [21]. This translated to an absolute increase in survival from 20% to 29% at 1 year. No clear differences in efficacy were observed with the cytotoxic agent (p=0.63), suggesting that platinum-based chemotherapy with any third-generation cytotoxic would be considered optimal.

### Cisplatin or carboplatin?

Cisplatin has serious toxicities including nausea, vomiting, myelosuppression, neurotoxicity and nephrotoxicity, and a long administration schedule. To overcome this, carboplatin was investigated due to its more favourable toxicity profile and lack of hydration requirement. Despite pre-clinical data suggesting similar mechanisms of action and efficacy between cisplatin and carboplatin, multiple trials investigating the therapeutic benefit of each platinum reported conflicting outcomes. A seminal individual patient meta-analysis of nine trials involving 2938 patients identified an improved response rate ($p<0.001$) for cisplatin without any significant benefit in overall survival ($p=0.100$) [22]. However, in nonsquamous NSCLC (nsNSCLC), patients treated with third-generation cytotoxics and carboplatin had inferior response rates (HR 1.37, 95% CI 1.16–1.61) and overall survival (HR 1.12, 95% CI 1.01–1.23).

## Does histology matter?

Age, performance status (PS), stage, sex and weight loss within 6 months were previously identified as significant prognostic factors [23]. However, histology is now an important predictive and prognostic variable due to customised systemic therapy contingent on somatic mutation status and histological subtype.

Pemetrexed is a third-generation, multitargeted antifolate cytotoxic that inhibits several enzymes involved in purine and pyrimidine synthesis, including thymidylate synthase, and the importance of histological NSCLC subtype characterisation has been firmly established though protocol-specified and *post hoc* analyses of pemetrexed trial data. In the JMEI registration noninferiority phase 3 trial in the second/third-line setting, pemetrexed was compared with docetaxel [24]. Noninferiority was confirmed with equivalent response rates (9.1% *versus* 8.8%, $p=0.105$), PFS and overall survival (8.3 *versus* 7.9 months, HR 0.99 (95% CI 0.82–1.2); $p=0.226$), with markedly increased toxicities observed for docetaxel, specifically neutropenia (40.2% *versus* 5.3%, $p<0.001$) and febrile neutropenia (12.7% *versus* 1.9%, $p<0.001$).

Having established pemetrexed for relapsed nsNSCLC, it was further evaluated in the first-line setting in the JMDB registration noninferiority phase III trial, comparing gemcitabine–cisplatin with pemetrexed–cisplatin [25]. Overall, noninferiority was confirmed for pemetrexed–cisplatin, with significantly improved grade 3/4 myelotoxicity. In a protocol-planned analysis, treatment-by-histology interaction was found to be a significant covariate ($p=0.0011$), with significant improvement in overall survival observed for pemetrexed–cisplatin in ADC over gemcitabine–cisplatin (12.6 *versus* 10.9 months, HR 0.82 (95% CI 0.70–0.94); $p=0.005$). In squamous tumours, pemetrexed–cisplatin was significantly inferior to gemcitabine–cisplatin (9.4 *versus* 10.8 months, HR 1.23; $p=0.05$). This efficacy data, the favourable toxicity profile and the 21-day scheduling helped establish cisplatin–pemetrexed as a standard of care for first-line treatment of nsNSCLC.

The histology findings prompted a *post hoc* analysis of JMEI [26] and, again, a significant treatment-by-histology interaction ($p=0.001$) was identified, with a greater overall survival for nsNSCLC (HR 0.758, 95% CI 0.61–1.00; $p=0.047$) and significantly worse overall survival in squamous tumours (HR 1.56, 95% CI 1.08–2.26; $p=0.18$). These findings prompted a label change by the FDA to exclude squamous tumours from pemetrexed indications.

Histology-guided treatment was the forerunner to personalised medicine. The discovery of individual actionable mutations, such as *EGFR* and *ALK* rearrangement, has led to targeted treatments. However, those patients without such actionable mutations are currently treated with histology-guided standard chemotherapies.

## What treatment duration is optimal?

Optimal treatment duration is an important question in the palliative setting as it influences quality of life, duration of hospital stay and cost. The 2003 American Society of Clinical Oncology (ASCO) guidelines on chemotherapy use recommended two to eight cycles for NSCLC based on limited evidence [27]. Early studies used older regimens and a meta-analysis of these published in 2009 [28] demonstrated that while PFS was longer with more treatment cycles (HR 0.75, 95% CI 0.69–0.81; p<0.0001), overall survival improvement was less meaningful (HR 0.92, 95% CI 0.86–0.99; p=0.003). Extending treatment also resulted in more treatment-related adverse events.

The first phase III study investigating the impact of treatment duration with a third-generation platinum-based regimen was in 2001 by Smith *et al.* [29]. 308 patients received either three or six cycles of mitomycin–vinblastine–cisplatin chemotherapy with no additional benefit seen in overall survival, 1-year survival (p=0.2) or symptom control (p=0.4). Furthermore, quality of life parameters were the same or improved in those receiving three cycles with significantly reduced fatigue (p=0.03). Further similar studies followed [30, 31] and results of these were combined in a recent individual patient meta-analysis including five trials [32]. While patients who received six cycles rather than fewer (three or four) had improved PFS (6.09 *versus* 5.33 months, HR 0.79 (95% CI 0.68–0.90); p=0.0007), this did not translate into a significant overall survival difference (9.54 *versus* 8.68 months, HR 0.94 (95% CI 0.83–1.07); p=0.33). There were no subgroups that benefited from extended treatment and haematological toxicity was more frequent in patients receiving extended treatment. Current ASCO chemotherapy use guidelines suggest no more than four cycles in nonresponders and six cycles in responders [33] while the European Society for Medical Oncology recommends four cycles in most patients, particularly if maintenance treatment is being considered, with a maximum of six cycles [34].

## Maintenance treatment

Extending treatment with maintenance therapy has had increasing interest in recent years due to low rates of patients suitable for chemotherapy on relapse, and has been developed through either continuation of an induction agent (continuation maintenance) or through switch to a different agent (switch maintenance). The landmark phase III study of 566 patients with NSCLC by Fidias *et al.* [35] demonstrated a median PFS improvement of 3 months (5.7 *versus* 2.7 months, p=0.001) when docetaxel was used as switch maintenance after induction gemcitabine/carboplatin compared to delayed docetaxel given at relapse, but failed short of meeting the primary end-point of overall survival (p=0.0853). However, only 31% of patients received delayed docetaxel, demonstrating the role of switch maintenance in ensuring patients receive second-line therapy prior to deterioration. Other phase III studies of maintenance schedules have failed to show a significant overall survival benefit with paclitaxel [36], gemcitabine [37] and vinorelbine [38].

By contrast, pemetrexed has demonstrated increased PFS and overall survival when used both as switch and continuous maintenance therapies. In the initial randomised phase III superiority trial of switch pemetrexed (JMEN), nonprogressors after four cycles of a cisplatin-based induction doublet were randomised to maintenance pemetrexed or placebo [39]. Pemetrexed improved PFS (4.3 *versus* 2.6 months, HR 0.50 (95% CI 0.42–0.61); p<0.0001) and overall survival (13.4 *versus* 10.6 months, HR 0.79 (95% CI 0.65–0.95);

p=0.012). The PARAMOUNT study investigated pemetrexed continuation maintenance after four cycles of cisplatin–pemetrexed induction *versus* placebo. Maintenance pemetrexed improved PFS (4.1 *versus* 2.8 months, HR 0.62 (95% CI 0.49–0.79); p<0.0001) and overall survival (13.9 *versus* 11.0 months, HR 0.78 (95% CI 0.64–0.96); p=0.0195) [40, 41]. However, fewer placebo patients received second-line pemetrexed or any type of anticancer systemic therapy, highlighting the inherent limitations of maintenance studies. Moreover, maintenance therapy commits patients to potentially long-term treatments, additional toxicities and frequent hospital visits, all of which can potentially impact on the normality of life. Thus, while maintenance therapy is approved by regulatory authorities, it may not be optimal for all patients, and such a strategy should be tailored to each individual patient.

Erlotinib is the only other agent that has shown activity in the maintenance setting. Erlotinib was given after four cycles of induction platinum doublet chemotherapy as part of the SATURN (Sequential Tarceva in Unresectable NSCLC) phase III trial. This increased PFS (12.3 *versus* 11.1 weeks, HR 0.79 (95% CI 0.51–0.82); p<0.0001) and overall survival only in the subgroup of patients with stable disease after induction treatment (11.9 *versus* 9.6 months, HR 0.72 (95% CI 0.59–0.89); p=0.0019) [42, 43].

Currently, maintenance therapy is only recommended in patients with nsNSCLC after tumour stabilisation or response to induction cisplatin/pemetrexed with maintenance pemetrexed [34]. Although these few positive trials suggest some benefit in the use of maintenance treatment and have led to regulatory approval, it has to be tailored to each individual patient based upon their response and tolerability of the toxicities of treatment.

## First-line treatment in patients with PS 2

It has long been established that PS is a key prognostic indicator in NSCLC [23] and patients with PS 2 have lower median (4.5 *versus* 8.9 months, p<0.01) and 1-year survival (10% *versus* 37%, p<0.01) when compared with PS 0–1 patients treated with a platinum-doublet chemotherapy [44]. Caution has been employed in using standard platinum doublets for PS 2 patients for fear of increased toxicities and reducing overall survival.

The first major randomised trial to evaluate the role of chemomonotherapy in PS 2 patients was the Elderly Lung Cancer Vinorelbine Italian Study [45]. Here, patients aged ⩾70 years were randomised to vinorelbine monotherapy or BSC. The trial was closed early due to poor accrual. Nevertheless, overall survival was significantly improved (median 21 *versus* 28 weeks, HR 0.65 (95% CI 0.45–0.93)). Supporting the role of chemomonotherapy, a multitude of phase 2 studies have demonstrated modest activity and expected toxicities [46].

Zukin *et al.* [47] assessed the role of platinum-doublet chemotherapy by randomising 205 patients with PS 2 to receive pemetrexed or pemetrexed-carboplatin. The doublet demonstrated significantly improved response rates (10.3% *versus* 23.8%, p=0.032), PFS (2.8 *versus* 5.8 months, p<0.001) and overall survival (5.3 *versus* 9.3 months, HR 0.62 (95% CI 0.46–0.83); p=0.001). Myelosuppression was more frequent in the combination group. These efficacy results were supported by a literature-based meta-analysis comparing single agents to combinations in PS 2 patients, analysing 12 trials [48]. A survival benefit was seen for platinum-based combination chemotherapy, at the expense of increased toxicities. Thus, platinum-based combination treatment should be considered in suitable PS 2 patients and, furthermore, has been shown to improve symptom control with a better quality of life improvement [44, 49].

### Treatment for relapsed NSCLC

Second- and subsequent-line treatment in patients with NSCLC and PS 0–2 is now considered the standard of care.

### Docetaxel

Docetaxel was the first agent approved for the use in the second-line setting for NSCLC and remains an international standard. In TAX317, 103 patients with PS 0–2 who had progressed after at least first-line platinum-based chemotherapy were randomised to docetaxel (100 mg·m$^{-2}$ every 3 weeks) or BSC [50]. 74% of patients were treated in the second-line setting. After excessive toxicity in the docetaxel 100 mg·m$^{-2}$ group (febrile neutropenia in 11 (22%) patients), docetaxel was amended to 75 mg·m$^{-2}$. Response rates for docetaxel were modest at 5.5%, with time to progression (TTP) (10.6 *versus* 6.7 weeks, p<0.001) and overall survival (7.0 *versus* 4.6 months, p=0.047) significantly longer for docetaxel. Neutropenia remained concerning at 67% but translated to a 1.8% febrile neutropenia rate.

Docetaxel registration was also supported by the TAX320 trial [51]. Here, docetaxel was shown to be superior to vinorelbine or ifosfomide (V/I) monotherapy in the second- or later-line setting. Again, response rates were modest, at 6.7% (docetaxel 75 mg·m$^{-2}$) *versus* 0.8% (V/I, p=0.036), and TTP was prolonged (p=0.046).

Attempting to improve the tolerability of 3-weekly docetaxel, several weekly administration schedules have been developed. A subsequent individual patient data meta-analysis of five trials of weekly *versus* 3-weekly therapy demonstrated no overall survival difference (p=0.24), with reduced neutropenia severity and febrile neutropenia (p<0.0001) [52].

### Pemetrexed

The data to underpin pemetrexed use in the first-line and maintenance settings have restricted its use in the second-line setting, as most pemetrexed-eligible patients receive it prior to their first relapse. These trials have been discussed above.

### Single agent or combination therapy?

Several phase 2 studies have subsequently identified activity for a number of other cytotoxics in relapsed NSCLC, including gemcitabine and vinorelbine. In good-PS patients, the role of single-agent or combination chemotherapy has been addressed with several studies demonstrating a potential efficacy advantage for combination therapy (table 1) [53–58].

In an important individual-patient meta-analysis, Di Maio *et al.* [59] pooled survival data from several trials of single-agent *versus* combination therapy, and demonstrated a small but significant PFS superiority for combination therapy (median 11.7 *versus* 14.0 weeks, p=0009) and a doubling of response rate (7.3% *versus* 15.1%, p=0.0004), but no improvement in

Table 1. Single-agent chemotherapy compared with combination chemotherapy in second-line treatment of advanced NSCLC

| First author [ref.] | Control arm | Additional agent# | Primary end-point | Patients n | PFS singlet *versus* doublet | OS singlet *versus* doublet |
|---|---|---|---|---|---|---|
| Takeda [53] | Docetaxel 60 $mg \cdot m^{-2}$ Day 1 Every 3 weeks | Gemcitabine 800 $mg \cdot m^{-2}$ Days 1 and 8 Every 3 weeks | OS | 130 | 2.1 *versus* 2.8 months (p=0.028) | 10.1 *versus* 10.3 months (p=0.36) |
| Georgoulias [54] | Irinotecan 300 $mg \cdot m^{-2}$ Day 1 Every 3 weeks | Gemcitabine 1000 $mg \cdot m^{-2}$ Days 1 and 8 | OS | 147 | 7.5 (range 2.5–19) months *versus* 5.0 (range 1.0–15.5) months (p=0.346) | 9 (range 0.5–29) months *versus* 7 (range 0.5–24) months (p=0.589) |
| Georgoulias [55] | Cisplatin 80 $mg \cdot m^{-2}$ Day 1 Every 3 weeks | Irinotecan 110 $mg \cdot m^{-2}$ Day 1 100 $mg \cdot m^{-2}$ Day 8 Every 3 weeks | OS | 139 | 2.6 (range 1–20.3) months *versus* 2.1 (range 1–17.6) months (TTP) (p=0.641) | 7.8 (range 0.5–25.2) months *versus* 8.8 (range 0.5–23.3) months (p=0.933) |
| Wachters [56] | Docetaxel 75 $mg \cdot m^{-2}$ Day 1 Every 3 weeks | Irinotecan 200 $mg \cdot m^{-2}$ Day 1 Every 3 weeks Docetaxel reduced to 60 $mg \cdot m^{-2} \cdot day^{-1}$ | RR | 108 | 18 (95% CI 16–21) weeks *versus* 15 (95% CI 12–18) weeks (p=0.42) | 32 (95% CI 25–40) weeks *versus* 27 (95% CI 8–46) weeks (p=0.69) |
| Gebbia [57] | Docetaxel 33.3 $mg \cdot m^{-2}$ Days 1, 8 and 15 Every 4 weeks | Capecitabine 1300 $mg \cdot m^{-2}$ Days 5–18 Every 4 weeks Docetaxel reduced to 30 $mg \cdot m^{-2} \cdot day^{-1}$ | OS | 84 | 12.4 (95% CI 11.6–23.6) weeks *versus* 11.9 (95% CI 8.9–26.6) weeks (p=0.60) | 40.0 (95% CI 25.0–58.7) weeks *versus* 39.7 (95% CI 24.9–NA) weeks (p=0.90) |
| Gebbia [57] | Docetaxel 33.3 $mg \cdot m^{-2}$ Days 1, 8 and 15 Every 4 weeks | Gemcitabine 800 $mg \cdot m^{-2}$ Days 1 and 8 Every 4 weeks Or vinorelbine 20 $mg \cdot m^{-2}$ Days 1 and 8 Every 4 weeks or docetaxel reduced to 30 $mg \cdot m^{-2} \cdot day^{-1}$ | OS | 84 | 12.4 (95% CI 11.6–23.6) weeks *versus* 13.1 (95% CI 11.4–44.9) weeks (p=0.44) | 40.0 (95% CI 25.0–58.7) weeks *versus* 32.6 (95% CI 13.9–50.9) weeks (p=0.18) |
| Smit [58] | Pemetrexed 500 $mg \cdot m^{-2}$ Every 3 weeks | Carboplatin AUC 5 | TTP | 240 | 2.8 (95% CI 2.5–3.0) months *versus* 4.2 (95% CI 3.7–4.6) months (HR 0.67, 95% CI 0.51–0.89; p=0.005) | 7.6 (95% CI 6.6–9.9) months *versus* 8.0 (95% CI 7.4–10.5) months (HR 0.85; 95% CI 0.63–1.2; p=NS) |

OS: overall survival; TTP: time to progression; RR: response rate; NA: not applicable; AUC: area under the curve; HR: hazard ratio; NS: nonsignificant. #: to control arm. Modified from [59].

overall survival (HR 0.92, 95% CI 0.79–1.08; p=0.32). Thus, single-agent therapy has become firmly established as a general standard.

## SCLC

SCLC was not recognised as an entity that required stratified treatments until the discovery of its differential propensity to aggressive behaviour and early metastases [60] supported by varied responses seen to cyclophosphamide monotherapy [4] and other single agents [61, 62]. Combination regimens were studied to improve outcomes and cyclophosphamide–doxorubicin–vincristine (CAV) became standard during the 1970–1980s, when this was shown to have response rates of 57% with an overall survival of 26 weeks in patients with extensive stage SCLC (ES-SCLC) [63].

## Etoposide–platinum chemotherapy in SCLC

Platinum-based agents were first investigated in the 1970s to a mixed reaction due to difficult-to-control nausea and vomiting [64]. Cisplatin and etoposide had synergistic activity in pre-clinical models [65], and were subsequently used in relapsed SCLC [66] and patients with anthracycline-contraindications [67]. Etoposide–cisplatin had response rates at induction of 71–94% with complete responses in 30–53% and overall survival of 43 weeks in ES-SCLC [67, 68]. Similar response rates to anthracycline combinations and favourable toxicities led to trials of CAV *versus* etoposide–platinum, demonstrating equivalent response rates (61% *versus* 51%, p=0.175) and overall survival (8.6 *versus* 8.3 months, p=0.662) [69].

An early literature-based meta-analysis of 4054 patients [70] suggested platinum-based combinations had significantly higher response rates and improved overall survival at 1 year (p=0.002) than alkylating regimens with no differences in toxic deaths. This was supported by a Norwegian randomised trial of 436 patients of etoposide–platinum or epirubicin–cyclophosphamide–vincristine (CEV). A significant overall survival benefit from etoposide–platinum chemotherapy was observed (10.2 *versus* 7.8 months, p<0.001), although this was primarily seen in the limited-stage cohort (overall survival 14.5 *versus* 9.7 months). A nonsignificant trend toward improved survival for etoposide–platinum was also seen in the extensive stage (overall survival 8.4 *versus* 6.5 months) [71].

### Cisplatin or carboplatin?

Head-to-head comparisons between cisplatin and carboplatin have failed to demonstrate differences in response rates or overall survival. However, increased rates of nausea, vomiting and neurotoxicity from cisplatin were observed [72]. These findings were supported in an elderly/poor-risk population [73] and also in a recent important meta-analysis of four trials [74]. While in this pooled analysis of 663 patients, no differences in response rate, PFS or overall survival were demonstrated between cisplatin and carboplatin, increased haematological toxicities were observed for carboplatin, and increased nonhaematological toxicities for cisplatin. Due to the limited number of patients pooled, there was insufficient power to draw meaningful conclusions for important subsets, such as young patients and those with limited-stage disease, and for these patients, cisplatin is recommended [75].

### Third-generation cytotoxics

Since etoposide–platinum has been established as standard first-line treatment for SCLC, there have been numerous studies investigating platinum-based doublets using etoposide–platinum as a control. Irinotecan, a topoisomerase I inhibitor, was studied in a Japanese phase III trial comparing etoposide–platinum with irinotecan–etoposide. This terminated early because of a significant overall survival benefit from irinotecan–etoposide (12.8 *versus* 9.4 months, p=0.002) on interim analysis [76]. These data led to irinotecan–etoposide being approved in Japan. Aiming to validate these results in non-Japanese patients, the US-based study by Hanna *et al.* [77] randomised 331 patients to modified irinotecan–etoposide or etoposide–platinum. Toxicities observed were as expected for these agents, but no differences in response rates (48% *versus* 43.6%), median TTP or overall survival (median 9.3 *versus* 10.2 months) were identified. Aiming to see if dosing differences may have accounted for this discrepancy, the US S0124 study [77, 78] randomised 671 patients between irinotecan–etoposide and etoposide–platinum using exactly the same design and schedule as the Japanese trial [76]. Again, no differences in response rate, PFS or overall survival (median 9.9 *versus* 9.1 months) were observed, perhaps due to pharmacogenomic differences between populations.

Pemetrexed has unfortunately demonstrated little impact in SCLC. A noninferiority phase III trial of pemetrexed–carboplatin in chemotherapy-naïve, extensive-stage SCLC was closed early after a planned interim analysis demonstrated inferior response rate, PFS and overall survival (median 8.1 *versus* 10.6 months, p<0.01) for pemetrexed [79].

Combination gemcitabine with carboplatin has been evaluated in a UK noninferiority phase III trial, randomising 241 patients with previously untreated SCLC and poor prognostic factors to either gemcitabine–carboplatin or cisplatin–etoposide [80]. PFS and overall survival were not different between gemcitabine–carboplatin and cisplatin–etoposide (median overall survival 8.0 *versus* 8.1 months, respectively), with less alopecia reported.

### Alternative chemotherapy strategies

To consolidate the benefit of platinum-based chemotherapy, a number of strategies have been employed. Duration of therapy and maintenance treatment have been assessed with no significant improvements [81]. Non-cross-resistant regimes have been trialled with conflicting results [69, 82], and rapid sequencing of treatment and dose intensification have also been attempted. All have failed to improve outcomes with a detrimental increased toxicity [83–86]. Maintaining dose intensity by haematopoietic growth factors usage has been trialled [87, 88] but not demonstrated a reproducible benefit [89–91]. High-dose chemotherapy with stem cell transplant was associated with high treatment-related mortality and no difference in overall survival [92].

### First-line treatment in patients with a poor PS

Limited trials have included patients with poor PS. Evidence to date demonstrates that using inferior chemotherapy regimens to limit toxicities has inferior response rates, PFS and overall survival, with little or no difference in toxicities observed. Accordingly, oral etoposide was compared with alternating CAV/etoposide–platinum and all outcome measures were inferior for etoposide [93]. Furthermore, no differences in outcome or palliation scores were observed for split-dose etoposide–platinum compared to carboplatin–etoposide in patients with poor PS [73]. Thus, for patients with poor PS due to SCLC where chemotherapy is considered, then an optimal regime to induce response is recommended, but needs to be balanced with the high mortality observed in poor-PS patients. Here, the use of prophylactic antibiotics and granulocyte colony-stimulating factor may reduce the frequency of febrile neutropenia [94].

## Second-line treatment

Patients progressing after first-line SCLC treatment have poor prognosis, with overall survival of 2–3 months without treatment. Use of cytotoxic chemotherapy in the second line is debateable, but has shown to be beneficial, although responses are short lived and survival still poor. Response to initial chemotherapy and PS are prognostic and predictive of chemotherapy outcomes [95]. Three categories of patients have been described, related to small historical observational studies based on responses to first-line treatment [96, 97] "Sensitive relapse" refers to patients with a treatment-free interval of >90 days, "resistant relapse" refers to patients who progress <90 days from completing first-line treatment and "refractory" patients are those who did not respond to first-line chemotherapy.

From a large systematic analysis pooling outcome data from 26 trials of chemotherapy based on 1692 patients with relapsed SCLC stratified by relapse before/after 90 days of completing first-line chemotherapy, significant response rate differences were observed for sensitive, resistant and refractory cases [98]. Response rates of 27.7% with an overall survival of 7.7 months were observed for sensitive relapse, while evidence of benefit for treating patients with refractory/resistant disease is debateable, with a response rate of 14.8% and an overall survival of 5.5 months [98].

Patients with a sensitive relapse and a treatment-free interval of at least 6 months may respond to first-line agent re-challenge, with response rates reported to be 34–62%, demonstrated by historical patient series and retrospective clinical dataset analyses, although prospective trial validation is lacking [99–101].

Given this poor prognostic group, the toxicity profile and its effect on quality of life are important considerations for chemotherapy. Several single agents (gemcitabine, irinotecan, paclitaxel and vinorelbine) have been investigated, with inferior outcomes compared with combination regimens [102–104]. The second-line results of an important crossover study [71] not only demonstrated the superiority of EP for first-line SCLC, but also established anthracycline-based therapy for relapsed SCLC. The second-line outcomes from this trial demonstrated that only 42% of patients were suitable for chemotherapy randomisation at relapse, and a benefit of chemotherapy over BSC for relapsed SCLC (median overall survival 5.3 *versus* 2.2 months, $p<0.0001$) [105].

An important single-arm, phase 2 study of the topoisomerase I inhibitor topotecan demonstrated activity in both sensitive and refractory relapsed SCLC [106], with response rates of 6.4% in refractory patients and 37.8% in sensitive patients. Developing topotecan further, a large trial randomising relapsed SCLC patients to either CAV or intravenous topotecan demonstrated equivalent response rates (24.3% *versus* 18.3%, $p=0.285$) and overall survival (25 *versus* 24.7 weeks, $p=0.795$) with superior palliation of symptoms, but increased myelosuppression, from topotecan [107]. With the development of an oral topotecan formulation, a randomised phase III trial [108] demonstrated equivalence of oral *versus* intravenous formulations (median overall survival 33 *versus* 35 weeks, respectively). A subsequent pivotal phase 3 trial of oral topotecan *versus* BSC in patients with relapsed SCLC [109] confirmed superiority of topotecan (overall survival 25.9 *versus* 13.9 weeks) irrespective of resistant or sensitive relapse and improved symptom control, at the expense of haematological toxicities. This study led to registration of topotecan for use in the second-line setting: the only licensed agent in this setting to date.

### Recent advances in SCLC

#### *Amrubicin*

Amrubicin is a noncardiotoxic, synthetic anthracycline-based topoisomerase II inhibitor. Developed in Japan, initial studies demonstrated encouraging efficacy for relapsed SCLC [110, 111]. Studies in the first-line setting were encouraging, although neutropenia rates were significant (95% grade 3/4 neutropenia) [112]. Aiming to develop amrubicin globally for relapsed SCLC, ACT1 was a large phase III trial randomising relapsed SCLC patients to either amrubicin or topotecan. The primary end-point of overall survival was not met (median overall survival 7.5 *versus* 7.8 months (amrubicin *versus* topotecan), p=0.17). Significantly increased treatment-related grade 3/4 myelosuppression, infections and febrile neutropenia were observed [113], and as a result, amrubicin has not been developed further in the USA or Europe.

#### *Picoplatin*

Picoplatin is an organic platinum analogue rationally designed to overcome acquired platinum resistance [114]. Initial evidence for efficacy came from a phase 2 study in platinum-refractory/resistant SCLC. However, the subsequent pivotal global phase III trial of resistant/refractory relapsed SCLC patients randomised to picoplatin or BSC failed to reach its primary end-point of overall survival (hazard ration 0.8, p=0.09) [115].

## Conclusion

There have been major advances in the cytotoxic management of patients with advanced NSCLC. Having seemed to reach a therapeutic plateau, the development of pemetrexed has caused major changes in NSCLC diagnosis, requiring pathologists now to subclassify NSCLC by histological subtype. Coupled with advances in molecular therapeutics, management of advanced NSCLC in 2015 is totally different to that 10 years previously. In the future, a better understanding of differing molecular subtypes will be gained as well as how best to integrate cytotoxic chemotherapy with molecular targeted therapy and the new immune checkpoint inhibitors.

For SCLC, a therapeutic impasse has been reached, with no major systemic advances since topotecan registration. Significantly active therapeutics for relapsed SCLC are lacking and a better understanding of SCLC biology is urgently required to implement scientifically rationalised studies for what is becoming a rarer disease in the West.

## References


1. Wolf J, Yesner R, Patno ME. Evaluation of nitrogen mustard in prolonging life of patients with bronchogenic carcinoma. *Cancer Chemother Rep* 1962; 16: 473–475.
2. Wolf J, Spear P, Yesner R, *et al.* Nitrogen mustard and the steroid hormones in the treatment of inoperable bronchogenic carcinoma. *Am J Med* 1960; 29: 1008–1016.
3. Levine B, Weisberger AS. The response of various types of bronchogenic carcinoma to nitrogen mustard. *Ann Intern Med* 1955; 42: 1089–1096.
4. Green RA, Humphrey E, Close H, *et al.* Alkylating agents in bronchogenic carcinoma. *Am J Med* 1969; 46: 516–525.
5. Alberto P, Brunner KW, Martz G, *et al.* Treatment of bronchogenic carcinoma with simultaneous or sequential combination chemotherapy, including methotrexate, cyclophosphamide, procarbazine and vincristine. *Cancer* 1976; 38: 2208–2216.
6. Eagan RT, Ingle JN, Frytak S, *et al.* Platinum-based polychemotherapy *versus* dianhydrogalactitol in advanced non-small cell lung cancer. *Cancer Treat Rep* 1977; 61: 1339–1345.
7. Rapp E, Pater JL, Willan A, *et al.* Chemotherapy can prolong survival in patients with advanced non-small-cell lung cancer – report of a Canadian multicenter randomized trial. *J Clin Oncol* 1988; 6: 633–641.
8. Laing AH, Berry RJ, Newman CR, *et al.* Treatment of inoperable carcinoma of bronchus. *Lancet* 1975; 2: 1161–1164.
9. Cormier Y, Bergeron D, La Forge J, *et al.* Benefits of polychemotherapy in advanced non-small-cell bronchogenic carcinoma. *Cancer* 1982; 50: 845–849.
10. Anderson G, Payne H. Response rate and toxicity of etoposide (VP-16) in squamous carcinoma of the lung: report from the Lung Cancer Treatment Study Group. *Semin Oncol* 1985; 12: Suppl. 2, 21–22.
11. Cellerino R, Tummarello D, Guidi F, *et al.* A randomized trial of alternating chemotherapy *versus* best supportive care in advanced non-small-cell lung cancer. *J Clin Oncol* 1991; 9: 1453–1461.
12. Kaasa S, Lund E, Thorud E, *et al.* Symptomatic treatment *versus* combination chemotherapy for patients with extensive non-small cell lung cancer. *Cancer* 1991; 67: 2443–2447.
13. Woods RL, Williams CJ, Levi J, *et al.* A randomised trial of cisplatin and vindesine *versus* supportive care only in advanced non-small cell lung cancer. *Br J Cancer* 1990; 61: 608–611.
14. De Mulder PHM. Ondansetron compared with high-dose metoclopramide in prophylaxis of acute and delayed cisplatin-induced nausea and vomiting. *Ann Intern Med* 1990; 113: 834.
15. Hainsworth J, Harvey W, Pendergrass K, *et al.* A single-blind comparison of intravenous ondansetron, a selective serotonin antagonist, with intravenous metoclopramide in the prevention of nausea and vomiting associated with high-dose cisplatin chemotherapy. *J Clin Oncol* 1991; 9: 721–728.
16. Non-Small Cell Lung Cancer Collaborative Group. Chemotherapy in non-small cell lung cancer: a meta-analysis using updated data on individual patients from 52 randomised clinical trials. *BMJ* 1995; 311: 899–909.
17. D'Addario G, Pintilie M, Leighl NB, *et al.* Platinum-based *versus* non-platinum-based chemotherapy in advanced non-small-cell lung cancer: a meta-analysis of the published literature. *J Clin Oncol [Internet]* 2005; 23: 2926–2936.
18. Pujol J-L, Barlesi F, Daurès J-P. Should chemotherapy combinations for advanced non-small cell lung cancer be platinum-based? A meta-analysis of phase III randomized trials. *Lung Cancer* 2006; 51: 335–345.
19. Schiller JH, Harrington D, Belani CP, *et al.* Comparison of four chemotherapy regimens for advanced non-small-cell lung cancer. *N Engl J Med* 2002; 346: 92–98.
20. Scagliotti GV, De Marinis F, Rinaldi M, *et al.* Phase III randomized trial comparing three platinum-based doublets in advanced non-small-cell lung cancer. *J Clin Oncol* 2002; 20: 4285–4291.
21. NSCLC Meta-Analyses Collaborative Group. Chemotherapy in addition to supportive care improves survival in advanced non-small-cell lung cancer: a systematic review and meta-analysis of individual patient data from 16 randomized controlled trials. *J Clin Oncol* 2008; 26: 4617–4625.
22. Ardizzoni A, Boni L, Tiseo M, *et al.* Cisplatin- *versus* carboplatin-based chemotherapy in first-line treatment of advanced non-small-cell lung cancer: an individual patient data meta-analysis. *J Natl Cancer Inst* 2007; 99: 847–857.
23. Stanley KE. Prognostic factors for survival in patients with inoperable lung cancer. *J Natl Cancer Inst* 1980; 65: 25–32.
24. Hanna N, Shepherd FA, Fossella FV, *et al.* Randomized phase III trial of pemetrexed *versus* docetaxel in patients with non-small-cell lung cancer previously treated with chemotherapy. *J Clin Oncol* 2004; 22: 1589–1597.
25. Scagliotti GV, Parikh P, von Pawel J, *et al.* Phase III study comparing cisplatin plus gemcitabine with cisplatin plus pemetrexed in chemotherapy-naive patients with advanced-stage non-small-cell lung cancer. *J Clin Oncol* 2008; 26: 3543–3551.
26. Scagliotti G, Hanna N, Fossella F, *et al.* The differential efficacy of pemetrexed according to NSCLC histology: a review of two Phase III studies. *Oncologist* 2009; 14: 253–263.
27. Azzoli CG, Baker S, Temin S, *et al.* American Society of Clinical Oncology Clinical Practice Guideline update on chemotherapy for stage IV non-small-cell lung cancer. *J Clin Oncol* 2009; 27: 6251–6266.

28. Soon YY, Stockler MR, Askie LM, *et al.* Duration of chemotherapy for advanced non-small-cell lung cancer: a systematic review and meta-analysis of randomized trials. *J Clin Oncol* 2009; 27: 3277–3283.
29. Smith IE, O'Brien ME, Talbot DC, *et al.* Duration of chemotherapy in advanced non-small-cell lung cancer: a randomized trial of three *versus* six courses of mitomycin, vinblastine, and cisplatin. *J Clin Oncol* 2001; 19: 1336–1343.
30. Von Plessen C, Bergman B, Andresen O, *et al.* Palliative chemotherapy beyond three courses conveys no survival or consistent quality-of-life benefits in advanced non-small-cell lung cancer. *Br J Cancer* 2006; 95: 966–973.
31. Park JO, Kim S-W, Ahn JS, *et al.* Phase III trial of two *versus* four additional cycles in patients who are nonprogressive after two cycles of platinum-based chemotherapy in non small-cell lung cancer. *J Clin Oncol* 2007; 25: 5233–5239.
32. Rossi A, Chiodini P, Sun J-M, *et al.* Six *versus* fewer planned cycles of first-line platinum-based chemotherapy for non-small-cell lung cancer: a systematic review and meta-analysis of individual patient data. *Lancet Oncol* 2014; 15: 1254–1262.
33. Azzoli CG, Temin S, Aliff T, *et al.* 2011 Focused update of 2009 American Society of Clinical Oncology clinical practice guideline update on chemotherapy for stage IV non-small-cell lung cancer. *J Clin Oncol* 2011; 29: 3825–3831.
34. Reck M, Popat S, Reinmuth N, *et al.* Metastatic non-small-cell lung cancer (NSCLC): ESMO Clinical Practice Guidelines for diagnosis, treatment and follow-up. *Ann Oncol* 2014; 25: Suppl. 3, iii27–iii39.
35. Fidias PM, Dakhil SR, Lyss AP, *et al.* Phase III study of immediate compared with delayed docetaxel after front-line therapy with gemcitabine plus carboplatin in advanced non-small-cell lung cancer. *J Clin Oncol* 2009; 27: 591–598.
36. Belani CP, Barstis J, Perry MC, *et al.* Multicenter, randomized trial for stage IIIB or IV non-small-cell lung cancer using weekly paclitaxel and carboplatin followed by maintenance weekly paclitaxel or observation. *J Clin Oncol* 2003; 21: 2933–2939.
37. Brodowicz T, Krzakowski M, Zwitter M, *et al.* Cisplatin and gemcitabine first-line chemotherapy followed by maintenance gemcitabine or best supportive care in advanced non-small cell lung cancer: a phase III trial. *Lung Cancer* 2006; 52: 155–163.
38. Westeel V, Quoix E, Moro-Sibilot D, *et al.* Randomized study of maintenance vinorelbine in responders with advanced non-small-cell lung cancer. *J Natl Cancer Inst* 2005; 97: 499–506.
39. Ciuleanu T, Brodowicz T, Zielinski C, *et al.* Maintenance pemetrexed plus best supportive care *versus* placebo plus best supportive care for non-small-cell lung cancer: a randomised, double-blind, phase 3 study. *Lancet* 2009; 374: 1432–1440.
40. Paz-Ares L, de Marinis F, Dediu M, *et al.* Maintenance therapy with pemetrexed plus best supportive care *versus* placebo plus best supportive care after induction therapy with pemetrexed plus cisplatin for advanced non-squamous non-small-cell lung cancer (PARAMOUNT): a double-blind, phase 3, random. *Lancet Oncol* 2012; 13: 247–255.
41. Paz-Ares LG, de Marinis F, Dediu M, *et al.* PARAMOUNT: final overall survival results of the phase III study of maintenance pemetrexed *versus* placebo immediately after induction treatment with pemetrexed plus cisplatin for advanced nonsquamous non-small-cell lung cancer. *J Clin Oncol* 2013; 31: 2895–2902.
42. Cappuzzo F, Ciuleanu T, Stelmakh L, *et al.* Erlotinib as maintenance treatment in advanced non-small-cell lung cancer: a multicentre, randomised, placebo-controlled phase 3 study. *Lancet Oncol* 2010; 11: 521–529.
43. Coudert B, Ciuleanu T, Park K, *et al.* Survival benefit with erlotinib maintenance therapy in patients with advanced non-small-cell lung cancer (NSCLC) according to response to first-line chemotherapy. *Ann Oncol* 2012; 23: 388–394.
44. Helbekkmo N, Aasebø U, Sundstrøm SH, *et al.* Treatment outcome in performance status 2 advanced NSCLC patients administered platinum-based combination chemotherapy. *Lung Cancer* 2008; 62: 253–260.
45. Effects of vinorelbine on quality of life and survival of elderly patients with advanced non-small-cell lung cancer. The Elderly Lung Cancer Vinorelbine Italian Study Group. *J Natl Cancer Inst* 1999; 91: 66–72.
46. Gridelli C, Maione P, Rossi A, *et al.* Chemotherapy of advanced NSCLC in special patient population. *Ann Oncol* 2006; 17: Suppl. 5, v72–v78.
47. Zukin M, Barrios CH, Pereira JR, *et al.* Randomized phase III trial of single-agent pemetrexed *versus* carboplatin and pemetrexed in patients with advanced non-small-cell lung cancer and Eastern Cooperative Oncology Group performance status of 2. *J Clin Oncol* 2013; 31: 2849–2853.
48. Mörth C, Valachis A. Single-agent *versus* combination chemotherapy as first-line treatment for patients with advanced non-small cell lung cancer and performance status 2: a literature-based meta-analysis of randomized studies. *Lung Cancer* 2014; 84: 209–214.
49. Leong SS, Toh CK, Lim WT, *et al.* A randomized phase II trial of single-agent gemcitabine, vinorelbine, or docetaxel in patients with advanced non-small cell lung cancer who have poor performance status and/or are elderly. *J Thorac Oncol* 2007; 2: 230–236.

50. Shepherd FA, Dancey J, Ramlau R, *et al.* Prospective randomized trial of docetaxel *versus* best supportive care in patients with non-small-cell lung cancer previously treated with platinum-based chemotherapy. *J Clin Oncol* 2000; 18: 2095–2103.
51. Fossella FV, DeVore R, Kerr RN, *et al.* Randomized phase III trial of docetaxel *versus* vinorelbine or ifosfamide in patients with advanced non-small-cell lung cancer previously treated with platinum-containing chemotherapy regimens. The TAX 320 Non-Small Cell Lung Cancer Study Group. *J Clin Oncol* 2000; 18: 2354–2362.
52. Di Maio M, Perrone F, Chiodini P, *et al.* Individual patient data meta-analysis of docetaxel administered once every 3 weeks compared with once every week second-line treatment of advanced non-small-cell lung cancer. *J Clin Oncol* 2007; 25: 1377–1382.
53. Takeda K, Negoro S, Tamura T, *et al.* Phase III trial of docetaxel plus gemcitabine *versus* docetaxel in second-line treatment for non-small-cell lung cancer: results of a Japan Clinical Oncology Group trial (JCOG0104). *Ann Oncol* 2009; 20: 835–841.
54. Georgoulias V, Kouroussis C, Agelidou A, *et al.* Irinotecan plus gemcitabine *vs* irinotecan for the second-line treatment of patients with advanced non-small-cell lung cancer pretreated with docetaxel and cisplatin: a multicentre, randomised, phase II study. *Br J Cancer* 2004; 91: 482–488.
55. Georgoulias V, Agelidou A, Syrigos K, *et al.* Second-line treatment with irinotecan plus cisplatin *vs* cisplatin of patients with advanced non-small-cell lung cancer pretreated with taxanes and gemcitabine: a multicenter randomised phase II study. *Br J Cancer* 2005; 93: 763–769.
56. Wachters FM, Groen HJM, Biesma B, *et al.* A randomised phase II trial of docetaxel *vs* docetaxel and irinotecan in patients with stage IIIb-IV non-small-cell lung cancer who failed first-line treatment. *Br J Cancer* 2005; 92: 15–20.
57. Gebbia V, Gridelli C, Verusio C, *et al.* Weekly docetaxel *vs.* docetaxel-based combination chemotherapy as second-line treatment of advanced non-small-cell lung cancer patients. The DISTAL-2 randomized trial. *Lung Cancer* 2009; 63: 251–258.
58. Smit EF, Burgers SA, Biesma B, *et al.* Randomized phase II and pharmacogenetic study of pemetrexed compared with pemetrexed plus carboplatin in pretreated patients with advanced non-small-cell lung cancer. *J Clin Oncol* 2009; 27: 2038–2045.
59. Di Maio M, Chiodini P, Georgoulias V, *et al.* Meta-analysis of single-agent chemotherapy compared with combination chemotherapy as second-line treatment of advanced non-small-cell lung cancer. *J Clin Oncol* 2009; 27: 1836–1843.
60. Watson WL, Berg JW. Oat cell lung cancer. *Cancer* 1962; 15: 759–768.
61. Joss RA, Cavalli F, Goldhirsch A, *et al.* New agents in non-small cell lung cancer. *Cancer Treat Rev* 1984; 11: 205–236.
62. Kokron O. Die Behandlung des kleinzelligen metastasierenden Bronchuskarzinoms mit Ifosfamid. Ergebnisse einer prospektiven randomisierten Studie. [Treatment of oat cell metastazing bronchial carcinoma with isofosfamide. Results of a prospective randomized study.] *Osterr Z Onkol* 1974; 5–6: 123–127.
63. Livingston RB, Moore TN, Heilbrun L, *et al.* Small-cell carcinoma of the lung: combined chemotherapy and radiation: a Southwest Oncology Group study. *Ann Intern Med* 1978; 88: 194–199.
64. Dombernowsky P, Sörenson S, Aisner J, *et al.* *cis*-Dichlorodiammineplatinum (II) in small cell anaplastic bronchogenic carcinoma: a phase II study. *Cancer Treat Rep* 1979; 63: 543–545.
65. Sierocki JS, Hilaris BS, Hopfan S, *et al.* *cis*-Dichlorodiammineplatinum(II) and VP-16-213: an active induction regimen for small cell carcinoma of the lung. *Cancer Treat Rep* 1979; 63: 1593–1597.
66. Evans WK, Osoba D, Feld R, *et al.* Etoposide (VP-16) and cisplatin: an effective treatment for relapse in small-cell lung cancer. *J Clin Oncol* 1985; 3: 65–71.
67. Evans WK, Shepherd FA, Feld R, *et al.* VP-16 and cisplatin as first-line therapy for small-cell lung cancer. *J Clin Oncol* 1985; 3: 1471–1477.
68. Evans WK, Feld R, Murray N, *et al.* The use of VP-16 plus cisplatin during induction chemotherapy for small-cell lung cancer. *Semin Oncol* 1986; 13: Suppl. 3, 10–16.
69. Roth BJ, Johnson DH, Einhorn LH, *et al.* Randomized study of cyclophosphamide, doxorubicin, and vincristine *versus* etoposide and cisplatin *versus* alternation of these two regimens in extensive small-cell lung cancer: a phase III trial of the Southeastern Cancer Study Group. *J Clin Oncol* 1992; 10: 282–291.
70. Pujol JL, Carestia L, Daurès JP. Is there a case for cisplatin in the treatment of small-cell lung cancer? A meta-analysis of randomized trials of a cisplatin-containing regimen *versus* a regimen without this alkylating agent. *Br J Cancer* 2000; 83: 8–15.
71. Sundstrøm S, Bremnes RM, Kaasa S, *et al.* Cisplatin and etoposide regimen is superior to cyclophosphamide, epirubicin, and vincristine regimen in small-cell lung cancer: results from a randomized phase III trial with 5 years' follow-up. *J Clin Oncol* 2002; 20: 4665–4672.
72. Skarlos DV, Samantas E, Kosmidis P, *et al.* Randomized comparison of etoposide-cisplatin *vs.* etoposide-carboplatin and irradiation in small-cell lung cancer. A Hellenic Co-operative Oncology Group study. *Ann Oncol* 1994; 5: 601–607.

73. Okamoto H, Watanabe K, Kunikane H, *et al.* Randomised phase III trial of carboplatin plus etoposide *vs* split doses of cisplatin plus etoposide in elderly or poor-risk patients with extensive disease small-cell lung cancer: JCOG 9702. *Br J Cancer* 2007; 97: 162–169.
74. Rossi A, Di Maio M, Chiodini P, *et al.* Carboplatin- or cisplatin-based chemotherapy in first-line treatment of small-cell lung cancer: the COCIS meta-analysis of individual patient data. *J Clin Oncol* 2012; 30: 1692–1698.
75. Früh M, De Ruysscher D, Popat S, *et al.* Small-cell lung cancer (SCLC): ESMO Clinical Practice Guidelines for diagnosis, treatment and follow-up. *Ann Oncol* 2013; 24: Suppl. 6, vi99–vi105.
76. Noda K, Nishiwaki Y, Kawahara M, *et al.* Irinotecan plus cisplatin compared with etoposide plus cisplatin for extensive small-cell lung cancer. *N Engl J Med* 2002; 346: 85–91.
77. Hanna N, Bunn PA, Langer C, *et al.* Randomized phase III trial comparing irinotecan/cisplatin with etoposide/cisplatin in patients with previously untreated extensive-stage disease small-cell lung cancer. *J Clin Oncol* 2006; 24: 2038–2043.
78. Lara PN, Natale R, Crowley J, *et al.* Phase III trial of irinotecan/cisplatin compared with etoposide/cisplatin in extensive-stage small-cell lung cancer: clinical and pharmacogenomic results from SWOG S0124. *J Clin Oncol* 2009; 27: 2530–2535.
79. Socinski MA, Smit EF, Lorigan P, *et al.* Phase III study of pemetrexed plus carboplatin compared with etoposide plus carboplatin in chemotherapy-naive patients with extensive-stage small-cell lung cancer. *J Clin Oncol* 2009; 27: 4787–4792.
80. Lee SM, James LE, Qian W, *et al.* Comparison of gemcitabine and carboplatin *versus* cisplatin and etoposide for patients with poor-prognosis small cell lung cancer. *Thorax* 2009; 64: 75–80.
81. Bleehen NM, Girling DJ, Machin D, *et al.* A randomised trial of three or six courses of etoposide cyclophosphamide methotrexate and vincristine or six courses of etoposide and ifosfamide in small cell lung cancer (SCLC). I: Survival and prognostic factors. Medical Research Council Lung Cancer Working Party. *Br J Cancer* 1993; 68: 1150–1156.
82. Fukuoka M, Furuse K, Saijo N, *et al.* Randomized trial of cyclophosphamide, doxorubicin, and vincristine *versus* cisplatin and etoposide *versus* alternation of these regimens in small-cell lung cancer. *J Natl Cancer Inst* 1991; 83: 855–861.
83. Murray N, Livingston RB, Shepherd FA, *et al.* Randomized study of CODE *versus* alternating CAV/EP for extensive-stage small-cell lung cancer: an Intergroup Study of the National Cancer Institute of Canada Clinical Trials Group and the Southwest Oncology Group. *J Clin Oncol* 1999; 17: 2300–2308.
84. Johnson DH, Einhorn LH, Birch R, *et al.* A randomized comparison of high-dose *versus* conventional-dose cyclophosphamide, doxorubicin, and vincristine for extensive-stage small-cell lung cancer: a phase III trial of the Southeastern Cancer Study Group. *J Clin Oncol* 1987; 5: 1731–1738.
85. Ihde DC, Mulshine JL, Kramer BS, *et al.* Prospective randomized comparison of high-dose and standard-dose etoposide and cisplatin chemotherapy in patients with extensive-stage small-cell lung cancer. *J Clin Oncol* 1994; 12: 2022–2034.
86. James LE, Gower NH, Rudd RM, *et al.* A randomised trial of low-dose/high-frequency chemotherapy as palliative treatment of poor-prognosis small-cell lung cancer: a Cancer research Campaign trial. *Br J Cancer* 1996; 73: 1563–1568.
87. Steward WP, von Pawel J, Gatzemeier U, *et al.* Effects of granulocyte-macrophage colony-stimulating factor and dose intensification of V-ICE chemotherapy in small-cell lung cancer: a prospective randomized study of 300 patients. *J Clin Oncol* 1998; 16: 642–650.
88. Thatcher N, Girling DJ, Hopwood P, *et al.* Improving survival without reducing quality of life in small-cell lung cancer patients by increasing the dose-intensity of chemotherapy with granulocyte colony-stimulating factor support: results of a British Medical Research Council Multicenter Randomized Trial. Medical Research Council Lung Cancer Working Party. *J Clin Oncol* 2000; 18: 395–404.
89. Sculier JP, Paesmans M, Lecomte J, *et al.* A three-arm phase III randomised trial assessing, in patients with extensive-disease small-cell lung cancer, accelerated chemotherapy with support of haematological growth factor or oral antibiotics. *Br J Cancer* 2001; 85: 1444–1451.
90. Ardizzoni A, Tjan-Heijnen VCG, Postmus PE, *et al.* Standard *versus* intensified chemotherapy with granulocyte colony-stimulating factor support in small-cell lung cancer: a prospective European Organization for Research and Treatment of Cancer-Lung Cancer Group Phase III Trial-08923. *J Clin Oncol* 2002; 20: 3947–3955.
91. Lorigan P, Woll PJ, O'Brien MER, *et al.* Randomized phase III trial of dose-dense chemotherapy supported by whole-blood hematopoietic progenitors in better-prognosis small-cell lung cancer. *J Natl Cancer Inst* 2005; 97: 666–674.
92. Humblet Y, Symann M, Bosly A, *et al.* Late intensification chemotherapy with autologous bone marrow transplantation in selected small-cell carcinoma of the lung: a randomized study. *J Clin Oncol* 1987; 5: 1864–1873.
93. Souhami RL, Spiro SG, Rudd RM, *et al.* Five-day oral etoposide2 treatment for advanced small-cell lung cancer: randomized comparison with intravenous chemotherapy. *J Natl Cancer Inst* 1997; 89: 577–580.

94. Timmer-Bonte JN, de Boo TM, Smit HJ, *et al.* Prevention of chemotherapy-induced febrile neutropenia by prophylactic antibiotics plus or minus granulocyte colony-stimulating factor in small-cell lung cancer: a Dutch Randomized Phase III Study. *J Clin Oncol* 2005; 23: 7974–7984.
95. Kim YH, Goto K, Yoh K, *et al.* Performance status and sensitivity to first-line chemotherapy are significant prognostic factors in patients with recurrent small cell lung cancer receiving second-line chemotherapy. *Cancer* 2008; 113: 2518–2523.
96. Vincent M, Evans B, Smith I. First-line chemotherapy rechallenge after relapse in small cell lung cancer. *Cancer Chemother Pharmacol* 1988; 21: 45–48.
97. Giaccone G, Donadio M, Bonardi G, *et al.* Teniposide in the treatment of small-cell lung cancer: the influence of prior chemotherapy. *J Clin Oncol* 1988; 6: 1264–1270.
98. Owonikoko TK, Behera M, Chen Z, *et al.* A systematic analysis of efficacy of second-line chemotherapy in sensitive and refractory small-cell lung cancer. *J Thorac Oncol* 2012; 7: 866–872.
99. Giaccone G, Ferrati P, Donadio M, *et al.* Reinduction chemotherapy in small cell lung cancer. *Eur J Cancer Clin Oncol* 1987; 23: 1697–1699.
100. Postmus PE, Berendsen HH, van Zandwijk N, *et al.* Retreatment with the induction regimen in small cell lung cancer relapsing after an initial response to short term chemotherapy. *Eur J Cancer Clin Oncol* 1987; 23: 1409–1411.
101. Garassino MC, Torri V, Michetti G, *et al.* Outcomes of small-cell lung cancer patients treated with second-line chemotherapy: a multi-institutional retrospective analysis. *Lung Cancer* 2011; 72: 378–383.
102. Smit EF, Fokkema E, Biesma B, *et al.* A phase II study of paclitaxel in heavily pretreated patients with small-cell lung cancer. *Br J Cancer* 1998; 77: 347–351.
103. Masuda N, Fukuoka M, Kusunoki Y, *et al.* CPT-11: a new derivative of camptothecin for the treatment of refractory or relapsed small cell lung cancer. *J Clin Oncol* 1992; 10: 1225–1229.
104. Furuse K, Kubota K, Kawahara M, *et al.* Phase II study of vinorelbine in heavily previously treated small cell lung cancer. Japan Lung Cancer Vinorelbine Study Group. *Oncology* 1996; 53: 169–172.
105. Sundstrøm S, Bremnes RM, Kaasa S, *et al.* Second-line chemotherapy in recurrent small cell lung cancer. Results from a crossover schedule after primary treatment with cisplatin and etoposide (EP-regimen) or cyclophosphamide, epirubicin, and vincristin (CEV-regimen). *Lung Cancer* 2005; 48: 251–261.
106. Ardizzoni A, Hansen H, Dombernowsky P, *et al.* Topotecan, a new active drug in the second-line treatment of small-cell lung cancer: a phase II study in patients with refractory and sensitive disease. The European Organization for Research and Treatment of Cancer Early Clinical Studies Group and New Dr. *J Clin Oncol* 1997; 15: 2090–2096.
107. Von Pawel J, Schiller JH, Shepherd FA, *et al.* Topotecan *versus* cyclophosphamide, doxorubicin, and vincristine for the treatment of recurrent small-cell lung cancer. *J Clin Oncol* 1999; 17: 658–667.
108. Eckardt JR, von Pawel J, Pujol J-L, *et al.* Phase III study of oral compared with intravenous topotecan as second-line therapy in small-cell lung cancer. *J Clin Oncol* 2007; 25: 2086–2092.
109. O'Brien MER, Ciuleanu T-E, Tsekov H, *et al.* Phase III trial comparing supportive care alone with supportive care with oral topotecan in patients with relapsed small-cell lung cancer. *J Clin Oncol* 2006; 24: 5441–5447.
110. Onoda S, Masuda N, Seto T, *et al.* Phase II trial of amrubicin for treatment of refractory or relapsed small-cell lung cancer: Thoracic Oncology Research Group Study 0301. *J Clin Oncol* 2006; 24: 5448–5453.
111. Hirose T, Nakashima M, Shirai T, *et al.* Phase II trial of amrubicin and carboplatin in patients with sensitive or refractory relapsed small-cell lung cancer. *Lung Cancer* 2011; 73: 345–350.
112. Ohe Y, Negoro S, Matsui K, *et al.* Phase I-II study of amrubicin and cisplatin in previously untreated patients with extensive-stage small-cell lung cancer. *Ann Oncol* 2005; 16: 430–436.
113. Von Pawel J, Jotte R, Spigel DR, *et al.* Randomized phase III trial of amrubicin *versus* topotecan as second-line treatment for patients with small-cell lung cancer. *J Clin Oncol* 2014; 32: 4012–4019.
114. Tang C-H, Parham C, Shocron E, *et al.* Picoplatin overcomes resistance to cell toxicity in small-cell lung cancer cells previously treated with cisplatin and carboplatin. *Cancer Chemother Pharmacol* 2010; 67: 1389–1400.
115. Ciuleanu T, Samarzjia M, Demidchik Y, *et al.* Randomized phase III study (SPEAR) of picoplatin plus best supportive care (BSC) or BSC alone in patients (pts) with SCLC refractory or progressive within 6 months after first line platinum-based chemotherapy. *J Clin Oncol* 2010; 28: Suppl. 15, 7002.

---

**Support statement:** S. Popat acknowledges UK National Health Service (NHS) funding to the Royal Marsden NHS Foundation Trust/The Institute of Cancer Research NIHR Biomedical Research Centre.

**Disclosures:** S. Popat has served as an uncompensated consultant to Eli Lilly and has received a grant from Pierre Fabre, outside the submitted work.

Chapter 16

# Systemic treatment of elderly patients

Charlotte Leduc and Elisabeth Quoix

Lung cancer incidence increases with age, with a median age at diagnosis between 63 and 72 years depending on the country and the diagnostic procedures performed.

The treatment of elderly patients, and especially systemic treatment, is of utmost importance. However, treating elderly patients has some caveats: geriatric syndromes, comorbidities and polypharmacy interfering with the metabolism of the drugs are frequent; and renal function may necessitate an adaptation of the doses. Finally, haematopoietic reserves are often reduced, needing more extensive use of granulocyte colony stimulating factors. Thus, there has been quite a long period of therapeutic nihilism regarding these patients, but studies dedicated to elderly patients have increased in number in the last 15 years, allowing for the development of recommendations regarding some clinical situations. For example, whereas there are no specific recommendations for peri-operative chemotherapy or locally advanced NSCLC, they do exist for metastatic-stage NSCLC and for first-line systemic treatment of SCLC.

Like many cancers, lung cancer is linked to ageing and the median age of patients diagnosed with lung cancer is now around 70 years in the USA [1], and between 63 and 72 years in Europe depending on whether only proven lung cancers are considered [2] or proven and presumed [3]. For quite a long time, until the end of the 1980s, the treatment of elderly patients was not the subject of much research. Inclusion of elderly patients in clinical trials was, at most, modest and did not at all reflect the frequency of elderly patients with lung cancer [4]. Moreover, the only data obtained were from clinical trials with either no age limit for inclusion or an age limit of 75 years. Such trials prevent of any generalisability of the results because, as can be expected, elderly patients included in trials designed for a majority of younger patients represent a selection of patients with favourable clinical characteristics. However, there have been considerable improvements in the outcomes of lung cancer due to the evolution of operative and peri-operative management (mini-invasive thoracotomies, anaesthesiology and post-operative care progresses) but also to radiation therapy techniques (reduction of radiation fields, tomotherapy, intensity modulation and development of stereotactic ablative radiation) and, finally, to more codified chemotherapy use, reducing toxicity and increasing survival. As a consequence, there has been considerable interest in the optimisation of treatment of elderly patients with lung cancer over the last two decades.

Service de Pneumologie, Hôpitaux Universitaires, Strasbourg, France.

Correspondence: Elisabeth Quoix, Service de Pneumologie, Hôpitaux Universitaires, 1 place de l'hôpital, 67091 Strasbourg cedex, France. E-mail: elisabeth.quoix@chru-strasbourg.fr

 Print ISBN: 978-1-84984-061-3. Online ISBN: 978-1-84984-062-0. Print ISSN: 2312-508X. Online ISSN: 2312-5098.

The expected demographic changes in upcoming years, with a substantial increase of elderly patients with lung cancer, will force the need to develop validated recommendations for treatment of lung cancer in elderly patients.

## Definition and characteristics of elderly patients with lung cancer

The cut-off used to define elderly patients is somewhat variable between studies. 65 years is often used in population-based or epidemiological studies [5, 6] and in some subgroup analyses of clinical trials [7–9], whereas 70 years is the limit usually used in trials dedicated to elderly patients [10–13]. This cut-off appears meaningful because it corresponds to a mandatory adaptation of systemic treatment.

Adaptation of systemic therapy in elderly patients must be done for various reasons. Comorbidity increases with age, especially in smokers, who are particularly susceptible to cardiovascular disease and COPD. These comorbidities may have a great impact on therapeutic decisions and chemotherapy toxicity. There is a number of physiological and biological alterations with age. First, renal function decline is common in the elderly, with renal mass shrinking, reduction in renal blood flow and gradual loss of functioning nephrons [14]. The modification of diet in renal disease method appears to be the closest representative of the true glomerular filtration rate and, thus, should be used in elderly patients [14]. Second, haematopoietic reserves are lower, and severe neutropenia and related infection are more frequent in the elderly than in their younger counterparts [15]. However, elderly patients have the same ability to respond to granulocyte stimulation as their younger counterparts [16]. Third, the body composition is different, with more fat, less lean tissue and less water in elderly patients [17], which may impact on the metabolism of drugs and be responsible for more toxicity.

### Geriatric assessment tools

Performance status, even if it is, as in younger patients, an important prognostic factor, cannot by itself predict outcome in elderly patients [18]. Performing a geriatric assessment may lead to a better appraisal of the fitness of an elderly patient. This geriatric assessment comprises several items (table 1) addressing cognition (Mini-Mental Score [20]) and daily

Table 1. Comprehensive geriatric assessment

| Parameters | Assessment methods |
|---|---|
| **Functional status** | PS, ADL, IADL, Timed Up and Go |
| **Comorbidity** | Charlson comorbidity index, CIRS-G |
| **Socioeconomic status** | Income, transport availibity, living conditions, domestic help |
| **Cognitive status** | Folstein Mini-Mental Score |
| **Nutritional status** | Body mass index, nutritional miniquestionnaire |
| **Emotional status** | Geriatric depression scale |
| **Medications** | Number, usefulness, interactions |
| **Geriatric syndromes** | Dementia, repeated falls, bone fractures, neglect, abuse |

PS: performance status; ADL: Activities of Daily Living; IADL: Instrumental ADL; CIRS-G: Geriatic Comorbidity Illness Rating Score. Reproduced and modified from [19] with permission from the publisher.

activities (Activity of Daily Living (ADL) and Instrumental ADL (IADL) [21]). The ADL checklist includes everything necessary for self-care (dressing, transfer, feeding, toilet, *etc.*). The IADL refers to the use of transport, use of the telephone, the ability to go shopping, proper medication intake and money management, *etc.* The timed Up and Go test is the time required to get up from a chair, walk 3 m and return to the chair. The depression scale, nutrition assessment and comorbidity (assessed by the Charlson index) are also part of geriatric tests. All these evaluations are part of the comprehensive geriatric assessment (CGA), which is a very time-consuming procedure. Screening tests have been developed in order to select patients who should really undergo a complete CGA [22].

After careful assessment, elderly patients may be classified in three groups according to Balducci and Extermann [23]: 1) patients who have no specific risk and who may be treated like their younger counterparts; 2) patients who have treatable comorbidities and may be treated with an adapted treatment; and 3) patients who have multiple untreatable comorbidities or dependent patients, for whom only best supportive care (BSC) should be proposed.

Although the prognostic role of geriatric index is well established, as is its predictive value for toxicity of chemotherapy, its potential role in treatment decisions is not established [24].

## Epidemiological features

NSCLC represent 85% of all lung cancer cases in the elderly [1, 25]. This is quite similar to what is observed in younger patients. However, the distribution of histological subtypes differs, as SCCs are more frequent in elderly than younger patients, in whom ADC is now the main subtype [1, 25]. This distribution may be linked to the modifications of smoking habits over time, with an increase of the use of filters and decrease of dark tobacco use, resulting in a more peripheral deposition of carcinogens of tobacco smoke.

The proportion of never-smokers is higher in elderly patients than their younger counterparts [26], reflecting a lower role of tobacco in the incidence of lung cancer, whereas ageing *per se* is more and more important as a risk factor.

## Systemic treatment of SCLC in the elderly

Chemotherapy is the cornerstone of the treatment of SCLC. Doublet platinum salt plus etoposide has now been used for more than 30 years and no other combination has demonstrated any superiority except for cisplatin–irinotecan in Japan [27], this superiority not being confirmed in Caucasian patients [28]. Induction therapy consists of four to six cycles [29] and there is no advantage to pursuing any treatment until relapse. Second-line treatment depends on the delay between the end of induction therapy and relapse. Rechallenging the initial combination should be all the more considered, as the treatment-free interval is ⩾3 months [30].

If the delay is less than 3 months or if relapse occurs during induction therapy (refractory disease), topotecan is the drug of choice [31, 32], either intravenously or orally [33], although the combination of cyclophosphamide, vincristine and adriamycin may also be used [34].

Regarding elderly patients, there have been very few dedicated studies, most of them mixing elderly and poor performance status patients. The inclusion rate in clinical trials is even less than in NSCLC and this trend is worsening with the fact that clinical trials in SCLC are now very few. Chemotherapy is often given at reduced doses and schedules to elderly patients with a consequently lower dose intensity [35].

In a population-based study, performed in patients aged ⩾75 years between 1997 and 2004 in the Netherlands [36], 945 patients were diagnosed with a SCLC, 577 of whom had extensive-stage disease. Among the patients with limited-stage disease, 23% aged between 75 and 79 years received a combination of chemo- and radiotherapy; this percentage decreased to 15% between 80 and 84 years, and 0% in those aged 80 years or more. In limited-stage patients, however, chemotherapy was administered alone to 40% of patients, irrespective of age. In extensive-stage disease, chemotherapy was administered to 55% of the patients aged between 75 and 79 years but only in 32% of those aged between 80 and 84 years, and 23% of those aged 85 years and more. Overall, 48% of all patients, irrespective of stage, did not receive chemotherapy.

Moreover, adaptations of dose, number of cycles, time between two cycles and type of chemotherapy were decided in 70% of patients with limited-stage disease and 62% of those with extensive disease stage either before beginning treatment or during the course of treatment.

Nevertheless, the role of age as a prognostic factor is not demonstrated. In a registry-based study performed in the Bas-Rhin department of France, age >70 years was an unfavourable prognostic factor only in crude survival analysis but not when a relative survival analysis was performed [37].

Carboplatin has been proposed as a replacement of cisplatin in elderly patients. In a study of 36 patients aged more than 70 years, response rate with carboplatin and etoposide was 75% and median survival was 10.8 months at the expense of important haematological toxicity (60% grade 3–4 leukopenia and 51% grade 3–4 thrombopenia) [38]. In an unselected series of 38 patients aged 70 years or more with extensive-stage disease treated with carboplatin and etoposide phosphate, a high percentage of early deaths was noted (seven before the second cycle, two of them being toxic). Median survival time was 7.6 months and 1 year survival probability 25% [39].

Carboplatin plus irinotecan has been specifically studied in elderly patients in Japan [40], and a phase II/III trial comparing carboplatin and irinotecan to carboplatin and etoposide is currently being conducted [41].

More aggressive chemotherapies have been evaluated [42] with the combination of cisplatin, doxorubicin, vincristine and etoposide in 66 patients aged more than 65 years. Response rate was 92% for limited-stage and 87% for extensive-stage disease. There were 18% febrile neutropenias resulting in one death.

However, attenuated regimens administered to elderly patients resulted in lower response and survival rates [43]. Therefore, age should not be a criterion for under-treatment; in particular, single-agent therapy is not an option [44, 45]. The combination with the best ratio of benefit to tolerance is carboplatin–etoposide [29].

Regarding radiation therapy in limited-stage disease, there has been unfortunately no specific study performed in elderly patients, to the best of our knowledge. Thus, only retrospective subgroup analyses of elderly patients included in broader age limit trials are available. All retrospective analyses show no difference regarding the outcomes but significantly more toxicity, especially regarding pneumonitis and treatment-related deaths [46–48].

In a community-based population analysis, performed on 174 patients referred to the Vancouver Island Centre of the British Columbia Cancer Agency (Victoria, BC, Canada) with limited SCLC [49], combined chemoradiotherapy was given in 86% of patients aged <65 years, 66% of those aged between 65 and 74 years, and 40% of those aged >75 years. With advancing age, chemotherapy was given in fewer cycles, less intensive regimens and lower total doses. Prophylactic cranial irradiation was given to 41 patients but only three were aged >70 years. There was a decrease in overall survival, with median survival being 17, 12 and 7 months for patients <65 years, aged between 65 and 74 years, and >75 years, respectively. However, on multivariate analysis, age was not an independent prognostic factor.

Thus, combined modalities of treatment should be proposed to elderly patients with careful assessment of benefit/risk ratio on an individualised basis.

## Chemotherapy in early stage NSCLC

Due to demographic trends and CT-based screening, the incidence of early stage NSCLC in elderly is expected to increase. Optimal treatment in this population remains controversial and frequently, elderly patients without significant comorbidities do not benefit from any treatment [50]. Surgical treatment is feasible in the elderly, as shown in recent series including octogenarians [51–53], and should be proposed in fit patients. Therefore, operable patients could benefit from peri-operative chemotherapy (adjuvant or neoadjuvant). Adjuvant chemotherapy seems to be associated with a survival benefit in the elderly. Nevertheless, data are limited, especially in patients over 80 years of age, and there is no study dedicated to this population. In the subgroup analysis of the Lung Adjuvant Cisplatin Evaluation meta-analysis [54], there was no interaction between age and chemotherapy effect, and patients ⩾70 years appeared to have the same benefit as their younger counterparts. However, it is important to highlight that elderly patients included in clinical trials are very selected and particularly fit. According to a Canadian population-based study [55] of 2763 patients ⩾70 years of age, uptake of adjuvant chemotherapy in the elderly increased from 3.3% (2001–2003) to 16.2% (2004–2006). Adjuvant chemotherapy administration was associated with a significant survival benefit (4-year survival increased from 47.1% to 49.9%, p=0.01). Nevertheless, the benefit was not verified in patients older than 80 years. The cisplatin–vinorelbine doublet was the most frequently used, but 28% of patients received carboplatin-based regimen. The likelihood of receiving chemotherapy significantly declined with advancing age (42.7% for those <70 years; 23.1%, 70–74 years; 13.3%, 75–79 years; and 4.6% ⩾80 years) (p=0.001). These results are comparable to those of another study in which adjuvant chemotherapy was administered to 44% of patients <65 years, 18% of patients between 65 to 75 years, and only 9% of patients >75 years [56]. However, tolerability and quality of life seem to be similar between elderly and younger patients [57]. A very recent analysis of the Surveillance, Epidemiology and End Results database showed that only 9% of 3289 elderly patients with a stage I NSCLC (tumour size ⩾4 cm) received platin-based adjuvant therapy after lobectomy [58]. There was a survival benefit for these patients that was not observed for the elderly patients with T4, N0 or N1 disease receiving adjuvant chemotherapy, who experienced higher rates of severe toxicity [59]. The low proportion of elderly patients receiving adjuvant chemotherapy reflects the fact that few of them are able to receive adjuvant chemotherapy (especially cisplatin-based) after surgery. Even in younger patients, compliance to adjuvant chemotherapy is only around 50%, *versus* 90% for neoadjuvant chemotherapy. Consequently, the induction chemotherapy benefit should be larger. In a recent meta-analysis of 15 randomised studies [60], neoadjuvant chemotherapy significantly improved survival (hazard ratio (HR) 0.87, 95% CI 0.78–0.96; p=0.007). 5-year survival increased from 40% to 45%. 2385 patients were included, with 468 (19.6%) ⩾70 years, and there was no interaction between age and chemotherapy benefit. If used, neoadjuvant chemotherapy should be administrated with caution, in selected elderly patients. Indeed, a case–control study reported by Rivera *et al.* [61] (81 patients ⩾75 years *versus* 81 patients <75 years) showed that post-operative morbidity (*i.e.* incidence and severity grade of post-operative complications) was higher in the elderly group, with no significant difference in the type of operation and post-operative mortality. In conclusion, peri-operative chemotherapy could be associated with survival benefit in the elderly and, therefore, should not be denied to these patients. Treatments decisions should take into account the estimated absolute benefit, life expectancy, treatment tolerance, presence of comorbidity and patient preferences.

## Locally advanced NSCLC

According to recent publications, elderly patients with inoperable, locally advanced NSCLC are more likely to receive no treatment [50, 62]. When they are treated, these patients may benefit from chemoradiotherapy [63].

Concurrent radiotherapy has been shown to result in longer survival than sequential radiotherapy [64] at the expense of a higher oesophageal toxicity rate. In subgroup analysis, the benefit was comparable regardless of the age, although age was a significant prognostic factor in multivariate analysis. Another retrospective analysis of two CALGB trials by subsets of age showed no difference regarding response and survival [65] when stratifying by age. However, there were no patients aged 80 years or more in this trial.

Two North Central Cancer Treatment Group randomised trials have studied the benefit of combined-modality therapy. The first compared once-daily radiotherapy alone, twice-daily radiotherapy alone and concurrent chemotherapy plus twice-daily radiotherapy in 246 patients between 1994 and 1999 [66]. Median age was 64 years and 83 (26%) patients were aged 70 years or more. Again, there was no difference regarding survival according to age at the expense of a higher rate of haematological toxicity. Analysis of this trial was combined with a second that compared three arms: once-daily radiotherapy alone, twice-daily radiotherapy alone and concurrent chemotherapy plus twice-daily radiotherapy [67]. The chemotherapy regimen of both trials was etoposide and cisplatin. Of the 166 elderly patients who were included in this analysis, 37 received radiotherapy alone and 129 chemoradiotherapy. There was a significant survival advantage for chemoradiotherapy: the median and 5-year survival rates were 10.5 months and 5.4% for the radiotherapy-only group compared with 13.7 months and 14.7% for the chemoradiotherapy group (log-rank p=0.05). Patients who received chemoradiotherapy experienced significantly more severe toxicity (grade ⩾3) compared with patients who received radiotherapy alone (89.9% *versus* 32.4%; p<0.01).

In a Hoosier Oncology Group study of docetaxel as a consolidation after chemoradiotherapy, retrospective analysis according to age did not show any significant survival difference [68], again at the expense of an increased haematological toxicity and fatigue. There was also a nonsignificantly higher oesophageal toxicity.

The first prospective randomised study conducted specifically in the elderly to prove the feasibility of chemoradiotherapy and its clinical benefit was a phase III trial by the Japan Clinical Oncology Group [69]. A total of 200 patients ⩾70 years with unresectable stage III NSCLC and good performance status (0 and 1) were randomly assigned to chemoradiotherapy (60 Gy plus concurrent low-dose carboplatin (30 mg·m$^{-2}$ per day, 5 days a week for 20 days)) or radiotherapy alone. Median overall survival was significantly longer in the chemoradiotherapy group: 22.4 months (95% CI 16.5–33.6 months) *versus* 16.9 months (95% CI 13.4–20.3 months) for the radiotherapy-only group (HR 0.68, p=0.0179). Regarding toxicity, more patients had grade 3–4 haematological toxic effects and grade 3 infections in the chemotherapy group. Incidences of grade 3–4 pneumonitis and late lung toxicity were similar between groups.

In conclusion, fit elderly patients appeared to gain a survival advantage from a combination of chemotherapy and concurrent radiotherapy, at the cost of additional toxicity. Treatment decisions should take into account patients' life expectancy, comorbidities, functional limitations and preferences [70].

## Treatment of elderly patients with metastatic-stage NSCLC

Although elderly patients represent the majority of patients with advanced NSCLC, they are significantly underrepresented in clinical trials. For example, among the 100 most cited phase III trials [71], 33% excluded elderly patients in their design (with age limits between 65 and 75 years). The median age was 60.9 years but, even more strikingly, the median age of patients included in clinical trials with no age limit was only 61 years.

### First-line chemotherapy

The question of chemotherapy in elderly metastatic NSCLC patients was first investigated by the Italian phase III Elderly Lung Cancer Vinorelbine Italian Group Study [10]. Survival was longer in the vinorelbine arm (median overall survival 28 *versus* 21 weeks for BSC, p=0.03). Patients receiving vinorelbine were significantly more likely to survive for at least 1 year (32% *versus* 14%) and the relative risk of death in the vinorelbine group was 0.65 (95% CI 0.45–0.93). The same authors then compared, in 698 elderly patients, either vinorelbine or gemcitabine to a vinorelbine–gemcitabine doublet. The combination of vinorelbine plus gemcitabine was not more effective than single-agent vinorelbine or gemcitabine [12].

Therefore, the American Society of Clinical Oncology and the European Organisation for Research and Treatment of Cancer (EORTC) have recommended single-agent therapy as the treatment of choice for elderly population [72, 73]. However, several subgroup analyses of elderly patients included in clinical trials not devoted to the elderly but with no upper age limit as a criteria of inclusion (table 2) were in favour of the use of platinum-based doublets (as in younger patients) rather than single-agent therapy, although these analyses were not pre-planned [8, 74–77].

In a phase III trial, the French Intergroup of Thoracic Oncology (IFCT) compared a monthly carboplatin and weekly paclitaxel doublet chemotherapy regimen with monotherapy (either vinorelbine or gemcitabine) in elderly patients with advanced NSCLC (IFCT 0501) [13]. 451 patients aged 70–89 years were randomised. Despite increased toxic effects (especially neutropenia and asthenia), platinum-based doublet chemotherapy was associated with survival benefits compared with vinorelbine or gemcitabine monotherapy: median overall survival (fig. 1) was 10.3 months for doublet chemotherapy *versus* 6.2 months for monotherapy (HR 0.64, 95% CI 0.52–0.78; p<0.0001); 1-year survival was 44.5% (95% CI 37.9–50.9%) *versus* 25.4% (19.9–31.3%), respectively. Quality of life assessment was similar in both arms. On the basis of these results, EORTC and the National Comprehensive Cancer Network now recommend the use of a carboplatin-based doublet in fit elderly patients. Single-agent treatment (gemcitabine, vinorelbine or taxanes) represents a valid option for less fit patients. No treatment has proved more effective than any other [70].

Ther use of bevacizumab in elderly patients is still a matter of debate. In a recent meta-analysis [78], there was no interaction with age; however, the cut-off was set at 65 years and for overall survival, the upper bound of 95% confidence intervals was >1. The authors mention that data were not available to study the effect and toxicity of bevacizumab in patients ≥70 years. In a subgroup analysis of the Eastern Cooperative Oncology Group

Table 2 Subgroup analyses of elderly patients in clinical trials comparing a single agent therapy to a platin-based doublet

| First author [ref.] | Total patients/ patients ≥70 years n | Treatment arms | Response rate <70/≥70 years % | Median survival time <70/≥70 years months | 1-year survival rate <70/≥70 years % |
|---|---|---|---|---|---|
| **Langer [74]** | 574/86 | CDDP+VP16 *versus* CDDP +Pacli | 21.5/23.3¶ | 9.1¶/8.5 | 38¶/29 |
| **Lilenbaum [75]** | 561/155 | Carbo+Pacli *versus* | 28¶/36 | 9¶/8 | 38¶/33 |
| | | Pacli | 15/21 | 6.8/5.8 | 35/31 |
| **Belani [8]** | 1218/401# | CDDP+Doc *versus* | | 11.0/12.6 | 44/52 |
| | | Carbo+doc *versus* | | 9.7/9 | 37/39 |
| | | CDDP + VNR | | 10.1/9.9 | 41/41 |
| **Ansari [76]** | 1135/338 | Carbo+Gem *versus* | 30.1/28.2 | 7.7/8.8/8.0/7.2 | |
| | | Pacli+Gem *versus* | 24.8/24.4 | 8.9/9.8/5.9/7.8 | |
| | | Carbo+Pacli | + | 9.4/8.4/6.1/7.9§ | |
| **Blanchard [77]** | 616/122 | CDDP+VNR *versus* Carbo+Pacli | 27/30 | 9 *versus* 7 (p=0.04) | 40/27 |

CDDP: cisplatin; VP16: etoposide; Pacli: paclitaxel; Carbo: carboplatin; Doc: docetaxel; VNR: vinorelbine; Gem: gemcitabine. #: 401 patients aged ≥65 years. ¶: global per cent or median survival time for the two arms together. +: response rate by categories of age, the three arms being combined (<70, 70–74, 75–79 and ≥80 years). §: median survival by arm and age categories; no significant difference. Reproduced and modified from [19] with permission from the publisher.

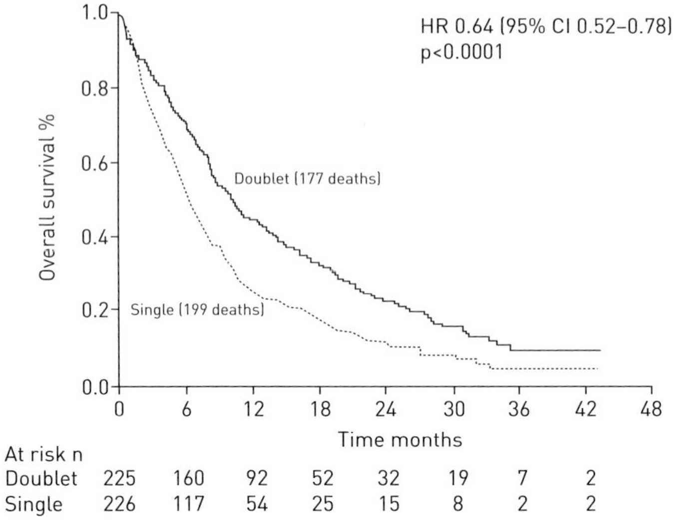


Figure 1. Overall survival of patients treated with the doublet carboplatin plus weekly paclitaxel *versus* single agent therapy (IFCT 0501). Single-arm (n=226): median survival (95% CI) 6.2 (5.3–7.4) months; 1-year survival 25.4% (19.9–31.3%). Doublet arm (n=225): median survival 1.03 (8.3–12.6) months; 1-year survival 44.5% (37.9–50.9%). HR: hazard ratio. Reproduced and modified from [14] with permission from the publisher.

4599 trial in patients aged more than 70 years, bevacizumab showed higher toxic effects and no improvement of survival [79]. Specifically, in a retrospective cohort study of 4168 patients aged more than 65 years, adding bevacizumab to carboplatin plus paclitaxel did not provide any survival benefit [80]. Given all these data, bevacizumab cannot be recommended in elderly patients at this time, and more specific studies are needed.

Regarding induction therapy in older patients with *EGFR* mutations, a subgroup analysis of a trial comparing carboplatin plus paclitaxel to gefitinib showed that older patients with *EGFR* mutations gained even more advantage in PFS than younger patients with gefitinib as first-line treatment, with a statistically significant interaction between age and treatment [81]. A subgroup analysis of a study comparing erlotinib as first line to cisplatin or carboplatin plus docetaxel or gemcitabine showed the same benefit of PFS in favour of erlotinib regardless of age [82].

## Maintenance therapy

Although maintenance is validated in stage IV NSCLC patients responding or stable after four cycles of induction chemotherapy [83], the question remains unclear in elderly because there is no trial specifically designed for this population. Old patients seem to receive the same benefit as younger patients in a subgroup analysis of the PARAMOUNT trial [84]. A phase III trial conducted by IFCT is currently ongoing to verify the interest of maintenance therapy in patients ⩾70 years (www.clinicaltrials.gov identifier number NCT01850303).

## Second-line therapy

There has been no dedicated study of second-line treatment for elderly patients with advanced NSCLC. A retrospective analysis of 461 patients did not observe any difference in either efficacy or toxicity of second-line treatment (chemotherapy and EGFR-TKI) in elderly or nonelderly patients [85]. The IFCT 0501 trial has also demonstrated the efficacy of EGFR-TKI in second-line therapy [86].

## Conclusion

The number of elderly patients is growing and they will constitute the majority of patients with lung cancer in upcoming years. These patients are an inhomogeneous population that must be carefully assessed before making therapeutic decisions and it is of paramount importance to correctly identify those patients who are eligible for aggressive treatment approaches like surgery, multimodal treatment or combined chemotherapy.

## References

1. Owonikoko TK, Ragin CC, Belani CP, *et al.* Lung cancer in elderly patients: an analysis of the surveillance, epidemiology, and end results database. *J Clin Oncol* 2007; 25: 5570–5577.
2. Quoix E. Therapeutic options in older patients with metastatic non-small cell lung cancer. *Ther Adv Med Oncol* 2012; 4: 247–254.
3. Khakwani A, Rich AL, Powell HA, *et al.* Lung cancer survival in England: trends in non-small-cell lung cancer survival over the duration of the National Lung Cancer Audit. *Br J Cancer* 2013; 109: 2058–2065.
4. Talarico L, Chen G, Pazdur R. Enrollment of elderly patients in clinical trials for cancer drug registration: a 7-year experience by the US Food and Drug Administration. *J Clin Oncol* 2004; 22: 4626–4631.
5. Caprario LC, Kent DM, Strauss GM. Effects of chemotherapy on survival of elderly patients with small-cell lung cancer: analysis of the SEER-Medicare database. *J Thorac Oncol* 2013; 8: 1272–1281.
6. Rajan SS, Cai Y, Yi M, *et al.* Use of hematopoietic growth factors in elderly lung cancer patients receiving chemotherapy: a SEER-Medicare-based study. *Am J Clin Oncol* 2014 [In press DOI: 10.1097/COC.0000000000000104].
7. Shepherd FA, Abratt RP, Anderson H, *et al.* Gemcitabine in the treatment of elderly patients with advanced non-small cell lung cancer. *Semin Oncol* 1997; 24: Suppl. 7, S7-50–S7-55.
8. Belani CP, Fossella F. Elderly subgroup analysis of a randomized phase III study of docetaxel plus platinum combinations versus vinorelbine plus cisplatin for first-line treatment of advanced nonsmall cell lung carcinoma (TAX 326). *Cancer* 2005; 104: 2766–2774.
9. Gridelli C, Brodowicz T, Langer CJ, *et al.* Pemetrexed therapy in elderly patients with good performance status: analysis of two phase III trials of patients with nonsquamous non-small-cell lung cancer. *Clin Lung Cancer* 2012; 13: 340–346.
10. Gridelli C. The ELVIS trial: a phase III study of single-agent vinorelbine as first-line treatment in elderly patients with advanced non-small cell lung cancer. Elderly Lung Cancer Vinorelbine Italian Study. *Oncologist* 2001; 6: Suppl. 1, 4–7.
11. Frasci G, Lorusso V, Panza N, *et al.* Gemcitabine plus vinorelbine *versus* vinorelbine alone in elderly patients with advanced non-small-cell lung cancer. *J Clin Oncol* 2000; 18: 2529–2536.
12. Gridelli C, Perrone F, Gallo C, *et al.* Chemotherapy for elderly patients with advanced non-small-cell lung cancer: the Multicenter Italian Lung Cancer in the Elderly Study (MILES) phase III randomized trial. *J Natl Cancer Inst* 2003; 95: 362–372.
13. Quoix E, Zalcman G, Oster JP, *et al.* Carboplatin and weekly paclitaxel doublet chemotherapy compared with monotherapy in elderly patients with advanced non-small-cell lung cancer: IFCT-0501 randomised, phase 3 trial. *Lancet* 2011; 378: 1079–1088.
14. Launay-Vacher V, Chatelut E, Lichtman SM, *et al.* Renal insufficiency in elderly cancer patients: International Society of Geriatric Oncology clinical practice recommendations. *Ann Oncol* 2007; 18: 1314–1321.
15. Balducci L, Carreca I. The role of myelopoietic growth factors in managing cancer in the elderly. *Drugs* 2002; 62: Suppl. 1, 47–63.
16. Aapro MS, Bohlius J, Cameron DA, *et al.* 2010 update of EORTC guidelines for the use of granulocyte-colony stimulating factor to reduce the incidence of chemotherapy-induced febrile neutropenia in adult patients with lymphoproliferative disorders and solid tumours. *Eur J Cancer* 2011; 47: 8–32.
17. Steen B. Body composition and aging. *Nutr Rev* 1988; 46: 45–51.
18. Extermann M, Overcash J, Lyman GH, *et al.* Comorbidity and functional status are independent in older cancer patients. *J Clin Oncol* 1998; 16: 1582–1587.

19. Quoix E, Westeel V, Zalcman G, *et al.* Chemotherapy in elderly patients with advanced non-small cell lung cancer. *Lung Cancer* 2011; 74: 364–368.
20. Folstein MF, Robins LN, Helzer JE. The Mini-Mental State Examination. *Arch Gen Psychiatry* 1983; 40: 812.
21. Spector WD, Katz S, Murphy JB, *et al.* The hierarchical relationship between activities of daily living and instrumental activities of daily living. *J Chronic Dis* 1987; 40: 481–489.
22. Extermann M. Basic assessment of the older cancer patient. *Curr Treat Options Oncol* 2011; 12: 276–285.
23. Balducci L, Extermann M. Management of cancer in the older person: a practical approach. *Oncologist* 2000; 5: 224–237.
24. Puts MTE, Santos B, Hardt J, *et al.* An update on a systematic review of the use of geriatric assessment for older adults in oncology. *Ann Oncol* 2014; 25: 307–315.
25. Piquet J, Blanchon F, Grivaux M, *et al.* Le cancer bronchique primitif du sujet âgé en France. Résultats de l'étude KBP-2000 du Collège des Pneumologues des Hôpitaux Généraux (CPHG). [Primary bronchial carcinoma in elderly subjects in France.] *Rev Mal Respir* 2003; 20: 691–699.
26. Piquet J, Blanchon F, Grivaux M, *et al.* Le cancer bronchique primitif du sujet âgé en France. Résultats de l'étude KBP-2000 du Collège des Pneumologues des Hôpitaux Généraux (CPHG). [Primary lung cancer in elderly subjects in France.] *Rev Mal Respir* 2004; 21: 8S70–8S78.
27. Noda K, Nishiwaki Y, Kawahara M, *et al.* Irinotecan plus cisplatin compared with etoposide plus cisplatin for extensive small-cell lung cancer. *N Engl J Med* 2002; 346: 85–91.
28. Hanna N, Bunn PA, Langer C, *et al.* Randomized phase III trial comparing irinotecan/cisplatin with etoposide/cisplatin in patients with previously untreated extensive-stage disease small-cell lung cancer. *J Clin Oncol* 2006; 24: 2038–2043.
29. Jett JR, Schild SE, Kesler KA, *et al.* Treatment of small cell lung cancer: diagnosis and management of lung cancer, 3rd ed: American College of Chest Physicians evidence-based clinical practice guidelines. *Chest* 2013; 143: e400S–e419S.
30. Eckardt JR. Second-line treatment of small-cell lung cancer. The case for systemic chemotherapy. *Oncol* 2003; 17: 181–188.
31. O'Brien MER, Ciuleanu TE, Tsekov H, *et al.* Phase III trial comparing supportive care alone with supportive care with oral topotecan in patients with relapsed small-cell lung cancer. *J Clin Oncol* 2006; 24: 5441–5447.
32. Von Pawel J, Jotte R, Spigel DR, *et al.* Randomized phase III trial of amrubicin *versus* topotecan as second-line treatment for patients with small-cell lung cancer. *J Clin Oncol* 2014; 32: 4012–4019.
33. Eckardt JR, von Pawel J, Pujol JL, *et al.* Phase III study of oral compared with intravenous topotecan as second-line therapy in small-cell lung cancer. *J Clin Oncol* 2007; 25: 2086–2092.
34. Von Pawel J, Schiller JH, Shepherd FA, *et al.* Topotecan *versus* cyclophosphamide, doxorubicin, and vincristine for the treatment of recurrent small-cell lung cancer. *J Clin Oncol* 1999; 17: 658–667.
35. Dajczman E, Fu LY, Small D, *et al.* Treatment of small cell lung carcinoma in the elderly. *Cancer* 1996; 77: 2032–2038.
36. Janssen-Heijnen MLG, Maas HA, van de Schans SA, *et al.* Chemotherapy in elderly small-cell lung cancer patients: yes we can, but should we do it? *Ann Oncol* 2011; 22: 821–826.
37. Lebitasy MP, Hédelin G, Purohit A, *et al.* Progress in the management and outcome of small-cell lung cancer in a French region from 1981 to 1994. *Br J Cancer* 2001; 85: 808–815.
38. Okamoto H, Watanabe K, Nishiwaki Y, *et al.* Phase II study of area under the plasma-concentration-*versus*-time curve-based carboplatin plus standard-dose intravenous etoposide in elderly patients with small-cell lung cancer. *J Clin Oncol* 1999; 17: 3540–3545.
39. Quoix E, Breton JL, Daniel C, *et al.* Etoposide phosphate with carboplatin in the treatment of elderly patients with small-cell lung cancer: a phase II study. *Ann Oncol* 2001; 12: 957–962.
40. Misumi Y, Nishio M, Takahashi T, *et al.* A feasibility study of carboplatin plus irinotecan treatment for elderly patients with extensive disease small-cell lung cancer. *Jpn J Clin Oncol* 2014; 44: 116–121.
41. Eba J, Shimokawa T, Nakamura K, *et al.* A phase II/III study comparing carboplatin and irinotecan with carboplatin and etoposide for the treatment of elderly patients with extensive-disease small-cell lung cancer (JCOG1201). *Jpn J Clin Oncol* 2015; 45: 115–118.
42. Quon H, Shepherd FA, Payne DG, *et al.* The influence of age on the delivery, tolerance, and efficacy of thoracic irradiation in the combined modality treatment of limited stage small cell lung cancer. *Int J Radiat Oncol Biol Phys* 1999; 43: 39–45.
43. Ardizzoni A, Favaretto A, Boni L, *et al.* Platinum-etoposide chemotherapy in elderly patients with small-cell lung cancer: results of a randomized multicenter phase II study assessing attenuated-dose or full-dose with lenograstim prophylaxis – a Forza Operativa Nazionale Italiana Carcinoma Polmonare and Gruppo Studio Tumori Polmonari Veneto (FONICAP-GSTPV) study. *J Clin Oncol* 2005; 23: 569–575.
44. White SC, Lorigan P, Middleton MR, *et al.* Randomized phase II study of cyclophosphamide, doxorubicin, and vincristine compared with single-agent carboplatin in patients with poor prognosis small cell lung carcinoma. *Cancer* 2001; 92: 601–608.

45. Souhami RL, Spiro SG, Rudd RM, *et al.* Five-day oral etoposide treatment for advanced small-cell lung cancer: randomized comparison with intravenous chemotherapy. *J Natl Cancer Inst* 1997; 89: 577–580.
46. Yuen AR, Zou G, Turrisi AT, *et al.* Similar outcome of elderly patients in intergroup trial 0096: Cisplatin, etoposide, and thoracic radiotherapy administered once or twice daily in limited stage small cell lung carcinoma. *Cancer* 2000; 89: 1953–1960.
47. Schild SE, Stella PJ, Brooks BJ, *et al.* Results of combined-modality therapy for limited-stage small cell lung carcinoma in the elderly. *Cancer* 2005; 103: 2349–2354.
48. Siu LL, Shepherd FA, Murray N, *et al.* Influence of age on the treatment of limited-stage small-cell lung cancer. *J Clin Oncol* 1996; 14: 821–828.
49. Ludbrook JJS, Truong PT, MacNeil MV, *et al.* Do age and comorbidity impact treatment allocation and outcomes in limited stage small-cell lung cancer? A community-based population analysis. *Int J Radiat Oncol Biol Phys* 2003; 55: 1321–1330.
50. Wang S, Wong ML, Hamilton N, *et al.* Impact of age and comorbidity on non-small-cell lung cancer treatment in older veterans. *J Clin Oncol* 2012; 30: 1447–1455.
51. Fanucchi O, Ambrogi MC, Dini P, *et al.* Surgical treatment of non-small cell lung cancer in octogenarians. *Interact Cardiovasc Thorac Surg* 2011; 12: 749–753.
52. Rivera C, Falcoz PE, Bernard A, *et al.* Surgical management and outcomes of elderly patients with early stage non-small cell lung cancer: a nested case-control study. *Chest* 2011; 140: 874–880.
53. Blanchard EM, Arnaoutakis K, Hesketh PJ. Lung cancer in octogenarians. *J Thorac Oncol* 2010; 5: 909–916.
54. Früh M, Rolland E, Pignon JP, *et al.* Pooled analysis of the effect of age on adjuvant cisplatin-based chemotherapy for completely resected non–small-cell lung cancer. *J Clin Oncol* 2008; 26: 3573–3581.
55. Cuffe S, Booth CM, Peng Y, *et al.* Adjuvant chemotherapy for non-small-cell lung cancer in the elderly: a population-based study in Ontario, Canada. *J Clin Oncol* 2012; 30: 1813–1821.
56. Younis T, Al-Fayea T, Virik K, *et al.* Adjuvant chemotherapy uptake in non-small cell lung cancer. *J Thorac Oncol* 2008; 3: 1272–1278.
57. Park S, Kim IR, Baek KK, *et al.* Prospective analysis of quality of life in elderly patients treated with adjuvant chemotherapy for non-small-cell lung cancer. *Ann Oncol* 2013; 24: 1630–1639.
58. Malhotra J, Mhango G, Gomez JE, *et al.* Adjuvant chemotherapy for elderly patients with stage I non-small-cell lung cancer ⩾4cm in size: an SEER-Medicare analysis. *Ann Oncol* 2015; 26: 768–773.
59. Sigel K, Mhango G, Cohen J, *et al.* Outcomes after adjuvant platinum-based chemotherapy in elderly NSCLC patients with T4 disease. *Ann Surg Oncol* 2013; 20: 1013–1019.
60. NSCLC Meta-analysis Collaborative Group. Preoperative chemotherapy for non-small-cell lung cancer: a systematic review and meta-analysis of individual participant data. *Lancet* 2014; 383: 1561–1571.
61. Rivera C, Jougon J, Dahan M, *et al.* Are postoperative consequences of neoadjuvant chemotherapy for non-small cell lung cancer more severe in elderly patients? *Lung Cancer Amst Neth* 2012; 76: 216–221.
62. Davidoff AJ, Gardner JF, Seal B, *et al.* Population-based estimates of survival benefit associated with combined modality therapy in elderly patients with locally advanced non-small cell lung cancer. *J Thorac Oncol* 2011; 6: 934–941.
63. Coate LE, Massey C, Hope A, *et al.* Treatment of the elderly when cure is the goal: the influence of age on treatment selection and efficacy for stage III non-small cell lung cancer. *J Thorac Oncol* 2011; 6: 537–544.
64. Curran WJ, Paulus R, Langer CJ, *et al.* Sequential *vs.* concurrent chemoradiation for stage III non-small cell lung cancer: randomized phase III trial RTOG 9410. *J Natl Cancer Inst* 2011; 103: 1452–1460.
65. Rocha Lima CMS, Herndon JE, Kosty M, *et al.* Therapy choices among older patients with lung carcinoma: an evaluation of two trials of the Cancer and Leukemia Group B. *Cancer* 2002; 94: 181–187.
66. Schild SE, Stella PJ, Geyer SM, *et al.* The outcome of combined-modality therapy for stage III non-small-cell lung cancer in the elderly. *J Clin Oncol* 2003; 21: 3201–3206.
67. Schild SE, Mandrekar SJ, Jatoi A, *et al.* The value of combined-modality therapy in elderly patients with stage III nonsmall cell lung cancer. *Cancer* 2007; 110: 363–368.
68. Jalal SI, Riggs HD, Melnyk A, *et al.* Updated survival and outcomes for older adults with inoperable stage III non-small-cell lung cancer treated with cisplatin, etoposide, and concurrent chest radiation with or without consolidation docetaxel: analysis of a phase III trial from the Hoosier Oncology Group (HOG) and US Oncology. *Ann Oncol* 2012; 23: 1730–1738.
69. Atagi S, Kawahara M, Yokoyama A, *et al.* Thoracic radiotherapy with or without daily low-dose carboplatin in elderly patients with non-small-cell lung cancer: a randomised, controlled, phase 3 trial by the Japan Clinical Oncology Group (JCOG0301). *Lancet Oncol* 2012; 13: 671–678.
70. Pallis AG, Gridelli C, Wedding U, *et al.* Management of elderly patients with NSCLC; updated expert's opinion paper: EORTC Elderly Task Force, Lung Cancer Group and International Society for Geriatric Oncology. *Ann Oncol* 2014; 25: 1270–1283.
71. Sacher AG, Le LW, Leighl NB, *et al.* Elderly patients with advanced NSCLC in phase III clinical trials: are the elderly excluded from practice-changing trials in advanced NSCLC? *J Thorac Oncol* 2013; 8: 366–368.

72. Pfister DG, Johnson DH, Azzoli CG, *et al.* American Society of Clinical Oncology treatment of unresectable non-small-cell lung cancer guideline: update 2003. *J Clin Oncol* 2004; 22: 330–353.
73. Pallis AG, Gridelli C, van Meerbeeck JP, *et al.* EORTC Elderly Task Force and Lung Cancer Group and International Society for Geriatric Oncology (SIOG) experts' opinion for the treatment of non-small-cell lung cancer in an elderly population. *Ann Oncol* 2010; 21: 692–706.
74. Langer CJ, Manola J, Bernardo P, *et al.* Cisplatin-based therapy for elderly patients with advanced non-small-cell lung cancer: implications of Eastern Cooperative Oncology Group 5592, a randomized trial. *J Natl Cancer Inst* 2002; 94: 173–181.
75. Lilenbaum RC, Herndon JEII, List MA, *et al.* Single-agent *versus* combination chemotherapy in advanced non-small-cell lung cancer: the Cancer and Leukemia Group B (study 9730). *J Clin Oncol* 2005; 23: 190–196.
76. Ansari RH, Socinski MA, Edelman MJ, *et al.* A retrospective analysis of outcomes by age in a three-arm phase III trial of gemcitabine in combination with carboplatin or paclitaxel *vs.* paclitaxel plus carboplatin for advanced non-small cell lung cancer. *Crit Rev Oncol Hematol* 2011; 78: 162–171.
77. Blanchard EM, Moon J, Hesketh PJ, *et al.* Comparison of platinum-based chemotherapy in patients older and younger than 70 years: an analysis of Southwest Oncology Group Trials 9308 and 9509. *J Thorac Oncol* 2011; 6: 115–120.
78. Soria JC, Mauguen A, Reck M, *et al.* Systematic review and meta-analysis of randomised, phase II/III trials adding bevacizumab to platinum-based chemotherapy as first-line treatment in patients with advanced non-small-cell lung cancer. *Ann Oncol* 2013; 24: 20–30.
79. Ramalingam SS, Dahlberg SE, Langer CJ, *et al.* Outcomes for elderly, advanced-stage non small-cell lung cancer patients treated with bevacizumab in combination with carboplatin and paclitaxel: analysis of Eastern Cooperative Oncology Group Trial 4599. *J Clin Oncol* 2008; 26: 60–65.
80. Zhu J, Sharma DB, Gray SW, *et al.* Carboplatin and paclitaxel with vs without bevacizumab in older patients with advanced non-small cell lung cancer. *JAMA* 2012; 307: 1593–1601.
81. Mok TS, Wu YL, Thongprasert S, *et al.* Gefitinib or carboplatin-paclitaxel in pulmonary adenocarcinoma. *N Engl J Med* 2009; 361: 947–957.
82. Rosell R, Carcereny E, Gervais R, *et al.* Erlotinib *versus* standard chemotherapy as first-line treatment for European patients with advanced *EGFR* mutation-positive non-small-cell lung cancer (EURTAC): a multicentre, open-label, randomised phase 3 trial. *Lancet Oncol* 2012; 13: 239–246.
83. Zhang X, Zang J, Xu J, *et al.* Maintenance therapy with continuous or switch strategy in advanced non-small cell lung cancer: a systematic review and meta-analysis. *Chest* 2011; 140: 117–126.
84. Gridelli C, de Marinis F, Thomas M, *et al.* Final efficacy and safety results of pemetrexed continuation maintenance therapy in the elderly from the PARAMOUNT phase III study. *J Thorac Oncol* 2014; 9: 991–997.
85. Wu CH, Fan WC, Chen YM, *et al.* Second-line therapy for elderly patients with non-small cell lung cancer who failed previous chemotherapy is as effective as for younger patients. *J Thorac Oncol* 2010; 5: 376–379.
86. Quoix E, Westeel V, Moreau L, *et al.* Second-line therapy in elderly patients with advanced nonsmall cell lung cancer. *Eur Respir J* 2014; 43: 240–249.


**Disclosures:** E. Quoix reports receiving personal fees and other support from Pfizer, AstraZeneca, Roche and Mundipharma, grants and other support from Lilly, personal fees from Boehringer Ingelheim, and other support from Amgen and GSK, outside the submitted work.

# Chapter 17

# Achievements in targeted therapies

Paolo Bironzo, Teresa Mele and Silvia Novello

Cytotoxic chemotherapy has historically been the cornerstone of advanced lung cancer treatment, but in recent years, new insights into the molecular pathways of this tumour have led to important therapeutic advances. The definition of different molecular profiles characterise some subpopulations that potentially will benefit from each target agent in terms of efficacy and quality of life. This landscape is evolving quickly as new oncogenic drivers are becoming the target for specific drugs. In this chapter, the state of the art will be presented together with perspectives on targeted therapies in lung cancer.

Targeted therapies are the perfect example of precision medicine and their role is rapidly emerging throughout different oncological diseases, including lung cancer. As opposed to traditional cytotoxic chemotherapy, which unselectively addresses rapidly dividing cells, targeted therapies are specific inhibitors of different molecules involved in cancer cell growth, survival or neoangiogenesis.

For many years, standard first-line systemic treatment for metastatic NSCLC has consisted of doublet chemotherapy (carboplatin or cisplatin, combined with a non-platinum-derived cytotoxic agent, such as taxanes, gemcitabine, vinorelbine or, more recently, pemetrexed). The introduction of targeted agents in the last few years has deeply changed the treatment paradigm in this setting and markedly modified the natural history of this disease.

The better understanding of molecular mechanisms underpinning oncogene addiction [1] has allowed, in the last 10 years, for the identification of different molecular subtypes of NSCLC, each dependent on a specific molecular driver, ultimately resulting in a constitutively active mutant signalling protein.

As depicted in figure 1, the most frequent molecular drivers described in NSCLC are *EGFR* mutations, *ALK* rearrangements, *FGFR* and Kirsten rat sarcoma viral oncogene homologue (*KRAS*) mutations.

However, to date, known and confirmed "druggable" mutations in everyday clinical practice are limited to lung ADCs (about 50% of all NSCLC). Outside these alterations, treatment

Oncology Dept, University of Turin, San Luigi Gonzaga University Hospital, Orbassano, Italy.

Correspondence: Silvia Novello, Dept of Oncology, University of Turin, San Luigi Gonzaga University Hospital, Regione Gonzole, 10, 10043 Orbassano, Italy. E-mail: silvia.novello@unito.it

 Print ISBN: 978-1-84984-061-3. Online ISBN: 978-1-84984-062-0. Print ISSN: 2312-508X. Online ISSN: 2312-5098.

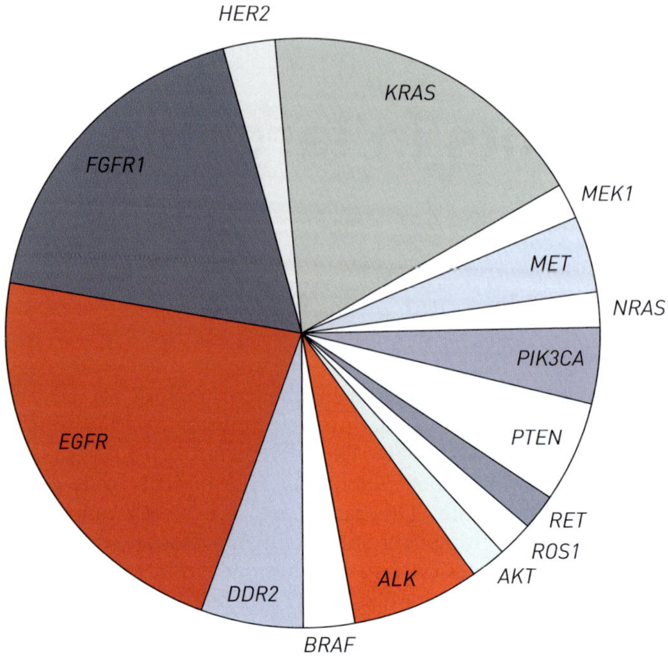


Figure 1. Frequency of known driver mutations in NSCLC. *KRAS*: Kirsten rat sarcoma viral oncogene homologue; *MEK1*: mitogen-activated protein kinase kinase 1; *MET*: Met; *NRAS*: neuroblastoma Ras viral oncogene homologue; *PIK3CA*: phosphatidylinositol-4,5-bisphosphate 3-kinase, catalytic subunit α; *PTEN*: phosphatase and tensin homologue; *RET*: Ret; *ROS1*: c-ros; *BRAF*: B-Raf; *DDR2*: discoidin domain receptor 2. Data from [2].

choice is still dependent on the histological subtype or clinical characteristics, and mainly limited to cytotoxic drugs.

The following sections will describe those targeted agents already approved by regulatory agencies in lung ADCs and some new ones that will enter clinical practice in the near future.

## EGFR and EGFR-directed agents

The *EGFR* gene is located on chromosome 7p12–13 and encodes a 170-kDa receptor tyrosine kinase [3]. EGFR (also known as HER1) is a transmembrane receptor, belonging to the ERBB family of cell-surface receptor tyrosine kinases together with HER2, HER3 and HER4, having an extracellular ligand-binding region, a single membrane-spanning region and a cytoplasmic tyrosine kinase-containing domain. Signalling through EGFR activation is pivotal to cell proliferation, evasion of apoptosis, angiogenesis and metastasis in various neoplasms, including NSCLC [4].

EGFR binding to EGF (its main ligand) triggers receptor homo- or heterodimerisation with other ERBB members on the cell surface, leading to activation of the intrinsic kinase domain and phosphorylation of tyrosine residues within the cytoplasmic tail. This process activates downstream effectors such as Ras/Raf/mitogen-activated protein kinase kinase (MEK)/extracellular signal-regulated kinase (ERK)/mitogen-activated protein kinase and phosphatidylinositol-4,5-bisphosphate 3-kinase (PI3K)/AKT/mTOR, with consequent cell survival and proliferation. Other EGFR ligands include TGF-α, amphiregulin, epigen, betacellulin, heparin-binding EGF and epiregulin [4, 5].

Under normal circumstances, EGFR signalling relies on ligand-dependent activation of the receptor. However, *EGFR* mutations can independently sustain cell growth and survival.

*EGFR* mutations are localised in exon 19, mainly consisting of an in-frame deletion (45–50%), and in exon 21, consisting of the L858R point mutation (40–45%); many other less common mutations have been also identified [6]. As far as clinical characteristics are concerned, *EGFR* mutations are known to be more commonly observed in never-smokers, ADC, women and Asian people [7]. In unselected NSCLC, this genetic alteration is found in about 10% of the Caucasian population, as opposed to 30% of the Asian population [8–10].

EGFR-directed agents can be divided into different subgroups presented in table 1. EGFR TKIs are the key drugs in the management of EGFR mutant NSCLC patients. The selection of cases cannot rely on clinical characteristics and mutation testing in this subset of patients drives treatment decisions. *EGFR* mutation analysis must be performed according to evidence-based recommendations [11].

EGFR-activating mutations cluster in the catalytic kinase domain; although over 100 mutations in the kinase domain have been identified in lung ADCs, most patients harbour one of seven major mutations (exon 19 deletion (del-19), L858R in exon 21, exon 20 insertions, G719X, L861X, exon 19 insertions and T790M [12], exon 19 deletion and L858R accounting for about 85% of EGFR mutations [13–15]).

## *EGFR* mutation detection

*EGFR* mutation testing is recommended in nonsquamous histology and never-smokers (independently of histotype) by a validated mutation test and it can be performed on the primary tumour or at a metastatic site. Several methods are currently available for this purpose, including direct sequencing and PCR [16].

These tests could be classified in two main groups: screening methods, *i.e.* those detecting all mutations in exons 18–21 including novel variants, and targeted methods, *i.e.* those identifying only already described mutations. IHC using mutation-specific antibodies has also been evaluated [17–22], but is not widely adopted due to concerns about its lower sensitivity and specificity compared with DNA-based molecular techniques. According to European Society for Medical Oncology guidelines, a wide coverage of mutations in exons 18–21 is strongly recommended, together with the identification of drug resistance-conferring mutations (such as exon 20 insertions or T790M substitution). *EGFR* mutation detection in peripheral blood has recently been shown to be highly predictive of the corresponding mutational status of the primary tumour [23].

## First-generation EGFR TKIs: gefitinib and erlotinib

First-generation TKIs were initially investigated in early phase II trials in previously treated, unselected patients [24, 25]: clinical benefit was observed within 3–4 weeks of treatment and responses (response rates ranging from 12% to 18%) were found to be higher in ADC histology, never-smokers and female patients.

Table 1. EGFR-directed agents

| Subgroup | Agents | Description |
|---|---|---|
| **First-generation, reversible TKIs** | Gefitinib<br>Erlotinib<br>Icotinib | Reversibly compete with ATP binding to tyrosine kinase domain of EGFR, inhibiting ligand-dependent receptor activation |
| **Second-generation, irreversible TKIs** | Afatinib<br>Dacomitinib<br>Neratinib<br>Canertinib | Pan-HER inhibitors that irreversibly bind the ATP-binding pocket of EGFR *via* covalent bonds, inducing permanent inhibition |
| **Third-generation TKIs** | Mutant-selective inhibitors (CO1686, AZD9291, HM61723) | Specifically target mutant forms of EGFR, exhibiting minimal activity toward the wild-type receptor |
| **Monoclonal antibodies** | Cetuximab<br>Panitumumab<br>Nimotuzumab<br>Necitumumab | Competitively inhibit ligand binding to EGFR, preventing ligand-induced activation and downstream signalling |

Subsequent phase III trials comparing platinum-based chemotherapy in association with a first-generation TKI *versus* chemotherapy alone in unselected patients did not show any significant difference in terms of survival (both in patients treated with gefitinib or erlotinib) [26–30]. A similar lack of success was reported in a large phase III trial (Iressa Survival Evaluation in Lung Cancer) comparing gefitinib with placebo as a second- or third-line treatment for locally advanced or metastatic NSCLC [31].

However, a trial by Shepherd *et al.* [32] demonstrated a survival benefit in unselected patients treated with erlotinib after failure of first- and second-line chemotherapy, and this led to the approval of erlotinib in NSCLC as a second- or third-line treatment (regardless of the mutational status).

As opposed to the early trials, different results were drawn from later studies in which patients were treated with EGFR-directed agents as a first-line treatment after being selected according to their clinical characteristics and, further on, according to specific molecular characteristics (*EGFR* mutational status).

In the Iressa Pan-Asia Study, Asian patients were selected according to their smoking history (never- or light smokers) and histology (ADC), and randomised to carboplatin–paclitaxel *versus* gefitinib as a first-line treatment. The primary end-point was PFS. Activating *EGFR* mutations were found in 60% of tested patients, and both overall response rate (ORR) and PFS favoured single-agent gefitinib in this subgroup. No significant difference in overall survival was observed and this was attributed to patient crossover from chemotherapy to gefitinib at the time of relapse [28]. In pointing out the role of *EGFR* mutations as predictive biomarkers in patients treated with gefitinib, this pivotal trial changed clinical practice. The beneficial role of a first-generation TKI in the Caucasian population was defined by the European Randomised Trial of Tarceva *versus* Chemotherapy, which compared erlotinib *versus* chemotherapy (cisplatin–gemcitabine or cisplatin–docetaxel) as a first-line treatment

[33]. As shown in table 2, other phase III trials on NSCLC patients selected on the basis of *EGFR* mutational status demonstrated a significant increase of PFS and led to a fundamental change in the approach to advanced NSCLC patients [34–37].

While evidence of an activating *EGFR* mutation is mandatory for first-line EGFR-TKI treatment, erlotinib is still registered and reimbursed, as previously reported, even in second- and third-line therapy, irrespectively of molecular characteristics, on the basis of the results of BR.21 trial [25]. Although rarely, even *EGFR* wild-type patients (or those supposed as such) respond to EGFR-TKI administration [40] and the mechanisms underlying this activity are still not completely clear. While in some cases such activity is due to rare mutations not assessed by commonly used targeted methods or could depend on false-negative results [41, 42], in other patients, TKI activity could rely on EGFR expression, amplification or phosphorylation, EGFR ligand expression, or other still unknown mechanisms [43–45].

Table 2. First-line TKIs in *EGFR*-mutated patients

| First author [ref.] | Study | Treatment | Patients n | Median PFS months | Median OS months |
|---|---|---|---|---|---|
| **Mok [28]** | IPASS | Gefitinib *versus* Carbo/Pacli | 261 | 9.8 *versus* 6.4 (HR 0.48, p<0.001) | 21.6 *versus* 21.9 (HR 1.00, p=0.99) |
| **Han [34]** | First-SIGNAL | Gefitinib *versus* Cis/Gem | 42 | 8.4 *versus* 6.7 (HR 0.61, p=0.084) | 30.6 *versus* 26.5 (HR 0.823, p=0.65) |
| **Mitsudomi [35]** | WJTOG | Gefitinib *versus* Cis/docetaxel | 172 | 9.2 *versus* 6.3 (HR 0.489, p<0.0001) | 35.5 *versus* 38.8 (HR 1.18) |
| **Maemondo [36]** | NEJ02 | Gefitinib *versus* Carbo/Pacli | 228 | 10.8 *versus* 5.4 (HR 0.32, p<0.001) | 27.7 *versus* 26.6 (HR 0.88, p=0.31) |
| **Zhou [37]** | OPTIMAL | Erlotinib *versus* Carbo/Gem | 154 | 13.1 *versus* 4.6 (HR 0.16, p<0.0001) | 22.7 *versus* 28.9 (HR 1.04) |
| **Rosell [33]** | EURTAC | Erlotinib *versus* platinum-based chemo | 173 | 9.7 *versus* 5.2 (HR 0.37, p<0.0001) | 19.3 *versus* 19.5 (HR 1.04, p=0.87) |
| **Sequist [38]** | LUX-Lung 3 | Afatinib *versus* Cis/Pem | 345 | 11.1 *versus* 6.9 (HR 0.59, p=0.0004) | Not reported |
| **Wu [39]** | LUX-Lung 6 | Afatinib *versus* Cis/Gem | 364 | 11.0 *versus* 5.6 (HR 0.28, p<0.0001) | 22.1 *versus* 22.2 (HR 0.95, p=0.76; immature data) |

OS: overall survival; IPASS: Iressa Pan-Asia Study; First-SIGNAL: First-Line Single-Agent Iressa *versus* Gemcitabine and Cisplatin Trial in Never-Smokers with Adenocarcinoma of the Lung; WJTOG: West Japan Thoracic Oncology Group; OPTIMAL: Erlotinib *versus* Standard Chemotherapy in the First-Line Treatment of Patients with Advanced *EGFR* Mutation-Positive NSCLC; EURTAC: European Randomised Trial of Tarceva *versus* Chemotherapy; Carbo: carboplatin; Pacli: paclitaxel; Cis: cisplatin; Gem: gemcitabine; chemo: chemotherapy; Pem: pemetrexed; HR: hazard ratio.

## Second-generation EGFR-TKIs: afatinib and dacomitinib

The LUX-Lung 3 phase III trial investigated the role of afatinib in the first-line setting of advanced NSCLC patients harbouring *EGFR* mutation. This trial was designed for 345 patients to compare the TKI with cisplatin–pemetrexed and a significant improvement in PFS was shown (11.1 *versus* 6.9 months). This effect was found to be even stronger (PFS 13.6 *versus* 6.9 months) in patients with common *EGFR* mutations (Del-19 and L858R) [38]. LUX-Lung 6 was conducted on Asian patients only, using cisplatin–gemcitabine as the standard arm and demonstrating similar results [39]. These trials led to afatinib approval in TKI-naïve patients with locally advanced or metastatic NSCLC harbouring *EGFR* mutations. The ongoing LUX-Lung 7 trial will provide data on afatinib *versus* gefitinib in first-line, *EGFR* mutation-positive patients (www.clinicaltrials.gov identifier number NCT01466660).

Dacomitinib did not show any significant improvement in PFS when used as a second- or third-line treatment in unselected patients [46]. Its role in *EGFR*-mutated patients is currently under evaluation in phase III trials comparing dacomitinib *versus* gefitinib in the first-line setting (ARCHER 1050 trial; NCT01774721).

## EGFR monoclonal antibodies

EGFR-directed monoclonal antibodies block receptor signalling through specific competitive binding to EGFR on the extracellular surface of cells. Their action on tumour cells is also enhanced by antibody-dependent cellular cytotoxicity. EGFR-directed monoclonal antibodies evaluated in NSCLC include cetuximab, panitumumab, nimotuzumab and necitumumab.

Cetuximab is a chimaeric monoclonal antibody (mAb) that selectively binds the extracellular domain of EGFR. The role of cetuximab in combination with first-line chemotherapy has been investigated in phase II and III trials [47–50] and within a subsequent meta-analysis [51], and a modest benefit in all efficacy end-points from the addition of cetuximab to standard platinum-based treatment in NSCLC was reported (table 3). Moreover, the addition of cetuximab to chemotherapy was characterised by an increased toxicity in terms of rash, diarrhoea, neutropenia and infusion reaction, and this is the main reason why (together with modest efficacy advantage) the First-Line Erbitux in Lung Cancer trial did not led to treatment approval by regulatory agencies.

Table 3. Combination of chemotherapy and cetuximab in advanced NSCLC

| First author [ref.] | Study | Treatment | Patients n | Median PFS months | Median OS months |
|---|---|---|---|---|---|
| **Butts [49]** | | Cis or Carbo/Gem ± Cet | 65 | 5.09 *versus* 4.21 | 11.99 *versus* 9.26 |
| **Rosell [50]** | | Cis/Vnb ± Cet | 86 | 5.0 *versus* 4.6 | 8.3 *versus* 7.3 |
| **Pirker [47]** | FLEX | Cis/Vnb ± Cet | 1125 | 4.8 *versus* 4.8 | 11.3 *versus* 10.1 |
| **Lynch [48]** | BMS099 | Taxane/Carbo ± Cet | 676 | 4.4 *versus* 4.24 | 9.69 *versus* 8.38 |

OS: overall survival; FLEX: First-Line Erbitux in Lung Cancer; Cis: cisplatin; Carbo: carboplatin; Gem: gemcitabine; Cet: cetuximab; Vnb: vinorelbine.

Necitumumab, a fully human mAb, has been evaluated in phase III trials in combination with cisplatin–pemetrexed in advanced nonsquamous NSCLC (INSPIRE trial, stopped early for unexpected toxicity) and with cisplatin–gemcitabine in squamous histology (SQUIRE trial). In the SQUIRE trial, the addition of necitumumab to cisplatin–gemcitabine statistically significantly improved overall survival (11.5 *versus* 9.9 months) and PFS (5.7 *versus* 5.5 months) [52].

Nimotuzumab (95% human antibody) is under investigation in phase II trials (NCT00983047 and NCT01393080).

None of the EGFR-directed monoclonal antibodies is currently part of the therapeutic armamentarium for NSCLC treatment, in any clinical setting.

### Toxicity

Despite the high selectivity of targeted therapies, a range of previously unknown and sometimes unpredictable side-effects have been described. Toxicity related to the aforementioned EGFR-directed agents mainly reflects their off-target effects, *i.e.* targeting wild-type EGFR in normal tissues. The most common toxicities are rash/dermatitis acneiform, diarrhoea, stomatitis, dry skin and pruritus [53, 54].

Skin disorders are generally mild or moderate in severity and can be managed by appropriate topical or systemic interventions, or by reducing the TKI dose [55]. As for other treatments, there is possibly an underestimation of toxicity by clinicians when compared with patients and this fact must be taken into account, especially if dealing with long-term therapies, which is the aim of these targeted drugs [56].

### Drug resistance

Despite the benefit that targeted agents brought to NSCLC treatment, not all *EGFR*-mutated patients exhibit durable responses, the median PFS is still less than 1 year and almost all patients develop resistance [33, 37, 38].

Primary resistance may occur in some patients not responding to TKIs from the very beginning and acquired resistance may also develop over time, due to several mechanisms. Secondary, acquired gatekeeper mutations in the EGFR kinase domain (such as T790M, L747S, D761Y and T854A) and PI3K mutations alter the binding kinetics of the receptor and its downstream effectors, representing a form of oncogenic drift [13, 14]. Other mechanisms of resistance include activation of second oncogenic drivers through different mechanisms, such as *MET* amplification, *EGFR* amplification, *HER2* upregulation and *ALK* amplification [57]. In addition, a shift towards SCLC histology and epithelial–mesenchymal transition have been described as additional mechanisms of acquired resistance [57, 58].

Clinically, TKI resistance can be classified into two categories: oligoprogression and systemic progression. Even without strong prospective data, in oligometastatic patients, local therapies (radiotherapy, surgery and local ablation) are feasible options together with continuation of the oral TKI beyond Response Evaluation Criteria In Solid Tumors (RECIST)-defined disease progression [59, 60]. The rationale of such approach is avoiding the flare-up phenomenon (rapid recurrence of symptoms and symptomatic decline) [61], taking advantage of the remaining drug sensitivity. Recent trials evaluated the role of TKI beyond progression. In the phase II ASPIRATION trial, Asian patients with advanced *EGFR* mutation-positive NSCLC received erlotinib beyond progression. The difference between PFS1 (calculated until RECIST progression) and PFS2 (calculated until progression assessed by doctor discretion) was 3.7 months [62]. The phase III Iressa Treatment Beyond Progression in Addition to Chemotherapy *versus* Chemotherapy Alone study explored the role of gefitinib beyond progression in addition to chemotherapy *versus* chemotherapy alone in *EGFR*-mutated NSCLC, but the study did not meet the primary end-point (PFS) and no benefit was seen in terms of survival or response rate from continuing the TKI with cytotoxic drugs [63].

The main therapeutic strategy to overcome EGFR-TKI resistance has been the development and introduction of third-line EGFR-TKIs. Combinatorial targeting of the EGFR pathway has been also investigated.

A single-arm, phase Ib trial investigated afatinib and cetuximab, in patients who developed acquired resistance to erlotinib or gefitinib, described a PFS of 4.7 months, but with some issues concerning the toxicity profile [64]. By contrast, a similar phase I/II trial of erlotinib and cetuximab did not demonstrate efficacy [65].

The identification of molecular drivers and the rapidly increasing development of corresponding new targeted agents led to an approach of cotargeting EGFR and further intracellular pathways as an alternative strategy to overcome EGFR-TKI resistance. In this setting, Met targeting has been thoroughly investigated (given its pivotal role both in *de novo* and acquired resistance) but combinatorial EFGR–Met targeting was discouraged by the results of phase III trials [66, 67]. No targeted-agent combination is currently recommended in EGFR-TKI-resistant NSCLC patients outside clinical trials and further data are warranted.

### Third-generation TKIs

Third-generation TKIs (CO1686, AZD9291 and HM61713) are oral, irreversible EGFR inhibitors that block mutated EGFR, including drug resistance mutations such as T790M. At therapeutic dose, they do not inhibit wild-type EGFR and such binding specificity deeply limits the observed toxicity [68, 69]. AZD9291 and CO1686 already showed very promising results in phase I/II trials reporting remarkable overall disease control rates (89% for CO1686 and 96% for AZD9291) [69, 70]. Phase II and III studies exploring these drugs in TKI-naïve and in TKI-resistant patients are currently ongoing. A recent phase I trial evaluated the role of HM61713 in EGFR-TKI-pre-treated patients, divided into two arms according to the time since prior EGFR-TKI treatment ($<4$ *versus* $\geqslant 4$ weeks), showing a good safety profile together with a disease control rate of 76.5% and 73.1% in the two arms, respectively [71].

## *ALK* rearrangements

The *EML4–ALK* fusion gene was first described as an oncogenic driver in lung ADC in 2007 [72]. This rearrangement is generated by an inversion in chromosome 2p that juxtaposes the 5′-end of *EML4* with the 3′-kinase domain of *ALK*, leading to constitutive ALK kinase activation.

Many variants of this fusion protein have been described to date [73] and other *ALK* partners emerged, including TRL-fused gene (*TFG*) [74], kinesin family member 5B (*KIF5B*) [75, 76], kinesin light chain 1 (*KLC1*) [77] and translocated promoter region (*TPR*) [78].

This genetic alteration is found in 2–7% of NSCLC patients, a percentage depending on the detection method used and on the screened population [79–82]. Typically, *EML4–ALK*-positive tumours are ADCs, mainly young nonsmoking patients, but not exclusively; the genetic alteration seems to be mutually exclusive to *KRAS* and *EGFR* mutations [83–87].

### *ALK* rearrangement detection

Currently, the gold standard and US Food and Drug Administration (FDA)-approved diagnostic test for *ALK* gene rearrangement detection is the break-apart FISH test [88]. However, this method is expensive, not always reproducible and not widely available.

For such reasons, clinical and preclinical research is evaluating alternative methods, such as real-time PCR, IHC with dedicated antibodies, and NGS techniques [89–92]. In Europe, IHC has recently been approved as one of the standard diagnostic tests to detect *ALK* rearrangements: in a paper by Marchetti *et al.* [93], an algorithm was proposed where ALK IHC is the first diagnostic step in EGFR- and KRAS-negative NSCLC, whereas FISH is reserved for IHC-positive patients only.

As for *EGFR* mutations, *ALK* rearrangement testing is recommended in all patients with advanced nonsquamous NSCLC at diagnosis and should be carried out in parallel with *EGFR* mutation analysis; moreover, *ALK* rearrangement testing should be considered even in SCC from patients with minimal or remote smoking history [23, 94].

### *ALK*-rearranged tumours: treatment

#### *Crizotinib*

In August 2011, crizotinib, an oral, small-molecule inhibitor of the Met, ALK and ROS1 tyrosine kinases, was approved by the FDA under an accelerated procedure for *ALK*-rearranged locally advanced and metastatic NSCLC patients on the basis of the results of phase I and II trials (PROFILE 1001 and PROFILE 1005) showing high response rates and a good tolerability profile [79, 95].

A phase III trial in previously treated patients [96] showed a statistically significant improvement in PFS (7.7 *versus* 3.3 months; hazard ratio (HR) 0.49 (95% CI 0.37–0.64), $p<0.001$) and response rate (65% *versus* 20%) with crizotinib, as compared with single-agent chemotherapy (pemetrexed or docetaxel) in advanced NSCLC, *ALK*-rearranged patients. More recently, preliminary data from a phase III, open-label, randomised trial comparing first-line platinum (either cisplatin or carboplatin)/pemetrexed chemotherapy *versus* crizotinib were presented, showing significant improvements in PFS (median 10.9 *versus* 7 months; HR 0.454 (95% CI 0.346–0.596), $p<0.0001$) and ORR (74% *versus* 45%; $p<0.0001$) with the TKI [97].

#### *Novel ALK inhibitors*

Ceritinib (LDK378), a novel ALK inhibitor with some activity on ROS1, insulin-like growth factor-1 receptor and insulin receptor, was evaluated in a phase I/II, open-label, randomised trial that enrolled 163 *ALK*-positive metastatic NSCLC patients progressing on or intolerant to crizotinib [98, 99]. Ceritinib led to an ORR of 58% (95% CI 48–67%) and, notably, an ORR of 56% in patients previously treated with crizotinib (95% CI 45–67%). Based on these data, on April 2014, the FDA granted accelerated approval of ceritinib for the treatment of metastatic, *ALK*-positive NSCLC previously treated with or intolerant to crizotinib.

Alectinib (RO5424802/CH5424802), another second-generation ALK inhibitor, demonstrated activity in both crizotinib-naïve [100] and pre-treated patients in phase I/II trials [101, 102]. The drug is currently approved in Japan for the treatment of *ALK*-positive, advanced NSCLC patients.

These novel ALK inhibitors can effectively cross the blood–brain barrier, also leading to good responses in patients harbouring central nervous system metastasis.

ASP3026 is also a novel ALK inhibitor showing activity in cases with the crizotinib-resistant gatekeeper mutation L1196M; preliminary results from a phase I trial demonstrated clinical activity in *ALK*-positive NSCLC that progressed on prior crizotinib [103]. AP26113 is a potent inhibitor of wild-type ALK that maintains activity against several crizotinib-resistant ALK mutants, as shown in a phase I/II, single-arm trial conducted by Gettinger *et al.* [104]. Due to these results, both agents, along with other compounds currently under active investigation (X-396, X-376, PF-06463922, TSR-011, RXDX-101, CEP-28122 and CEP-37440) could lead to further progress in *ALK*-positive NSCLC treatment [105].

### *Toxicity*

Crizotinib is usually well tolerated. The most common toxicities are neutropenia, diarrhoea, nausea, abdominal pain, transaminase elevation (especially alanine transaminase) and visual disorders; rare but potentially fatal drug-related pneumonia and hepatic insufficiency could also occur. Male patients could develop symptomatic hypogonadism [106].

Ceritinib could induce gastrointestinal toxicity, fatigue and transaminase alteration [107], while alectinib was reported to be associated with fluid retention and fatigue [108]. The most frequent ASP3026 adverse events are fatigue, vomiting, nausea and constipation, while AP26113, in addition, induced cough, headache and pulmonary symptoms such as dyspnoea and hypoxia.

### *Drug resistance*

Similarly to the *EGFR* population, in *ALK*-rearranged patients, after an initial response, progression occurs: the three main mechanisms of ALK resistance are mutation of the ALK tyrosine kinase domain (accounting for approximately 25% of cases), amplification of the *EML4–ALK* gene and activation of alternative signalling pathways [109–113].

Clinical research is currently focussing on evaluating second-generation ALK inhibitors in this context (see earlier). Moreover, interesting results come from heat shock protein (Hsp) inhibition [114]. Drugs inhibiting this target have been investigated in *ALK*-rearranged patients with low response rates, when used alone and compared with ALK inhibitors, but other trials are currently combining an ALK-TKI with and Hsp90 inhibitor, in order to prevent resistance development or overcome it [115] (NCT01579994 and NCT01772797).

An intriguing aspect, although still debated, is the activity of pemetrexed in *ALK*-rearranged patients, as observed in subgroup analyses and retrospective trials [96, 116].

## Angiogenesis inhibition

Neoangiogenesis, which promotes tumour growth and metastasis, is characterised by the formation of abnormal and chaotic vessels leading to an altered tumour microenvironment, which increases VEGF production, causing an autonomous proangiogenic and promitogenic loop. Currently available antiangiogenic drugs are directed against circulating VEGF or VEGFR.

Bevacizumab is a humanised mAb that targets circulating VEGF, approved for nonsquamous, advanced NSCLC first-line treatment, in addition to platinum doublet chemotherapy.

The registration of this drug was based on two phase III trials, which evaluated platinum-based doublet chemotherapy *versus* the same doublet plus bevacizumab. The Eastern Cooperative Oncology Group E4599 trial enrolled 878 patients with stage IIIB/IV nonsquamous NSCLC randomised to six cycles of carboplatin and paclitaxel with or without bevacizumab 15 $mg \cdot kg^{-1}$. Overall survival was significantly greater in the experimental arm (12.3 *versus* 10.3 months, $p=0.003$), as well as PFS (6.2 *versus* 4.5 months, $p<0.001$) and response rate (35% *versus* 15%, $p<0.001$) [117]. The Avastin in Lung Cancer trial randomised the same population to cisplatin and gemcitabine chemotherapy plus bevacizumab at two different doses (7.5 or 15 $mg \cdot kg^{-1}$) or placebo. Compared with the placebo group, the risk of progression or death at any time was reduced by 25% in the evacizumab 7.5 $mg \cdot kg^{-1}$ group (HR 0.75, 95% CI 0.64–0.87; $p=0.0003$) and by 15% in the bevacizumab 15 $mg \cdot kg^{-1}$ group (HR 0.85, 95% CI 0.73–1.00; $p=0.0456$), while no significant improvement was shown for overall survival [118]. The main toxicities of bevacizumab are arterial hypertension, haemorrhagic events, proteinuria and neutropenia [119].

Nintedanib is an oral inhibitor of VEGFR, platelet-derived growth factor and FGFR. This agent was added to docetaxel in second-line setting in a phase III randomised placebo-controlled trial (LUME-Lung 1). The combination significantly prolonged PFS in the whole population (median 3.4 *versus* 2.7 months, $p=0.0019$); moreover, overall survival was increased at a pre-planned subgroup analysis in ADC patients, especially in those who progressed within 9 months after starting first-line chemotherapy (10.9 *versus* 7.9 months, $p=0.0073$) [120].

A second study investigated nintedanib plus pemetrexed *versus* placebo plus pemetrexed in advanced nonsquamous NSCLC as second-line therapy. The trial was stopped after an interim analysis that suggested lack of improvement from the addition of nintedanib. The final analysis of the intention-to-treat population showed a significant although modest improvement of PFS with the experimental combination (median PFS 4.4 *versus* 3.6 months, $p=0.04$) [121].

Ramucirumab, an IgG1 mAb against the extracellular domain of VEGFR2, has been evaluated in a double-blind, placebo-controlled, phase III trial in association with docetaxel in second-line treatment of stage IV NSCLC. The addition of the mAb significantly improved ORR (22.9% *versus* 13.6%, $p<0.001$), PFS (median PFS 4.5 *versus* 3.0 months; HR 0.762, $p<0.0001$) and overall survival (median overall survival 10.5 *versus* 9.1 months; HR 0.857 (95% CI 0.751–0.98), $p=0.0235$), with only a slight increase of grade 3–4 neutropenia, fatigue and hypertension, while grade 5 adverse events were comparable between the two arms [122].

## Promising new targets and agents

*BRAF* somatic mutations occur in 1–2% of NSCLC, mainly in ADC and former/current smokers. V600E point mutation represents the most common, even if other sites of mutations are reported in lung cancer. Dabrafenib, a B-Raf inhibitor, showed clinical activity in a phase II study in 78 *BRAF* V600E-mutated NSCLC patients, with an ORR of 32% and a disease control rate of 56% after 12 weeks of treatment [123].

PI3K inhibitors are of interest in SCC where *PIK3CA*, *PTEN* (a phosphatase and tensin homologue) and *AKT* mutations are more frequent [124]. Currently, buparlisib (BKM-120) and pictilisib (GCD-0941) are under investigation in association with chemotherapy, and data are awaited (NCT01911325 and NCT01493843).

Met protein overexpression is found in approximately 25–75% of early-stage NSCLC and such alteration, along with gene amplification, is associated with poor prognosis [125–127]. While only 4–7% of untreated NSCLCs harbour *MET* amplification, 20% of patients previously treated with EGFR-TKIs show this alteration, possibly mediating EGFR-directed agent resistance [128, 129]. Moreover, elevated serum levels of HGF, which binds the Met tyrosine kinase receptor, have been associated with poor prognosis and aggressiveness in both NSCLC and SCLC, along with primary and secondary resistance to EGFR-TKIs [130–133].

mAbs binding HGF are currently being tested. Of these, ficlatuzumab seems to confer some benefit in *EGFR*-mutated patients with low c-Met expression when associated with gefinitib, possibly by delaying resistance onset [134].

In contrast, onartuzumab, a mAb against Met, after promising results in a phase II trial [135], was deemed ineffective, with the early closure of the phase III trial (MetLung) in Met-positive (IHC detection), advanced NSCLC patients [136]. Small molecules inhibiting Met include tivantinib (ARQ-197), cabozantinib (XL-184) and crizotinib. Two phase III trials investigating tivantinib, a non-ATP-competitive Met inhibitor, in association with erlotinib were both prematurely stopped because of either futility (MARQUEE trial) [66] or toxicity (ATTENTION trial) [67]. Cabozantinib and crizotinib are currently under investigation as Met inhibitors. Interestingly, cabozantinib is also a potent inhibitor of VEGFR2, AXL and Ret, showing activity in tumours positive for the *RET* fusion gene [137], which account for approximately 1.7% of lung ADCs [138].

*ROS1* rearrangement, which is detected in about 1% of ADCs [139], is actively targeted by crizotinib, with an ORR of 72% (95% CI 58–84%) and a median PFS of 19.2 months (95% CI 14.5 months–not reached) [140]; second-generation ALK inhibitors are also being investigated in clinical trials in this subset of patients.

A unique class of patients is represented by those carrying *HER2* mutations or amplification. While some data suggest activity of HER2-targeted agents such as trastuzumab and dacomitinib [141, 142], further studies are warranted to explore treatment opportunities actively in this subpopulation.

*KRAS* is the most common mutated gene in NSCLC, and is frequently detected in patients with smoking history (25% *versus* 6% in former/current smokers and nonsmokers, respectively) [143] and ADC (34%) [144]. Selumetinib inhibits MEK1/MEK2, downstream kinases of the Ras/Raf/MEK/ERK signalling pathway. This small molecule has been investigated with docetaxel in a phase II trial in patients who had progressed to first-line therapy, showing a statistically significant improvement in ORR (37% *versus* 0%, $p<0.0001$) and PFS (HR 0.58, 80% CI 0.42–0.79; one-sided $p=0.0014$), and numerically superior, although not statistically significant, overall survival (9.4 *versus* 5.2 months). However, the combination regimen was more toxic: higher rates of neutropenia, febrile neutropenia and serious adverse events leading to hospitalisation (48% *versus* 19%) [145]. Currently, a phase III trial is ongoing testing docetaxel plus selumetinib *versus* docetaxel plus placebo (NCT01933932).

## Conclusion

The introduction of targeted drugs in the clinical management of lung cancer patients is undoubtedly a step forward in tailored therapy. The current treatment choice relies on a careful assessment of histological and molecular features (*EGFR* mutations and *ALK* translocation are already part of routine diagnostic work-up), in order to identify those patients who may benefit more from a certain therapeutic approach.

This assessment is important both at diagnosis and at relapse, since cancer cells may dynamically change their features over time. Such modifications can occur for intrinsic cancer changes due to progression or they can be enhanced by selective pressure superimposed by treatment, ultimately leading to drug resistance (*i.e.* T790M mutation in patients who received EGFR-TKIs and *ALK* amplification in crizotinib treated patients).

One of the main hurdles underpinning disease progression and drug resistance is tumour heterogeneity and drug adaptation. Heterogeneous subclonal events caused by genetic drift may account for drug resistance and different clinical behaviour of the disease at different sites or diverse biological responses within the same lesion.

Liquid biopsies have recently been introduced as a tool to overcome limitations in collecting tissue samples, by genotyping circulating cell-free DNA or circulating cell DNA.

In current clinical practice, a single-gene testing approach is mainly used to identify variants (*e.g.* *EGFR* mutation or *ALK* rearrangement) to guide treatment decisions, and such serial testing takes time and depletes tumour tissue. In addition, the cost of single-gene methods scales linearly with the number of genes interrogated and targeted NGS of cancer-related genes could be a future method to detect commonly altered genes on a single platform.

The introduction of targeted drugs in the therapeutic armamentarium has also revolutionised the way in which clinical trials are designed in thoracic oncology. As opposed to previous clinical trials exploring the role of chemotherapy in wide, unselected groups of patients, those on targeted therapies are run on selected patient populations and, consequently, on small sample sizes. The so-called basket trials are designed to explore treatment efficacy in a quick and safe way: patients with multiple diseases and one or more targets are enrolled in small cohorts, according to their biomolecular features. Cohorts with good responses can be expanded, whereas cohorts with poor responses can be closed rapidly, allowing patients to shift to a new drug.

Finally, even though the identification of new active molecules is rapidly speeding up, the actual introduction of these compounds to clinical practice is not straightforward. This is due to the need for approval by regulatory agencies, which often lead to different scenarios across the world, depending on local approvals and regulations, which is inevitably stressful for both the patients and the physicians taking care of them.

## References


1. Weinstein IB. Addiction to oncogenes – the Achilles heal of cancer. *Science* 2002; 297: 63–64.
2. Lovly C, Horn L, Pao W. Molecular Profiling of Lung Cancer 2014. www.mycancergenome.org/content/disease/lung-cancer Date last accessed: November 10, 2014. Date last updated: February 6, 2015.
3. Mitsudomi T, Yatabe Y. Epidermal growth factor receptor in relation to tumor development: *EGFR* gene and cancer. *FEBS J* 2010; 277: 301–308.
4. Ciardiello F, Tortora G. EGFR antagonists in cancer treatment. *N Engl J Med* 2008; 358: 1160–1174.
5. Hynes NE, Lane HA. ERBB receptors and cancer: the complexity of targeted inhibitors. *Nature Rev Cancer* 2005; 5: 341–354.
6. Pao W, Miller V, Zakowski M, *et al.* EGF receptor gene mutations are common in lung cancers from "never smokers" and are associated with sensitivity of tumors to gefitinib and erlotinib. *Proc Natl Acad Sci USA* 2004; 101: 13306–13311.
7. Tokumo M, Toyooka S, Kiura K, *et al.* The relationship between epidermal growth factor receptor mutations and clinicopathologic features in non-small cell lung cancers. *Clin Cancer Res* 2005; 11: 1167–1173.
8. Rosell R, Moran T, Queralt C, *et al.* Screening for epidermal growth factor receptor mutations in lung cancer. *N Engl J Med* 2009; 361: 958–967.
9. Marchetti A, Martella C, Felicioni L, *et al. EGFR* mutations in non-small-cell lung cancer: analysis of a large series of cases and development of a rapid and sensitive method for diagnostic screening with potential implications on pharmacologic treatment. *J Clin Oncol* 2005; 23: 857–865.
10. Kawaguchi T, Matsumura A, Fukai S, *et al.* Japanese ethnicity compared with Caucasian ethnicity and never-smoking status are independent favorable prognostic factors for overall survival in non-small cell lung cancer: a collaborative epidemiologic study of the National Hospital Organization Study Group for Lung Cancer (NHSGLC) in Japan and a Southern California Regional Cancer Registry databases. *J Thorac Oncol* 2010; 5: 1001–1010.
11. Lindeman NI, Cagle PT, Beasley MB, *et al.* Molecular testing guideline for selection of lung cancer patients for EGFR and ALK tyrosine kinase inhibitors: guideline from the College of American Pathologists, International Association for the Study of Lung Cancer, and Association for Molecular Pathology. *J Thorac Oncol* 2013; 8: 823–859.
12. Yun CH, Boggon TJ, Li Y, *et al.* Structures of lung cancer-derived *EGFR* mutants and inhibitor complexes: mechanism of activation and insights into differential inhibitor sensitivity. *Cancer Cell* 2007; 11: 217–227.
13. Kobayashi S, Boggon TJ, Dayaram T, *et al.* EGFR mutation and resistance of non-small-cell lung cancer to gefitinib. *N Engl J Med* 2005; 352: 786–792.
14. Pao W, Miller VA, Politi KA, *et al.* Acquired resistance of lung adenocarcinomas to gefitinib or erlotinib is associated with a second mutation in the EGFR kinase domain. *PLoS Med* 2005; 2: e73.
15. Oxnard GR, Arcila ME, Sima CS, *et al.* Acquired resistance to EGFR tyrosine kinase inhibitors in *EGFR*-mutant lung cancer: distinct natural history of patients with tumors harboring the T790M mutation. *Clin Cancer Res* 2011; 17: 1616–1622.
16. Ellison G, Zhu G, Moulis A, *et al. EGFR* mutation testing in lung cancer: a review of available methods and their use for analysis of tumour tissue and cytology samples. *J Clin Pathol* 2013; 66: 79–89.
17. Kozu Y, Tsuta K, Kohno T, *et al.* The usefulness of mutation-specific antibodies in detecting epidermal growth factor receptor mutations and in predicting response to tyrosine kinase inhibitor therapy in lung adenocarcinoma. *Lung Cancer* 2011; 73: 45–50.
18. Brevet M, Arcila M, Ladanyi M. Assessment of *EGFR* mutation status in lung adenocarcinoma by immunohistochemistry using antibodies specific to the two major forms of mutant *EGFR*. *J Mol Diagn* 2010; 12: 169–176.
19. Ilie MI, Hofman V, Bonnetaud C, *et al.* Usefulness of tissue microarrays for assessment of protein expression, gene copy number and mutational status of *EGFR* in lung adenocarcinoma. *Virchows Arch* 2010; 457: 483–495.
20. Kato Y, Peled N, Wynes MW, *et al.* Novel epidermal growth factor receptor mutation-specific antibodies for non-small cell lung cancer: immunohistochemistry as a possible screening method for epidermal growth factor receptor mutations. *J Thorac Oncol* 2010; 5: 1551–1558.
21. Nakamura H, Mochizuki A, Shinmyo T, *et al.* Immunohistochemical detection of mutated epidermal growth factor receptors in pulmonary adenocarcinoma. *Anticancer Res* 2010; 30: 5233–5237.
22. Simonetti S, Molina MA, Queralt C, *et al.* Detection of *EGFR* mutations with mutation-specific antibodies in stage IV non-small-cell lung cancer. *J Transl Med* 2010; 8: 135.
23. Kerr KM, Bubendorf L, Edelman MJ, *et al.* Second ESMO consensus conference on lung cancer: pathology and molecular biomarkers for non-small-cell lung cancer. *Ann Oncol* 2014; 25: 1681–1690.
24. Fukuoka M, Yano S, Giaccone G, *et al.* Multi-institutional randomized phase II trial of gefitinib for previously treated patients with advanced non-small-cell lung cancer (The IDEAL 1 Trial). *J Clin Oncol* 2003; 21: 2237–2246.

25. Kris MG, Natale RB, Herbst RS, *et al.* Efficacy of gefitinib, an inhibitor of the epidermal growth factor receptor tyrosine kinase, in symptomatic patients with non-small cell lung cancer: a randomized trial. *JAMA* 2003; 290: 2149–2158.
26. Giaccone G, Herbst RS, Manegold C, *et al.* Gefitinib in combination with gemcitabine and cisplatin in advanced non-small-cell lung cancer: a phase III trial-INTACT 1. *J Clin Oncol* 2004; 22: 777–784.
27. Herbst RS, Giaccone G, Schiller JH, *et al.* Gefitinib in combination with paclitaxel and carboplatin in advanced non-small-cell lung cancer: a phase III trial-INTACT 2. *J Clin Oncol* 2004; 22: 785–794.
28. Mok TS, Wu YL, Thongprasert S, *et al.* Gefitinib or carboplatin-paclitaxel in pulmonary adenocarcinoma. *N Engl J Med* 2009; 361: 947–957.
29. Herbst RS, Prager D, Hermann R, *et al.* TRIBUTE: a phase III trial of erlotinib hydrochloride (OSI-774) combined with carboplatin and paclitaxel chemotherapy in advanced non-small-cell lung cancer. *J Clin Oncol* 2005; 23: 5892–5899.
30. Gatzemeier U, Pluzanska A, Szczesna A, *et al.* Phase III study of erlotinib in combination with cisplatin and gemcitabine in advanced non-small-cell lung cancer: the Tarceva Lung Cancer Investigation Trial. *J Clin Oncol* 2007; 25: 1545–1552.
31. Thatcher N, Chang A, Parikh P, *et al.* Gefitinib plus best supportive care in previously treated patients with refractory advanced non-small-cell lung cancer: results from a randomised, placebo-controlled, multicentre study (Iressa Survival Evaluation in Lung Cancer). *Lancet* 2005; 366: 1527–1537.
32. Shepherd FA, Rodrigues Pereira J, Ciuleanu T, *et al.* Erlotinib in previously treated non-small-cell lung cancer. *N Engl J Med* 2005; 353: 123–132.
33. Rosell R, Carcereny E, Gervais R, *et al.* Erlotinib *versus* standard chemotherapy as first line treatment for European patients with advanced *EGFR* mutation-positive non-small-cell lung cancer (EURTAC): a multicentre, open-label, randomised phase 3 trial. *Lancet Oncol* 2012; 13: 239–246.
34. Han JY, Park K, Kim SW, *et al.* First-SIGNAL: first-line single-agent Iressa *versus* gemcitabine and cisplatin trial in never-smokers with adenocarcinoma of the lung. *J Clin Oncol* 2012; 30: 1122–1128.
35. Mitsudomi T, Morita S, Yatabe Y, *et al.* Gefitinib *versus* cisplatin plus docetaxel in patients with non-small-cell lung cancer harbouring mutations of the epidermal growth factor receptor (WJTOG3405): an open label, randomised phase 3 trial. *Lancet Oncol* 2010; 11: 121–128.
36. Maemondo M, Inoue A, Kobayashi K, *et al.* Gefitinib or chemotherapy for non-small-cell lung cancer with mutated *EGFR*. *N Engl J Med* 2010; 362: 2380–2388.
37. Zhou C, Wu YL, Chen G, *et al.* Erlotinib *versus* chemotherapy as first-line treatment for patients with advanced *EGFR* mutation-positive non-small-cell lung cancer (OPTIMAL, CTONG-0802): a multicentre, open-label, randomised, phase 3 study. *Lancet Oncol* 2011; 12: 735–742.
38. Sequist LV, Yang JC, Yamamoto N, *et al.* Phase III study of afatinib or cisplatin plus pemetrexed in patients with metastatic lung adenocarcinoma with EGFR mutations. *J Clin Oncol* 2013; 31: 3327–3334.
39. Wu YL, Zhou C, Hu CP, *et al.* Afatinib *versus* cisplatin plus gemcitabine for first-line treatment of Asian patients with advanced non-small-cell lung cancer harbouring EGFR mutations (LUX-Lung 6): an open-label, randomised phase 3 trial. *Lancet Oncol* 2014; 15: 213–222.
40. Kobayashi T, Koizumi T, Agatsuma T, *et al.* A phase II trial of erlotinib in patients with *EGFR* wild-type advanced non-small-cell lung cancer. *Cancer Chemother Pharmacol* 2012; 69: 1241–1246.
41. Matsumoto Y, Maemondo M, Ishii Y, *et al.* A phase II study of erlotinib monotherapy in pre-treated non-small cell lung cancer without EGFR gene mutation who have never/light smoking history: re-evaluation of EGFR gene status (NEJ006/TCOG0903). *Lung Cancer* 2014; 86: 195–200.
42. Ulivi P, Delmonte A, Chiadini E, *et al.* Gene mutation analysis in *EGFR* wild type NSCLC responsive to erlotinib: are there features to guide patient selection? *Int J Mol Sci* 2015; 16: 747–757.
43. Wang F, Fu S, Shao Q, *et al.* High *EGFR* copy number predicts benefits from tyrosine kinase inhibitor treatment for non-small cell lung cancer patients with wild-type EGFR. *J Transl Med* 2013; 11: 90.
44. Lee Y, Shim HS, Park MS, *et al.* High *EGFR* gene copy number and skin rash as predictive markers for EGFR tyrosine kinase inhibitors in patients with advanced squamous cell lung carcinoma. *Clin Cancer Res* 2012; 18: 1760–1768.
45. Laurie SA, Goss GD. Role of epidermal growth factor receptor inhibitors in epidermal growth factor receptor wild-type non-small-cell lung cancer. *J Clin Oncol* 2013; 31: 1061–1069.
46. Ramalingam S, Janne P, Mok T, *et al.* Randomized, double-blinded study of dacomitinib, an irreversible pan-human epidermal growth factor receptor (HER) inhibitor, *versus* erlotinib for second-line/third-line therapy of locally advanced/metastatic non-small cell lung cancer (ARCHER 1009). *J Clin Oncol* 2014; 32: Suppl., 8018.
47. Pirker R, Pereira JR, Szczesna A, *et al.* Cetuximab plus chemotherapy in patients with advanced non-small-cell lung cancer (FLEX): an open-label randomised phase III trial. *Lancet* 2009; 373: 1525–1531.
48. Lynch TJ, Patel T, Dreisbach L, *et al.* Cetuximab and first-line taxane/carboplatin chemotherapy in advanced non-small-cell lung cancer: results of the randomized multicenter phase III trial BMS099.*J Clin Oncol* 2010; 28: 911–917.

49. Butts CA, Bodkin D, Middleman EL, *et al.* Randomized phase II study of gemcitabine plus cisplatin or carboplatin, with or without cetuximab, as first-line therapy for patients with advanced or metastatic non small-cell lung cancer. *J Clin Oncol* 2007; 25: 5777–5784.
50. Rosell R, Robinet G, Szczesna A, *et al.* Randomized phase II study of cetuximab plus cisplatin/vinorelbine compared with cisplatin/vinorelbine alone as first-line therapy in EGFR-expressing advanced non-small-cell lung cancer. *Ann Oncol* 2008; 19: 362–369.
51. Pujol JL, Pirker R, Lynch TJ, *et al.* Meta-analysis of individual patient data from randomized trials of chemotherapy plus cetuximab as first-line treatment for advanced non-small cell lung cancer. *Lung Cancer* 2014; 83: 211–218.
52. Thatcher N, Hirsch F, Szczesna A, *et al.* SQUIRE: A randomized, multicenter, open-label, phase III study of gemcitabine-cisplatin (GC) chemotherapy plus necitumumab (IMC-11F8/LY3012211) *versus* GC alone in the first-line treatment of patients (pts) with stage IV squamous non-small cell lung cancer (sq-NSCLC). *J Clin Oncol* 2014; 32: Suppl., 8008.
53. Robert C, Soria JC, Spatz A, *et al.* Cutaneous side-effects of kinase inhibitors and blocking antibodies. *Lancet Oncol* 2005; 6: 491–500.
54. Lacouture ME. Mechanisms of cutaneous toxicities to EGFR inhibitors. *Nat Rev Cancer* 2006; 6: 803–812.
55. Passaro A, Di Maio M, Del Signore E, *et al.* Management of nonhematologic toxicities associated with different EGFR-TKIs in advanced NSCLC: a comparison analysis. *Clin Lung Cancer* 2014; 15: 307–312.
56. Novello S, Capelletto E, Cortinovis D, *et al.* Italian multicenter survey to evaluate the opinion of patients and their reference clinicians on the "tolerance" to targeted therapies already available for non-small cell lung cancer treatment in daily clinical practice. *Transl Lung Cancer Res* 2014; 3: 173–180.
57. Sequist LV, Waltman BA, Dias-Santagata D, *et al.* Genotypic and histological evolution of lung cancers acquiring resistance to EGFR inhibitors. *Sci Transl Med* 2011; 3: 75ra26.
58. Morinaga R, Okamoto I, Furuta K, *et al.* Sequential occurrence of non-small cell and small cell lung cancer with the same *EGFR* mutation. *Lung Cancer* 2007; 58: 411–413.
59. Yu HA, Sima CS, Huang J, *et al.* Local therapy with continued EGFR tyrosine kinase inhibitor therapy as a treatment strategy in *EGFR*-mutant advanced lung cancers that have developed acquired resistance to EGFR tyrosine kinase inhibitors. *J Thorac Oncol* 2013; 8: 346–351.
60. Weickhardt AJ, Scheier B, Burke JM, *et al.* Local ablative therapy of oligoprogressive disease prolongs disease control by tyrosine kinase inhibitors in oncogene-addicted non-small-cell lung cancer. *J Thorac Oncol* 2012; 7: 1807–1814.
61. Chaft JE, Oxnard GR, Sima CS, *et al.* Disease flare after tyrosine kinase inhibitor discontinuation in patients with *EGFR*-mutant lung cancer and acquired resistance to erlotinib or gefitinib: implications for clinical trial design. *Clin Cancer Res* 2011; 17: 6298–6303.
62. Park K, Ahn M, Yu C, *et al.* ASPIRATION: first-line erlotinib until and beyond RECIST disease progression in Asian patients with EGFR mutation positive NSCLC. *Ann Oncol* 2014; 25: Suppl. 4, iv426–iv427.
63. Mok T, Wu Y, Nakagawa K, *et al.* Gefitinib/chemotherapy *vs* chemotherapy in epidermal growth factor receptor (EGFR) mutation-positive non-small-cell lung cancer (NSCLC) after progression on first-line gefitinib: the phase III, randomised IMPRESS study. *Ann Oncol* 2014; 25: Suppl. 4, LBA2_PR.
64. Janjigian YY, Smit EF, Groen HJ, *et al.* Dual inhibition of EGFR with afatinib and cetuximab in kinase inhibitor-resistant *EGFR*-mutant lung cancer with and without T790M mutations. *Cancer Discov* 2014; 4: 1036–1045.
65. Janjigian YY, Azzoli CG, Krug LM, *et al.* Phase I/II trial of cetuximab and erlotinib in patients with lung adenocarcinoma and acquired resistance to erlotinib. *Clin Cancer Res* 2011; 17: 2521–2527.
66. Scagliotti GV, Novello S, Schiller JH, *et al.* Rationale and design of MARQUEE: a phase III, randomized, double-blind study of tivantinib plus erlotinib *versus* placebo plus erlotinib in previously treated patients with locally advanced or metastatic, nonsquamous, non-small-cell lung cancer. *Clin Lung Cancer* 2012; 13: 391–395.
67. Azuma K, Yoshioka H, Yamamoto N, *et al.* Tivantinib plus erlotinib *versus* placebo plus erlotinib in Asian patients with previously treated nonsquamous NSCLC with wild-type *EGFR*: first report of a phase III ATTENTION trial. *J Clin Oncol* 2014; 32: Suppl., 8044.
68. Cross DA, Ashton SE, Ghiorghiu S, *et al.* AZD9291, an irreversible EGFR TKI, overcomes T790M-mediated resistance to EGFR inhibitors in lung cancer. *Cancer Discov* 2014; 4: 1046–1061.
69. Sequist L, Soria J, Gadgeel S, *et al.* First-in-human evaluation of CO-1686, an irreversible, highly selective tyrosine kinase inhibitor of mutations of EGFR (activating and T790M). *J Clin Oncol* 2014; 32: Suppl., 8010.
70. Janne P, Ramalingam S, Yang J, *et al.* Clinical activity of the mutant-selective EGFR inhibitor AZD9291 in patients (pts) with EGFR inhibitor–resistant non-small cell lung cancer (NSCLC). *J Clin Oncol* 2014; 32: Suppl., 8009.
71. Kim D, Lee D, Kang J, *et al.* Clinical activity and safety of HM61713, an *EGFR*-mutant selective inhibitor, in advanced non-small cell lung cancer (NSCLC) patients (pts) with *EGFR* mutations who had received EGFR tyrosine kinase inhibitors (TKIs). *J Clin Oncol* 2014; 32: Suppl., 8011.

72. Soda M, Choi YL, Enomoto M, *et al.* Identification of the transforming *EML4–ALK* fusion gene in non-small-cell lung cancer. *Nature* 2007; 448: 561–566.
73. Sasaki T, Rodig SJ, Chirieac LR, *et al.* The biology and treatment of *EML4–ALK* non-small cell lung cancer. *Eur J Cancer* 2010; 46: 1773–1780.
74. Rikova K, Guo A, Zeng Q, *et al.* Global survey of phosphotyrosine signaling identifies oncogenic kinases in lung cancer. *Cell* 2007; 131: 1190–1203.
75. Takeuchi K, Choi YL, Togashi Y, *et al.* KIF5B-ALK, a novel fusion oncokinase identified by an immunohistochemistry-based diagnostic system for *ALK*-positive lung cancer. *Clin Cancer Res* 2009; 15: 3143–3149.
76. Wong DW, Leung EL, Wong SK, *et al.* A novel *KIF5B–ALK* variant in nonsmall cell lung cancer. *Cancer* 2011; 117: 2709–2718.
77. Togashi Y, Soda M, Sakata S, *et al.* *KIF5B–ALK*: a novel fusion in lung cancer identified using a formalin-fixed paraffin-embedded tissue only. *PLoS One* 2012; 7: e31323.
78. Choi YL, Lira ME, Hong M, *et al.* A novel fusion of *TPR* and *ALK* in lung adenocarcinoma. *J Thorac Oncol* 2014; 9: 563–566.
79. Kwak EL, Bang YJ, Camidge DR, *et al.* Anaplastic lymphoma kinase inhibition in non-small-cell lung cancer. *N Engl J Med* 2010; 363: 1693–1703.
80. Camidge DR, Kono SA, Flacco A, *et al.* Optimizing the detection of lung cancer patients harboring anaplastic lymphoma kinase (*ALK*) gene rearrangements potentially suitable for ALK inhibitor treatment. *Clin Cancer Res* 2010; 16: 5581–5590.
81. Shaw AT, Yeap BY, Mino-Kenudson M, *et al.* Clinical features and outcome of patients with non-small-cell lung cancer who harbor *EML4–ALK*. *J Clin Oncol* 2009; 27: 4247–4253.
82. Solomon B, Varella-Garcia M, Camidge DR. *ALK* gene rearrangements: a new therapeutic target in a molecularly defined subset of non-small cell lung cancer. *J Thorac Oncol* 2009; 4: 1450–1454.
83. Scagliotti G, Stahel RA, Rosell R, *et al.* ALK translocation and crizotinib in non-small cell lung cancer: an evolving paradigm in oncology drug development. *Eur J Cancer* 2012; 48: 961–973.
84. Blackhall FH, Peters S, Bubendorf L, *et al.* Prevalence and clinical outcomes for patients with ALK-positive resected stage I to III adenocarcinoma: results from the European Thoracic Oncology Platform Lungscape Project. *J Clin Oncol* 2014; 32: 2780–2787.
85. Fallet V, Cadranel J, Doubre H, *et al.* Prospective screening for *ALK*: clinical features and outcome according to *ALK* status. *Eur J Cancer* 2014; 50: 1239–1246.
86. Ou SH, Bartlett CH, Mino-Kenudson M, *et al.* Crizotinib for the treatment of *ALK*-rearranged non-small cell lung cancer: a success story to usher in the second decade of molecular targeted therapy in oncology. *Oncologist* 2012; 17: 1351–1375.
87. Peters S, Taron M, Bubendorf L, *et al.* Treatment and detection of *ALK*-rearranged NSCLC. *Lung Cancer* 2013; 81: 145–154.
88. US Food and Drug Administration. Vysis ALK Break Apart FISH Probe Kit; Vysis Paraffin Pretreatment IV and Post Hybridization Wash Buffer Kit; ProbeChek ALK Negative Control Slides; and ProbeChek ALK Positive Control Slides - P110012. www.accessdata.fda.gov/scripts/cdrh/cfdocs/cftopic/pma/pma.cfm?num=p110012 Date last accessed: November 6, 2014. Date last updated: September 6, 2011.
89. Wang J, Cai Y, Dong Y, *et al.* Clinical characteristics and outcomes of patients with primary lung adenocarcinoma harboring *ALK* rearrangements detected by FISH, IHC, and RT-PCR. *PLoS One* 2014; 9: e101551.
90. Wu YC, Chang IC, Wang CL, *et al.* Comparison of IHC, FISH and RT-PCR methods for detection of *ALK* rearrangements in 312 non-small cell lung cancer patients in Taiwan. *PLoS One* 2013; 8: e70839.
91. Hutarew G, Hauser-Kronberger C, Strasser F, *et al.* Immunohistochemistry as a screening tool for *ALK* rearrangement in NSCLC: evaluation of five different ALK antibody clones and *ALK* FISH. *Histopathology* 2014; 65: 398–407.
92. Ali G, Proietti A, Pellicciioni S, *et al.* ALK rearrangement in a large series of consecutive non-small cell lung cancers: comparison between a new immunohistochemical approach and fluorescence *in situ* hybridization for the screening of patients eligible for crizotinib treatment. *Arch Pathol Lab Med* 2014; 138: 1449–1458.
93. Marchetti A, Ardizzoni A, Papotti M, *et al.* Recommendations for the analysis of *ALK* gene rearrangements in non-small-cell lung cancer: a consensus of the Italian Association of Medical Oncology and the Italian Society of Pathology and Cytopathology. *J Thorac Oncol* 2013; 8: 352–358.
94. Reck M, Popat S, Reinmuth N, *et al.* Metastatic non-small-cell lung cancer (NSCLC): ESMO Clinical Practice Guidelines for diagnosis, treatment and follow-up. *Ann Oncol* 2014; 25: Suppl. 3, iii27–iii39.
95. Camidge DR, Bang YJ, Kwak EL, *et al.* Activity and safety of crizotinib in patients with *ALK*-positive non-small-cell lung cancer: updated results from a phase 1 study. *Lancet Oncol* 2012; 13: 1011–1019.
96. Shaw AT, Kim DW, Nakagawa K, *et al.* Crizotinib *versus* chemotherapy in advanced *ALK*-positive lung cancer. *N Engl J Med* 2013; 368: 2385–2394.

97. Mok T, Kim D, Wu Y, *et al.* First-line crizotinib *versus* pemetrexed–cisplatin or pemetrexed–carboplatin in patients (pts) with advanced ALK-positive non-squamous non-small cell lung cancer (NSCLC): results of a phase III study (PROFILE 1014). *J Clin Oncol* 2014; 32: Suppl., 8002.
98. Shaw AT, Kim DW, Mehra R, *et al.* Ceritinib in ALK-rearranged non-small-cell lung cancer. *N Engl J Med* 2014; 370: 1189–1197.
99. Kim D, Mehra R, Tan D, *et al.* Ceritinib in advanced anaplastic lymphoma kinase (*ALK*) rearranged ($ALK^+$) non-small cell lung cancer (NSCLC): results of the ASCEND-1 trial. *J Clin Oncol* 2014; 32: Suppl., 8003.
100. Seto T, Kiura K, Nishio M, *et al.* CH5424802 (RO5424802) for patients with *ALK*-rearranged advanced non-small-cell lung cancer (AF-001JP study): a single-arm, open-label, phase 1-2 study. *Lancet Oncol* 2013; 14: 590–598.
101. Seto T, Hida T, Nakagawa K, *et al.* Anti-tumor activity of alectinib in crizotinib pre-treated *ALK*-rearranged NSCLC in JP8927 study. *Ann Oncol* 2014; 25: iv426–iv70.
102. Ou S, Gadgeel S, Chiappori A, *et al.* Safety and efficacy analysis of RO5424802/Ch5424802 in anaplastic lymphoma kinase (ALK)-positive non-small cell lung cancer (NSCLC) patients who have failed crizotinib in a dose-finding phase I study (AF-002JG, NCT01588028). *Eur J Cancer* 2013; 49: Suppl. 3, 44.
103. Maitland M, Ou S, Tolcher A, *et al.* Safety, activity, and pharmacokinetics of an oral anaplastic lymphoma kinase (ALK) inhibitor, ASP3026, observed in a "fast follower" phase 1 trial design. *J Clin Oncol* 2014; 32: Suppl., 2624.
104. Gettinger S, Bazhenova L, Salgia R, *et al.* Updated efficacy and safety of the ALK inhibitor AP26113 in patients (pts) with advanced malignancies, including $ALK^+$ non-small cell lung cancer (NSCLC). *J Clin Oncol* 2014; 32: Suppl., 8047.
105. Awad MM, Shaw AT. ALK inhibitors in non-small cell lung cancer: crizotinib and beyond. *Clin Adv Hematol Oncol* 2014; 12: 429–439.
106. Weickhardt AJ, Doebele RC, Purcell WT, *et al.* Symptomatic reduction in free testosterone levels secondary to crizotinib use in male cancer patients. *Cancer* 2013; 119: 2383–2390.
107. Felip E, Dong-Wang K, Mehra R, *et al.* Efficacy and safety of Ceritinib in patients with advanced Anaplastic Lymphoma Kinase (ALK)-rearranged (ALK +) Non-small Cell Lung Cancer (NSCLC): an update of ASCEND-1. *Ann Oncol* 2014; 25: Suppl. 4, iv456–iv457.
108. Gadgeel SM, Gandhi L, Riely GJ, *et al.* Safety and activity of alectinib against systemic disease and brain metastases in patients with crizotinib-resistant *ALK*-rearranged non-small-cell lung cancer (AF-002JG): results from the dose-finding portion of a phase 1/2 study. *Lancet Oncol* 2014; 15: 1119–1128.
109. Choi YL, Soda M, Yamashita Y, *et al.* *EML4–ALK* mutations in lung cancer that confer resistance to ALK inhibitors. *N Engl J Med* 2010; 363: 1734–1739.
110. Katayama R, Khan TM, Benes C, *et al.* Therapeutic strategies to overcome crizotinib resistance in non-small cell lung cancers harboring the fusion oncogene *EML4–ALK*. *Proc Natl Acad Sci USA* 2011; 108: 7535–7540.
111. Kim S, Kim TM, Kim DW, *et al.* Heterogeneity of genetic changes associated with acquired crizotinib resistance in *ALK*-rearranged lung cancer. *J Thorac Oncol* 2013; 8: 415–422.
112. Perez CA, Velez M, Raez LE, *et al.* Overcoming the resistance to crizotinib in patients with non-small cell lung cancer harboring *EML4/ALK* translocation. *Lung Cancer* 2014; 84: 110–115.
113. Doebele RC, Pilling AB, Aisner DL, *et al.* Mechanisms of resistance to crizotinib in patients with *ALK* gene rearranged non-small cell lung cancer. *Clin Cancer Res* 2012; 18: 1472–1482.
114. Sang J, Acquaviva J, Friedland JC, *et al.* Targeted inhibition of the molecular chaperone Hsp90 overcomes ALK inhibitor resistance in non-small cell lung cancer. *Cancer Discov* 2013; 3: 430–443.
115. Besse B, Bertino E, Pennell N, *et al.* A study of Hsp90 inhibitor AT13387 alone and in combination with crizotinib (CTZ) in the treatment of non-small cell lung cancer (NSCLC). *Ann Oncol* 2014; 25: Suppl. 4, iv430.
116. Shaw AT, Varghese AM, Solomon BJ, *et al.* Pemetrexed-based chemotherapy in patients with advanced, *ALK*-positive non-small cell lung cancer. *Ann Oncol* 2013; 24: 59–66.
117. Sandler A, Gray R, Perry MC, *et al.* Paclitaxel-carboplatin alone or with bevacizumab for non-small-cell lung cancer. *N Engl J Med* 2006; 355: 2542–2550.
118. Reck M, von Pawel J, Zatloukal P, *et al.* Overall survival with cisplatin–gemcitabine and bevacizumab or placebo as first-line therapy for nonsquamous non-small-cell lung cancer: results from a randomised phase III trial (AVAiL). *Ann Oncol* 2010; 21: 1804–1809.
119. Soria JC, Mauguen A, Reck M, *et al.* Systematic review and meta-analysis of randomised, phase II/III trials adding bevacizumab to platinum-based chemotherapy as first-line treatment in patients with advanced non-small-cell lung cancer. *Ann Oncol* 2013; 24: 20–30.
120. Reck M, Kaiser R, Mellemgaard A, *et al.* Docetaxel plus nintedanib *versus* docetaxel plus placebo in patients with previously treated non-small-cell lung cancer (LUME-Lung 1): a phase 3, double-blind, randomised controlled trial. *Lancet Oncol* 2014; 15: 143–155.
121. Hanna N, Kaiser R, Sullivan R, *et al.* LUME-lung 2: a multicenter, randomized, double-blind, phase III study of nintedanib plus pemetrexed *versus* placebo plus pemetrexed in patients with advanced nonsquamous non-small cell lung cancr (NSCLC) after failure of first-line chemotherapy. *J Clin Oncol* 2013; 31: Suppl., 8034.

122. Perol M, Ciuleanu T, Arrieta O, *et al.* REVEL: a randomized, double-blind, phase III study of docetaxel (DOC) and ramucirumab (RAM; IMC-1121b) *versus* DOC and placebo (PL) in the second-line treatment of stage IV non-small cell lung cancer (NSCLC) following disease progression after one prior platinum-based therapy. *J Clin Oncol* 2014; 32: Suppl., LBA8006.
123. Planchard D, Kim T, Mazieres J, *et al.* Dabrafenib in patients with BRAF V600E-mutant advanced non-small cell lung cancer (NSCLC): A multicenter, open-label, phase II trial (BRF113928). *Ann Oncol* 2014; 25: Suppl. 4, pLBA38_PR.
124. Cancer Genome Atlas Research Network. Comprehensive genomic characterization of squamous cell lung cancers. *Nature* 2012; 489: 519–525.
125. Ichimura E, Maeshima A, Nakajima T, *et al.* Expression of c-met/HGF receptor in human non-small cell lung carcinomas *in vitro* and *in vivo* and its prognostic significance. *Jpn J Canc Res* 1996; 87: 1063–1069.
126. Ma PC, Jagadeeswaran R, Jagadeesh S, *et al.* Functional expression and mutations of c-Met and its therapeutic inhibition with SU11274 and small interfering RNA in non-small cell lung cancer. *Cancer Res* 2005; 65: 1479–1488.
127. Benedettini E, Sholl LM, Peyton M, *et al.* Met activation in non-small cell lung cancer is associated with *de novo* resistance to EGFR inhibitors and the development of brain metastasis. *Am J Pathol* 2010; 177: 415–423.
128. Cappuzzo F, Janne PA, Skokan M, *et al.* *MET* increased gene copy number and primary resistance to gefitinib therapy in non-small-cell lung cancer patients. *Ann Oncol* 2009; 20: 298–304.
129. Bean J, Brennan C, Shih JY, *et al.* *MET* amplification occurs with or without T790M mutations in *EGFR* mutant lung tumors with acquired resistance to gefitinib or erlotinib. *Proc Natl Acad Sci USA* 2007; 104: 20932–20937.
130. Ujiie H, Tomida M, Akiyama H, *et al.* Serum hepatocyte growth factor and interleukin-6 are effective prognostic markers for non-small cell lung cancer. *Anti Res* 2012; 32: 3251–3258.
131. Hosoda H, Izumi H, Tukada Y, *et al.* Plasma hepatocyte growth factor elevation may be associated with early metastatic disease in primary lung cancer patients. *Ann Thorac Cardiovasc Surg* 2012; 18: 1–7.
132. Masago K, Togashi Y, Fujita S, *et al.* Clinical significance of serum hepatocyte growth factor and epidermal growth factor gene somatic mutations in patients with non-squamous non-small cell lung cancer receiving gefitinib or erlotinib. *Med Oncol* 2012; 29: 1614–1621.
133. Han JY, Kim JY, Lee SH, *et al.* Association between plasma hepatocyte growth factor and gefitinib resistance in patients with advanced non-small cell lung cancer. *Lung Cancer* 2011; 74: 293–299.
134. Mok T, Park K, Geater SL, *et al.* A randomized phase (PH) 2 study with exploratory biomarker analysis of ficlatuzumab (F) a humanized hepatocyte growth factor (HGF) inhibitory mAb in combination with gefitinib (G) *versus* G in Asian patients (pts) with lung adenocarcinoma (LA). *Ann Oncol* 2012; 23: Suppl. 9, ix391.
135. Spigel DR, Ervin TJ, Ramlau RA, *et al.* Randomized phase II trial of Onartuzumab in combination with erlotinib in patients with advanced non-small-cell lung cancer. *J Clin Oncol* 2013; 31: 4105–4114.
136. Spigel D, Edelman M, O'Byrne K, *et al.* Onartuzumab plus erlotinib *versus* erlotinib in previously treated stage IIIb or IV NSCLC: results from the pivotal phase III randomized, multicenter, placebo-controlled METLung (OAM4971g) global trial. *J Clin Oncol* 2014; 32: Suppl., 800.
137. Drilon A, Wang L, Hasanovic A, *et al.* Response to Cabozantinib in patients with *RET* fusion-positive lung adenocarcinomas. *Cancer Discov* 2013; 3: 630–635.
138. Wang R, Hu H, Pan Y, *et al.* *RET* fusions define a unique molecular and clinicopathologic subtype of non-small-cell lung cancer. *J Clin Oncol* 2012; 30: 4352–4359.
139. Bergethon K, Shaw AT, Ou SH, *et al.* *ROS1* rearrangements define a unique molecular class of lung cancers. *J Clin Oncol* 2012; 30: 863–870.
140. Shaw AT, Ou SH, Bang YJ, *et al.* Crizotinib in *ROS1*-rearranged non-small-cell lung cancer. *N Engl J Med* 2014; 371: 1963–1971.
141. Kelly RJ, Carter CA, Giaccone G. *HER2* mutations in non-small-cell lung cancer can be continually targeted. *J Clin Oncol* 2012; 30: 3318–3319.
142. Kris M, Camidge D, Giaccone G, *et al.* Results with dacomitinib (PF-00299804), an irreversible pan-HER tyrosine kinase inhibitor, in a phase II cohort of patients with HER2-mutant or amplified lung cancers. http://abstracts.webges.com/myitinerary/publication-2237.html?congress=wclc2013
143. Mao C, Qiu LX, Liao RY, *et al.* *KRAS* mutations and resistance to EGFR-TKIs treatment in patients with non-small cell lung cancer: a meta-analysis of 22 studies. *Lung Cancer* 2010; 69: 272–278.
144. Shepherd FA, Domerg C, Hainaut P, *et al.* Pooled analysis of the prognostic and predictive effects of *KRAS* mutation status and *KRAS* mutation subtype in early-stage resected non-small-cell lung cancer in four trials of adjuvant chemotherapy. *J Clin Oncol* 2013; 31: 2173–2181.
145. Janne PA, Shaw AT, Pereira JR, *et al.* Selumetinib plus docetaxel for KRAS-mutant advanced non-small-cell lung cancer: a randomised, multicentre, placebo-controlled, phase 2 study. *Lancet Oncol* 2013; 14: 38–47.


---

Disclosures: None declared.

Chapter 18

# Can we expect progress from targeted therapy of SCLC?

Nevin Murray[1] and Krista L. Noonan[2]

The success of cancer genomics research in transforming the clinical care of patients with advanced ADC of the lung has been a powerful incentive to identify molecular abnormalities in SCLC that can be treated with targeted agents. A considerable number of drugs have already been tried in SCLC clinical trials without notable success. Efforts to identify molecular targets for SCLC have been impeded by a paucity of adequate tissue for translational research in a disease in which resections are uncommon. Molecular abnormalities are extremely complex in this tobacco hyper-mutated tumour. Additionally, the circumstances for clinical research are difficult where patients with recurrent disease are frequently in rapid decline during the window of opportunity for biopsies, genomic studies, identification of a suitable target, and administration of novel agents. Despite these challenges, interesting work is moving forward with newly identified molecular targets emerging from comprehensive genomic profiling efforts. There is also the intriguing possibility that a high antigenic load from many mutations may be an asset for immunotherapy studies.

At the peak of the lung cancer epidemic in North America in the 1980s, ~20% of all lung cancers were SCLC. The proportion with SCLC has progressively declined and now stands below 13% [1]. SCLC in life-time nonsmokers is rare. Compared with NSCLC, SCLC has a more virulent natural history characterised by rapid growth and early widespread metastases. However, early investigators observed that SCLC responded better to both chemotherapy and radiotherapy [2]. Because of this biology of responsiveness, years ago, investigators had high hopes that SCLC would become a curable neoplasm. Despite considerable basic and clinical research over the past 30 years, the efficacy of systemic therapy has not improved [3].

For medical oncologists, the discovery of treatable molecular targets in ADCs with approved drugs is the most conspicuous and exciting development in the systemic treatment of advanced lung cancer [4]. However, no molecular targets that can be treated with drugs with proven efficacy have as yet been described for SCLC [5].

[1]Dept of Medical Oncology, British Columbia Cancer Agency, University of British Columbia, Vancouver, BC, Canada. [2]Dept of Medical Oncology, Memorial University, St John's, NL, Canada.

Correspondence: Nevin Murray, Dept of Medical Oncology, British Columbia Cancer Agency, 600 West 10th Avenue, Vancouver, BC, Canada V5Z 4E6. E-mail: nmurray@bccancer.bc.ca

 Print ISBN: 978-1-84984-061-3. Online ISBN: 978-1-84984-062-0. Print ISSN: 2312-508X. Online ISSN: 2312-5098.

The therapeutic landscape in SCLC is in stark contrast to NSCLC, where a number of mutations and gene fusions have been identified that drive cancer growth. These oncogenic targets guide treatment selection for specific patient subsets. Predictive biomarkers detect the presence of the target. Well-conducted clinical trials have confirmed treatment efficacy of drugs for a number of targets [4, 6]. Because of the success of targeted therapies in NSCLC patients with drugable mutations, the survival with metastatic NSCLC in these groups is approximately double that of patients without them [7]. The success of cancer genomics research in transforming the clinical care of patients with lung ADC is an incentive for similar attempts in SCLC. The remainder of this chapter focuses on whether we can expect progress from molecular-targeted therapy of SCLC.

## Pathology and genetic molecular hallmarks of SCLC

The World Health Organization (WHO) recognises three high-grade lung cancers of neuroendocrine origin [8]. These include SCLC, LCNEC, and combined SCLC and NSCLC. LCNEC is a subset of NSCLC large cell anaplastic type. However, similarities have been demonstrated at the protein and messenger RNA levels between SCLC and LCNEC, suggesting a biological relationship [9, 10]. SCLC and LCNEC are distinct in their epidemiology, molecular biology and clinical behaviour from atypical carcinoid and typical carcinoid tumours.

SCLC is a genetically complex cancer. Karyotypic studies show modal chromosome numbers, typically in the triploid range [11, 12]. Whang-Peng *et al.* [13] were the first to report non-random losses of chromosome 3, known as "3p deletions", as frequent genetic abnormalities in SCLC. Allelic loses of 3p are almost always observed in loss-of-heterozygosity studies of SCLC, supporting the hypothesis that tumour-suppressor genes relevant to the pathogenesis of the tumour reside in this chromosomal region [14–16]. Candidate genes in the 3p locus include FHIT (fragile histidine triad) [17], RARβ (retinoic acid receptor beta in >90%) [15] and RASSF1 (RAS effector homologue) [18]. Several of these genes can also be silenced by methylation. Studies with higher resolution of chromosomal abnormalities, using the high-throughput technology of comparative genomic hybridisation to characterise SCLC, indicate that the most frequent sites of chromosome loss are 3p, 5q and 13q (90% of samples). Additional sites of chromosome loss are 4q, 10q and 16q. Sites of chromosome gain are 3q and 5p (60–70% of SCLC samples) [19, 20].

SCLC is characterised by a nearly universal loss of TP53 (tumour protein 53) in 75–90% of patients [21–23], and RB1 (retinoblastoma 1) loss approaches 100% [24]. Beyond these shared molecular features, increased expression of c-Kit, amplification of MYC (v-*myc* avian myelocytomatosis viral homologue) family members (MYC and MYCN (MYC lung carcinoma-derived homologue 1) [25] and loss of PTEN (phosphatase and tensin homologue) have been described in some reports. Recently, these molecular hallmarks of SCLC were confirmed in two comprehensive genomic profiling studies [24, 26]. These independent studies reported exome, whole-genome, transcriptome and copy-number alteration data obtained from primary human SCLCs (together analysing >100 samples). Loss of the tumour suppressors TP53 and RB1 were the two most common events observed in both datasets [24, 26]. These studies also identified mutations with established roles in multiple cancer types (MYC family genes (16%), PTEN (10%), and FGFR1 (6%)). Rudin *et al.* [24] also report SOX2 (SRY-box 2) amplification and the presence of a recurrent RLF-MYCL1 (zinc finger protein-myelocytomatosis viral homologue lung) fusion in 27% and 9% of SCLCs, respectively.

Amplified FGFR1 and amplified SOX2 were first discovered and validated as driver oncogenes in squamous lung cancer [26, 27]. At least a subset of SCLC cases show genomic changes that overlap with those of squamous lung carcinoma, and this may be linked to their common origin from stem cells of the large central airways. A pattern of shared *versus* histological subtype-associated genes in the lung cancer subtypes is emerging (fig. 1) [28].

## Targets already investigated and reported as unsuccessful in SCLC treatment

A large number of molecularly targeted agents have already been studied in SCLC treatment without sufficient signal of activity to continue development (table 1). The rationale for some of these agents was based on preclinical studies and some knowledge of SCLC biology. Others are agents that have been used in NSCLC clinical trials and were tried for SCLC. A number of them are drugs that target molecular pathways of interest in other cancers and were simply available for an exploratory SCLC phase II effort. Some studies selected patients with a predictive biomarker but most did not. Some investigations were phase I and II with modest cost but others were large phase III studies with considerable expenditure of patient, investigator and financial resources (anti-idiotypic antibody mimicking GD3, a ganglioside antigen (BEC2)/ bacille Calmette–Guerin adjuvant vaccine [30], thalidomide [31, 32], matrix metalloproteinase inhibitors [33], pravastatin [34] and pemetrexed [35]).

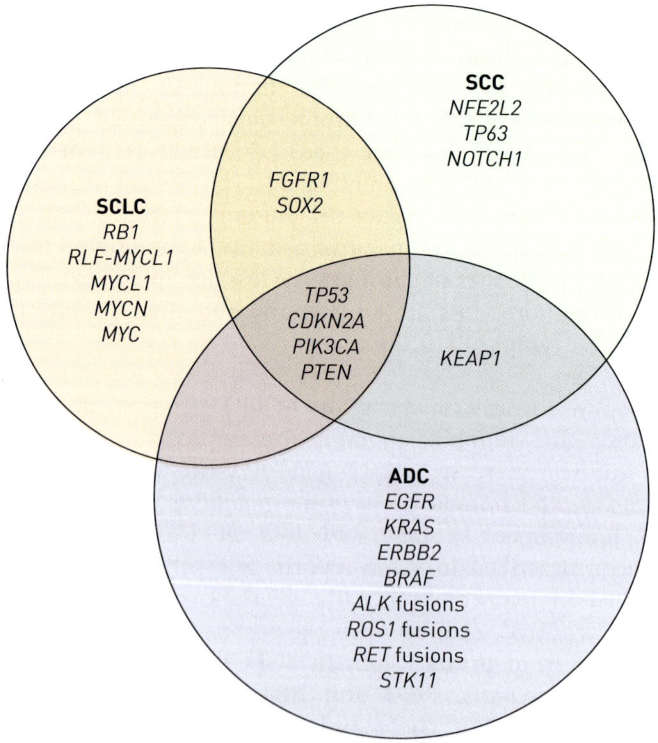


Figure 1. Major shared *versus* subtype-associated cancer-related genes in the three common subtypes of lung cancer. The relationships shown are relative, not absolute, and other cancer-associated genes for which this information is incomplete are not shown. Reproduced and modified from [28] with permission from the publisher.

Table 1. Molecular targeted agents investigated for treatment of SCLC

| Target | Agent | Clinical trial phase | Further studies |
|---|---|---|---|
| **Immune conjugates and vaccines** | | | |
| CD56 | BB-10901 | II | No |
| GD3 | BEC2/BCG adjuvant vaccine | III | No |
| P53 | Autologous dendritic cell adenovirus | II | No |
| **Multidrug-resistance modification** | | | |
| P-glycoprotein, MDR-1 | Biricoder | II | No |
| **Inhibitors of angiogenesis** | | | |
| VEGF-A | Bevacizumab | II | No |
| VEGFR-1, 2, 3 | Cediranib | II | No |
| VEGFR, EGFR | Anti-vandetanib | II | No |
| VEGFR, PDGFR, Raf-1 | Sorafenib | I, II | No |
| Undefined anti-angiogenic | Thalidomide | II, III | No |
| VEGFR, PDGFR, FLT-3, RET, KIT | Sunitinib | I, II | No |
| VEGF-A,B | Aflibercept | II | No |
| MMPs | Marimastat | II, III | No |
| | Tanomastat | II, III | No |
| **Apoptosis promoters** | | | |
| Bcl-2 | Oblimersen | II | No |
| Bcl-2 | AT-101 (R-(-) gossypo) | I, II | No |
| Bcl-2, Mcl-1, Bcl-w, Bcl-XL, A-1 | Obatoclax mesylate | I, II | No |
| Bcl-2, Bcl, Bcl-XL | Navitoclax | I | No |
| 26S proteasome | Bortezomib | II | No |
| PlK 1 serine/threonine kinase | PIK1 inhibitor BI 2536 | II | No |
| HDAC | Vorinostat | I, II | No |
| HDAC | Belinostat | I | No |
| HDAC | Entinostat | I | No |
| Hydroxymethylglutaryl Co-A reductase | Pravastatin | III | No |
| Multi-targeted antifolate | Pemetrexed | III | No |
| **Inhibitors of cell signalling pathways controlling inhibition** | | | |
| c-kit | Imatinib | II | No |
| Src | Saracatinib | II | No |
| Src | Dasatinib | II | No |
| EGFR | Gefitinib | II | No |
| Farnesyltranferase | Tipifarnib | II | No |
| mTOR | Temsirolimus | II | No |
| mTOR | Everolimus | I, II | No |
| IGFR | Cixutumumab | I | No |
| IGFR | CP-751, 871 | I | No |
| IGFR | Ganitumab | I, II | No |
| c-MET | Rilotumab | I, II | No |
| Hedgehog | Vismodegib | I, II | No |
| Hedgehog | Saridegib | I | No |

BEC2: anti-idiotypic antibody mimicking GD3, a ganglioside antigen; BCG: bacille Calmette-Guerin; MDR-1: multidrug-resistance associated protein-1; PDGFR: platelet-derived growth factor receptor; MMP: matrix metalloproteinase; IGFR: insulin-like growth factor receptor. Reproduced and modified from [29] with permission from the author.

The common theme of the agents cited in table 1 is that they did not work well enough for investigation to continue. Some of these drugs may be re-examined in patient subsets with development of a predictive biomarker. New drugs with potential superior efficacy for particular targets may be developed. However, there is no escaping the fact that the trials reported to date are disappointing. Different approaches to target selection and evaluation are required to make progress in SCLC.

The GALES (Global Analysis of Pemetrexed in SCLC Extensive Stage) phase III randomised trial of pemetrexed and cisplatin *versus* etoposide and cisplatin deserves special mention in a chapter on targeted therapy for SCLC [35]. Based on a phase II randomised study for extensive-stage SCLC patients comparing cisplatin-pemetrexed and carboplatin-pemetrexed [36], the carboplatin-pemetrexed arm had a median survival of 10.4 months. This survival outcome appeared similar to historical controls treated with etoposide-platinum doublets. The GALES phase III study compared pemetrexed plus carboplatin with etoposide plus carboplatin in chemotherapy-naïve patients with extensive SCLC [35]. The primary objective was non-inferiority of pemetrexed-carboplatin for overall survival with a 15% margin. Accrual was terminated with 908 of 1820 patients enrolled because of inferior overall survival (8.1 months for pemetrexed-carboplatin *versus* 10.6 months for etoposide-cisplatin; $p<0.01$). PFS was inferior in the pemetrexed-carboplatin arm (hazard ratio (HR) 1.85, 95% CI 1.58–1.92; log-rank $p<0.01$). Additionally, objective response rates were lower for pemetrexed-carboplatin (31% *versus* 52% for etoposide-carboplatin; $p<0.001$). The results of the study are remarkable because although it is easy to show worse survival for single agents *versus* combination chemotherapy for extensive SCLC [37, 38], when considering an inventory of randomised trials of chemotherapy combinations for extensive SCLC [39], it is unusual to see a statistically significant decrease in overall survival that requires that the trial be terminated by the data and safety monitoring committee. Pemetrexed is truly a bad drug for SCLC and efforts have been made to relate this to the molecular biology of this tumour.

The varying sensitivity of thoracic tumours to pemetrexed could be due to differing levels of thymidylate synthase (TS) expression. This mechanism was postulated as an explanation of the differential sensitivity of pemetrexed among NSCLC histological subtypes [40]. Preclinical data have shown that overexpression of TS correlates with reduced sensitivity to pemetrexed [41]. Studies evaluating TS expression using real-time PCR and IHC found high TS expression levels in SCLC tumour biopsies [42]. Although TS levels in lung cancer histological subtypes overlap, the average quantity is reported to be highest in SCLC, intermediate in squamous cancers and lower in ADCs [43]. However, when the GALES study investigators examined tumour biomarkers, including folate pathway biomarkers (TS, glycinamide ribonucleotide formyltransferase and folylpolyglutamate synthetase (FPGS)), in an attempt to gain evidence supporting the pemetrexed-TS hypothesis, the folate biomarker levels failed to predict any outcome in either study arm [44]. In the pemetrexed-carboplatin arm, the median survival for the high TS score was 7.6 (95% CI 6.2–9.4) months and for the low TS score it was 7.9 (95% CI 6.1–10) months.

For other thoracic tumours, TS and FPGS are not clinically useful markers of response to pemetrexed in patients with malignant pleural mesothelioma [45]. In NSCLC, a modestly better survival result for nonsquamous tumours was seen in a nonstratified subset analysis [40]. However, five prospective randomised trials of advanced NSCLC have since been reported that only included nonsquamous histology patients and compared pemetrexed-platinum with another platinum doublet; they did not show any hint of a greater efficacy for the pemetrexed-platinum combination [46–51]. Given the technical and reproducibility challenges involved in measuring TS, as well as the veracity of the predictive value of TS levels in individual patients, the predictive utility of TS for pemetrexed efficacy remains in serious doubt. An alternative hypothesis for the detrimental effect of pemetrexed-platinum in SCLC is that the folic acid supplementation that is routinely administered has an adverse effect on the growth of this poorly differentiated tumour, as was clearly shown by Sidney Farber in children with acute lymphoblastic leukaemia in 1947 [52]. TS level as a predictive test of pemetrexed sensitivity in SCLC is irrelevant as pemetrexed is contraindicated in this disease.

## Targets for the treatment of SCLC in ongoing clinical trials

### MYC alterations and targeting

About 20% of SCLC patient tumours have alterations in MYC family members. MYC family members are oncogenes in SCLC rather than tumour suppressors like TP53 and RB1. Although MYC was first described many years ago [53], designing a drug to directly inhibit its activity has been difficult. Recently, it was determined that MYC-amplified or -driven tumours may be more sensitive to certain targeted drugs, such as Aurora kinase or bromodomain inhibitors [54, 55].

At the 2014 meeting of the American Society of Clinical Oncology (ASCO), a phase II clinical trial of single-agent alisertib (a selective Aurora kinase A inhibitor) produced a response rate of 21% in 47 patients with recurrent or progressive SCLC [56]. The highest response rates were seen in the platinum refractory group relapsing within <3 months of completing front-line platinum-based chemotherapy. Single-agent alisertib activity in this difficult group is notable. Aurora kinase A has a key role in the mitotic spindle assembly, so these inhibitors may have a rationale for combination with taxanes chemotherapy.

### Overexpression of PARP1 protein and the potential role of DNA repair inhibitors

Some proteins in SCLC tumours or changes at the epigenetic level may represent another type of therapeutic target. For example, proteomic profiling of a panel of SCLC cell lines led to the identification of the DNA repair proteins (PARP1 (poly(ADP-ribose) polymerase 1)) and overexpression appears to be independent of the corresponding PARP gene [57]. Several PARP inhibitors (olaparib, rucaparib, BMN-673) have been investigated in preclinical models [57]. The first data on PARP inhibitors in SCLC patients were presented at the 2014 ASCO meeting showing that BMN-673 exhibited single agent activity [58]. On a larger scale, an ongoing randomised trial is currently studying temozolamide alone *versus* temozolamide plus veliparib for previously treated SCLC (fig. 2). The Eastern Cooperative Oncology Group trial E2511 is a first-line unpublished study of platinum-etoposide *versus* platinum-etoposide plus veliparib (fig. 3).

### Fibroblast growth factor inhibitors

FGFR is another potential target in SCLC. Amplification or mutations in the FGFR genes have been observed in 6% of SCLC tumours and some SCLC models with amplification have demonstrated sensitivity to FGFR inhibitors [54]. Drugs targeting FGFR (JNJ-42756493 and BIBF1120) are now in the early phase of clinical investigation in SCLC patients.

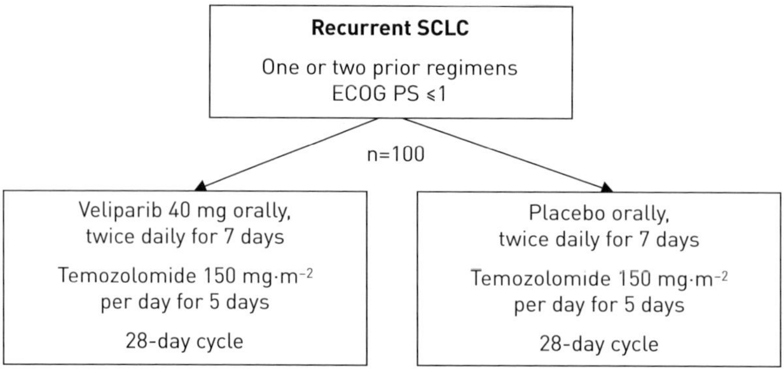


Figure 2. Phase II randomised trial of temozolamide alone *versus* temozolamide plus veliparib for previously treated SCLC. ECOG PS: Eastern Cooperative Oncology Group performance status. Reproduced and modified with kind permission from the author, Charles Rudin (Memorial Sloan Kettering Cancer Center, New York, NY, USA).

## Checkpoint antibody immunotherapy

Immune checkpoint blockade, either alone or in combination with chemotherapy, represents a very different approach to the treatment of this disease, with many mutations and numerous potential antigenic targets. In a randomised phase II study, ipilimumab, a monoclonal antibody targeting CTLA4 was combined with paclitaxel and carboplatin [59]. 130 patients with previously untreated metastatic SCLC were randomised to one of three treatment arms: 1) concurrent ipilimumab plus chemotherapy for four cycles followed by two cycles of chemotherapy plus placebo; 2) phased ipilimumab (chemotherapy plus placebo for two cycles followed by chemotherapy plus ipilimumab for four cycles); or 3) six cycles of chemotherapy plus placebo. In patients who received phased ipilimumab, an improvement was seen in PFS based on immune-related response criteria (HR 0.64; p=0.03) with a trend to

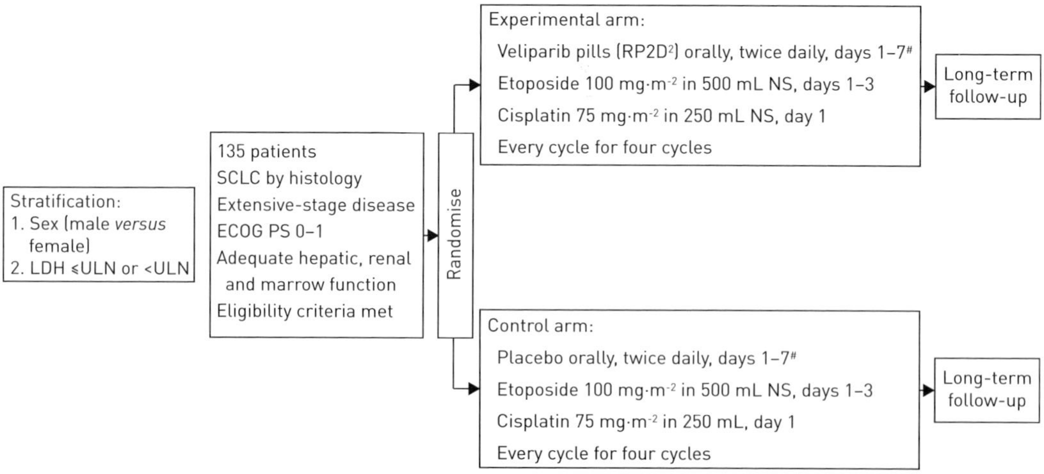


Figure 3. The Eastern Cooperative Oncology Group (ECOG) phase II trial of platinum-etoposide *versus* platinum-etoposide plus veliparib. The accrual goal was 150. The cycle was 3 weeks. Intravenous doses were based on actual weight. LDH: lactate dehydrogenase; ULN: upper limit of normal; PS: performance status. Reproduced and modified with kind permission from the author, Charles Rudin (Memorial Sloan Kettering Cancer Center, New York, NY, USA).

improved overall survival (12.4 for chemotherapy plus phased ipilimumab *versus* 9.1 months for chemotherapy plus placebo). A phase III study is underway (fig. 4).

Several trials of immunotherapy in the relapsed and previously treated setting are now ongoing with the programmed cell death protein 1 inhibitor nivolumab alone or combined with ipilimumab.

## The optimistic view of progress in targeted therapies of SCLC

It must be acknowledged that >40 phase III trials performed since the 1970s have failed to show progress with cytotoxic chemotherapy [39] and the list of failed targeted therapy is long (table 1); however, past performance may not be an indicator of future results. One could similarly cite a previous roster of long-standing therapeutic failure attempts for renal cell carcinoma and melanoma, both of which have been transformed with modern targeted therapy.

It can be argued that molecular targeted research in SCLC has not really been given a proper chance. Investment in SCLC research in recent years has been very low compared with NSCLC, and out of proportion with the number of patients with this disease. For example, in the fiscal year 2012, the American National Cancer Institute (NCI) research portfolio included 745 projects involving lung cancer research, but only 17 (~2%) focussed on SCLC. Remarkably, as few as around 100 interventional clinical trials in SCLC have been registered at ClinicalTrials.gov (https://www.clinicaltrials.gov) since December 2007. In addition, molecular profiling of SCLC has been greatly impeded by a lack genomic sequencing specimens. To date, whole-exome sequencing data (DNA sequencing of protein-coding regions of the genome) have only been published for ~100 SCLC tumours [26, 60]. This contrasts with NSCLC for which data from >1000 tumours have been published [61, 62]. The genomic studies of SCLC performed to date have been insufficiently powered to reliably identify recurrent mutations present in <10% of patients.

In order to make progress in these areas, several barriers to SCLC research should be addressed. First and foremost, the lack of adequate tissue for molecular profiling is linked to the fact that surgical resections are rare (3% of cases) for SCLC and diagnostic biopsies usually have few cancer cells. Although resection of a large quantity of the primary tumour is difficult, patients

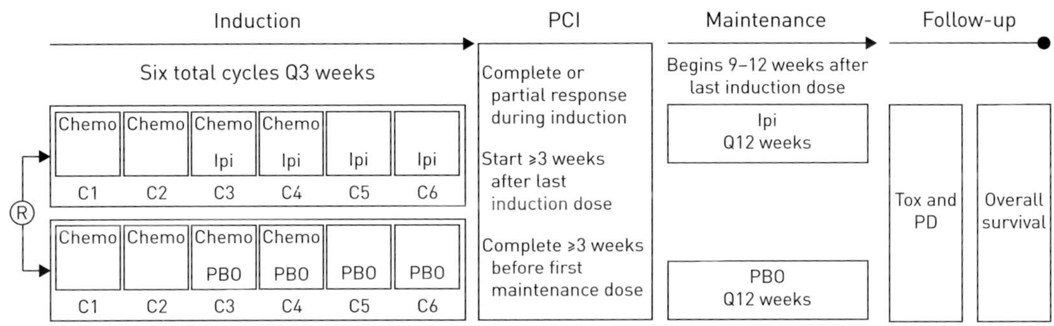


Figure 4. Phase III trial of platinum-etoposide with or without ipilumumab (Ipi). Chemotherapy (Chemo) is etoposide and cisplatin or carboplatin (investigator's choice). PCI: prophylactic cranial irradiation; Q3: every 3 weeks; Q12: every 12 weeks; R: randomised; C: cycle; PBO: placebo; Tox: toxicity assessment; PD: pharmacodynamic. Reproduced and modified with kind permission from the author, Charles Rudin (Memorial Sloan Kettering Cancer Center, New York, NY, USA).

do frequently have accessible lymph nodes in the supraclavicular station that could be biopsied for tissue quantities that are adequate for systematic genomic studies without requiring an unduly invasive procedure. Moreover, investigators have demonstrated the potential of "liquid biopsies" that obtain SCLC cells from a patient's circulation, which can be propagated in mouse models for subsequent molecular profiling and drug-sensitivity screening [63].

Recently invigorated research has yielded a number of new and potentially tractable targets. These include PARP overexpression, embryonic pathways (including notch 3) and the high antigenic load of SCLC. This heavily mutated tumour may provide many antigenic targets for the immune system unleashed by checkpoint inhibition. In addition, novel bioinformatic approaches have created new ways of exploring available data, including the identification of existing drugs that could be repurposed for SCLC treatment (*e.g.* tricyclic antidepressants) [64, 65]. Online resources, such as mycancergenome.org (http://www.mycancergenome.org), allow medical professionals to explore the most recent data for a given target and ongoing clinical trials for drugs directed against the target or associated pathway.

## The pessimistic view of progress in targeted therapies of SCLC

The molecular abnormalities of SCLC are complex in the extreme. At chromosomal level, the damage is extensive, with a roughly triploid karyotype and numerous areas of individual chromosomal loss and gain. Sequencing studies have shown a bewildering array of abnormalities in this tobacco hyper-mutated cancer. When Pleasance *et al.* [66] completed the first full sequencing of a SCLC cell line, they identified 22910 somatic substitutions, 65 indels, 334 copy number segments and 58 structural variants. Since SCLCs are almost always associated with smoking and the typical patient has 50 pack-years of tobacco exposure, the investigators extrapolated that an average of one mutation would occur for every 15 cigarettes smoked. On average, SCLC tumors have more than four times the number of mutations observed in breast cancer and almost 10 times the number in prostate cancer [60]. Pharmacological targeting of the relevant abnormalities is a daunting task even if mathematical modelling indicates that most mutations occurring in coding and promoter regions of the genome are passenger events. This makes it more difficult to definitively identify those mutations that are drivers of cancer growth and invasion, including those for which drugs may be used.

The checklist approach for molecular targeted therapy has tried many things and a Bayesian interpretation of the probability of future success gives little realistic hope. Regardless of the molecular biology of SCLC, the molecular targets in table 1 include most of the promising treatable pathways in cancer medicine; that so many have been tried empirically and failed is discouraging. Even for the more successful model of lung cancer-targeted therapy in NSCLC, the familiar pie chart of druggable driver mutations, has not recently changed. Although it may be an overstatement to say that discovery of new molecular targets for NSCLC has "hit the wall", it is clear that the rate of progress has stalled. In 2015, the most exciting research in targeted therapy of NSCLC is not identification of new targets but better treatment of known targets, such as EGFR mutations with third-generation inhibitors and ALK mutations with second-generation drugs. The low hanging fruit has been picked. For SCLC, the molecular abnormalities identified to date are mainly tumour-suppressor genes. Loss-of-function genetic alterations do not provide the clear opportunity for rapid clinical translation offered by an activating mutation in a known receptor tyrosine kinase. Some counterexamples may exist, like the MYC family, but designing a drug to directly inhibit MYC activity has been challenging.

Like squamous carcinomas, the molecular battlefield in SCLC is complex and bleak with little opportunity of even temporary respite by identification of mutually exclusive oncogenic drivers that can be treated to proven patient benefit.

Patients with SCLC are inherently difficult to investigate with novel therapies. Typically, this patient is old chronologically with a median age of >70 years, and has a physiological age of considerably older because of the premature ageing and comorbidities linked with heavy smoking. Furthermore, the rapid pace of tumour progression and the tempo of patient deterioration associated with it creates a logistical nightmare for a multidisciplinary team intending to expedite biopsies and molecular profiling in time to identify molecular targets for treatment initiation before it is too late.

Parenthetically, there is no evidence that current technology can detect early curable SCLC. For NSCLC, the promise of screening to detect early curable cancers was demonstrated in the National Lung Screening Trial [67]. However, early detection of SCLC did not reduce the number of patients who were diagnosed with extensive-stage disease, nor did it have an evident impact on survival.

## Conclusion

A more successful translational approach for the advancement of SCLC treatment must have a number of key elements. Adequate biopsy material must be made available from treatment-naïve and treatment-refractory patients in order for an appropriately funded multidisciplinary scientific community of SCLC investigators to perform molecular profiling/biomarker analyses for the identification of new targets suitable for drug trials. Clinical trial options for all stages of disease must be made available through clinical trial consortiums, basket studies and SCLC master protocols. These initiatives will require a considerable increase in SCLC funding.

## References

1. Govindan R, Page N, Morgensztern D, *et al.* Changing epidemiology of small-cell lung cancer in the United States over the last 30 years: analysis of the surveillance, epidemiologic, and end results database. *J Clin Oncol* 2006; 24: 4539–4544.
2. Watson WL, Berg JW. Oat cell lung cancer. *Cancer* 1962; 15: 759–768.
3. Johnson DH, Schiller JH, Bunn PA, Recent clinical advances in lung cancer management. *J Clin Oncol* 2014; 32: 973–982.
4. Reck M, Heigener DF, Mok T, *et al.* Management of non-small-cell lung cancer: recent developments. *Lancet* 2013; 382: 709–719.
5. Byers LA, Rudin CM. Small cell lung cancer: where do we go from here? *Cancer* 2015; 121: 664–672.
6. Mok TS. Personalized medicine in lung cancer: what we need to know. *Nat Rev Clin Oncol* 2011; 8: 661–668.
7. Pao W, Iafrate AJ, Su Z. Genetically informed lung cancer medicine. *J Pathol* 2011; 223: 230–240.
8. Hirsch FR, Matthews MJ, Aisner S, *et al.* Histopathologic classification of small cell lung cancer. Changing concepts and terminology. *Cancer* 1988; 62: 973–977.
9. Jones MH, Virtanen C, Honjoh D, *et al.* Two prognostically significant subtypes of high-grade lung neuroendocrine tumours independent of small-cell and large-cell neuroendocrine carcinomas identified by gene expression profiles. *Lancet* 2004; 363: 775–781.
10. Peng WX, Shibata T, Katoh H, *et al.* Array-based comparative genomic hybridization analysis of high-grade neuroendocrine tumors of the lung. *Cancer Sci* 2005; 96: 661–667.
11. Sozzi G, Bertoglio MG, Borrello MG, *et al.* Chromosomal abnormalities in a primary small cell lung cancer. *Cancer Genet Cytogenet* 1987; 27: 45–50.

12. Miura I, Graziano SL, Cheng JQ, *et al.* Chromosome alterations in human small cell lung cancer: frequent involvement of 5q. *Cancer Res* 1992; 52: 1322–1328.
13. Whang-Peng J, Kao-Shan CS, Lee EC, *et al.* Specific chromosome defect associated with human small-cell lung cancer; deletion 3p(14–23). *Science* 1982; 215: 181–182.
14. Brauch H, Johnson B, Hovis J, *et al.* Molecular analysis of the short arm of chromosome 3 in small-cell and non-small-cell carcinoma of the lung. *N Engl J Med* 1987; 317: 1109–1113.
15. Kok K, Osinga J, Carritt B, *et al.* Deletion of a DNA sequence at the chromosomal region 3p21 in all major types of lung cancer. *Nature* 1987; 330: 578–581.
16. Naylor SL, Johnson BE, Minna JD, *et al.* Loss of heterozygosity of chromosome 3p markers in small-cell lung cancer. *Nature* 1987; 329: 451–454.
17. Sozzi G, Veronese ML, Negrini M, *et al.* The FHIT gene 3p14.2 is abnormal in lung cancer. *Cell* 1996; 85: 17–26.
18. Dammann R, Li C, Yoon JH, *et al.* Epigenetic inactivation of a RAS association domain family protein from the lung tumour suppressor locus 3p21.3. *Nat Genet* 2000; 25: 315–319.
19. Levin NA, Brzoska PM, Warnock ML, *et al.* Identification of novel regions of altered DNA copy number in small cell lung tumors. *Genes Chromosomes Cancer* 1995; 13: 175–185.
20. Ried T, Petersen I, Holtgreve-Grez H, *et al.* Mapping of multiple DNA gains and losses in primary small cell lung carcinomas by comparative genomic hybridization. *Cancer Res* 1994; 54: 1801–1806.
21. Miller CW, Simon K, Aslo A, *et al.* P53 mutations in human lung tumors. *Cancer Res* 1992; 52: 1695–1698.
22. Takahashi T, Takahashi T, Suzuki H, *et al.* The p53 gene is very frequently mutated in small-cell lung cancer with a distinct nucleotide substitution pattern. *Oncogene* 1991; 6: 1775–1778.
23. D'Amico D, Carbone D, Mitsudomi T, *et al.* High frequency of somatically acquired p53 mutations in small-cell lung cancer cell lines and tumors. *Oncogene* 1992; 7: 339–346.
24. Rudin CM, Durinck S, Stawiski EW, *et al.* Comprehensive genomic analysis identifies SOX2 as a frequently amplified gene in small-cell lung cancer. *Nat Genet* 2012; 44: 1111–1116.
25. Wistuba II, Gazdar AF, Minna JD. Molecular genetics of small cell lung carcinoma. *Semin Oncol* 2001; 28; Suppl. 4, 3–13.
26. Peifer M, Fernandez-Cuesta L, Sos ML, *et al.* Integrative genome analyses identify key somatic driver mutations of small-cell lung cancer. *Nat Genet* 2012; 44: 1104–1110.
27. Bass AJ, Watanabe H, Mermel CH, *et al.* SOX2 is an amplified lineage-survival oncogene in lung and esophageal squamous cell carcinomas. *Nat Genet* 2009; 41: 1238–1242.
28. Pietanza MC, Ladanyi M. Bringing the genomic landscape of small-cell lung cancer into focus. *Nat Genet* 2012; 44: 1074–1075.
29. Abidin AZ, Garassino MC, Califano R, *et al.* Targeted therapies in small call lung cancer: a review. *Ther Adv Med Oncol* 2010; 2: 25–37.
30. Giaccone G, Debruyne C, Felip E, *et al.* Phase III study of adjuvant vaccination with Bec2/Bacille Calmette-Guerin in responding patients with limited-disease small-cell lung cancer (European Organisation for Research and Treatment of Cancer 08971–08971B; Silva Study). *J Clin Oncol* 2005; 23: 6854–6864.
31. Pujol JL, Breton JL, Gervais R, *et al.* Phase III double-blind, placebo-controlled study of thalidomide in extensive-disease small-cell lung cancer after response to chemotherapy: an intergroup study FNCLCC cleo04 IFCT 00–01. *J Clin Oncol* 2007; 25: 3945–3951.
32. Lee SM, Woll PJ, Rudd R, *et al.* Anti-angiogenic therapy using thalidomide combined with chemotherapy in small cell lung cancer: a randomized, double-blind, placebo-controlled trial. *J Natl Cancer Inst* 2009; 101: 1049–1057.
33. Shepherd FA, Giaccone G, Seymour L, *et al.* Prospective, randomized, double-blind, placebo-controlled trial of marimastat after response to first-line chemotherapy in patients with small-cell lung cancer: a trial of the National Cancer Institute of Canada-Clinical Trials Group and the European Organization for Research and Treatment of Cancer. *J Clin Oncol* 2002; 20: 4434–4439.
34. Seckl M, Ottensmeier C, Cullen MH, *et al.* A multicenter phase III randomized double-blind placebo controlled trial of pravastatin added to first-line standard chemotherapy in patients with small cell lung cancer (SCLC). *ASCO Meeting Abstracts* 2013; 31: Suppl. 15, 7595.
35. Socinski MA, Smit EF, Lorigan P, *et al.* Phase III study of pemetrexed plus carboplatin compared with etoposide plus carboplatin in chemotherapy-naive patients with extensive-stage small-cell lung cancer. *J Clin Oncol* 2009; 27: 4787–4792.
36. Socinski MA, Weissman C, Hart LL, *et al.* Randomized phase II trial of pemetrexed combined with either cisplatin or carboplatin in untreated extensive-stage small-cell lung cancer. *J Clin Oncol* 2006; 24: 4840–4847.
37. Souhami RL, Spiro SG, Rudd RM, *et al.* Five-day oral etoposide treatment for advanced small-cell lung cancer: randomized comparison with intravenous chemotherapy. *J Natl Cancer Inst* 1997; 89: 577–580.
38. Girling DJ. Comparison of oral etoposide and standard intravenous multidrug chemotherapy for small-cell lung cancer: a stopped multicentre randomised trial. Medical Research Council Lung Cancer Working Party. *Lancet* 1996; 348: 563–566.
39. Oze I, Hotta K, Kiura K, *et al.* Twenty-seven years of phase III trials for patients with extensive disease small-cell lung cancer: disappointing results. *PLoS One* 2009; 4: e7835.

40. Scagliotti GV, Parikh P, von Pawel J, *et al.* Phase III study comparing cisplatin plus gemcitabine with cisplatin plus pemetrexed in chemotherapy-naive patients with advanced-stage non-small-cell lung cancer. *J Clin Oncol* 2008; 26: 3543–3551.
41. Schultz RM, Chen VJ, Bewley JR, *et al.* Biological activity of the multitargeted antifolate, MTA (LY231514), in human cell lines with different resistance mechanisms to antifolate drugs. *Semin Oncol* 1999; 26: Suppl. 6, 68–73.
42. Ceppi P, Volante M, Ferrero A, *et al.* Thymidylate synthase expression in gastroenteropancreatic and pulmonary neuroendocrine tumors. *Clin Cancer Res* 2008; 14: 1059–1064.
43. Ceppi P, Volante M, Saviozzi S, *et al.* Squamous cell carcinoma of the lung compared with other histotypes shows higher messenger RNA and protein levels for thymidylate synthase. *Cancer* 2006; 107: 1589–1596.
44. Smit EF, Socinski MA, Mullaney BP, *et al.* Biomarker analysis in a phase III study of pemetrexed-carboplatin *versus* etoposide-carboplatin in chemonaive patients with extensive-stage small-cell lung cancer. *Ann Oncol* 2012; 23: 1723–1729.
45. Lustgarten DE, Deshpande C, Aggarwal C, *et al.* Thymidylate synthase and folyl-polyglutamate synthase are not clinically useful markers of response to pemetrexed in patients with malignant pleural mesothelioma. *J Thorac Oncol* 2013; 8: 469–477.
46. Rodrigues-Pereira J, Kim JH, Magallanes M, *et al.* A randomized phase 3 trial comparing pemetrexed/carboplatin and docetaxel/carboplatin as first-line treatment for advanced, nonsquamous non-small cell lung cancer. *J Thorac Oncol* 2011; 6: 1907–1914.
47. Bennouna J, Zatloukal P, Krzakowski MJ, *et al.* Prospective randomized phase II trial of oral vinorelbine (NVBo) and cisplatin (P) or pemetrexed (Pem) and P in first-line metastatic or locally advanced non-small cell lung cancer (M or LA NSCLC) patients (pts) with nonsquamous (non SCC) histologic type: NAVoTRIAL01 Preliminary results. *ASCO Meeting Abstracts* 2012; 30: Suppl. 15, 7575.
48. Patel JD, Socinski MA, Garon EB, *et al.* PointBreak: a randomized phase III study of pemetrexed plus carboplatin and bevacizumab followed by maintenance pemetrexed and bevacizumab *versus* paclitaxel plus carboplatin and bevacizumab followed by maintenance bevacizumab in patients with stage IIIB or IV nonsquamous non-small-cell lung cancer. *J Clin Oncol* 2013; 31: 4349–4357.
49. Zinner RG, Obasaju CK, Spigel DR, *et al.* PRONOUNCE: randomized, open-label, phase III study of first-line pemetrexed + carboplatin followed by maintenance pemetrexed *versus* paclitaxel + carboplatin + bevacizumab followed by maintenance bevacizumab in patients with advanced nonsquamous non-small-cell lung cancer. *J Thorac Oncol* 2015; 10: 134–142.
50. Kim Y, Oh I, Kim K, *et al.* A randomized phase III study of docetaxel plus cisplatin *versus* pemetrexed plus cisplatin in first line non-squamous non-small cell lung cancer (NSQ-NSCLC). *Ann Oncol* 2014; 25: Suppl. 4, LBA41_PR.
51. Murray N. Reality check for pemetrexed and maintenance therapy in advanced non-small-cell lung cancer. *J Clin Oncol* 2014; 32: 482–483.
52. Farber S, Cutler EC, Hawkins JW, *et al.* The action of pteroylglutamic conjugates on man. *Science* 1947; 106: 619–621.
53. Little CD, Nau MM, Carney DN, *et al.* Amplification and expression of the c-myc oncogene in human lung cancer cell lines. *Nature* 1983; 306: 194–196.
54. Sos ML, Dietlein F, Peifer M, *et al.* A framework for identification of actionable cancer genome dependencies in small cell lung cancer. *Proc Natl Acad Sci USA* 2012; 109: 17034–17039.
55. Mertz JA, Conery AR, Bryant BM, *et al.* Targeting MYC dependence in cancer by inhibiting BET bromodomains. *Proc Natl Acad Sci USA* 2011; 108: 16669–16674.
56. Melichar B, Adenis A, Havel L, *et al.* Phase (Ph) I/II study of investigational Aurora A kinase (AAK) inhibitor MLN8237 (alisertib): updated ph II results in patients (pts) with small cell lung cancer (SCLC), non-SCLC (NSCLC), breast cancer (BrC), head and neck squamous cell carcinoma (HNSCC), and gastroesophageal cancer (GE). *ASCO Meeting Abstracts* 2013; 31: Suppl. 15, 605.
57. Byers LA, Wang J, Nilsson MB, *et al.* Proteomic profiling identifies dysregulated pathways in small cell lung cancer and novel therapeutic targets including PARP1. *Cancer Discov* 2012; 2: 798–811.
58. Wainberg ZA, Rafii S, Ramanathan RK, *et al.* Safety and antitumor activity of the PARP inhibitor BMN673 in a phase 1 trial recruiting metastatic small-cell lung cancer (SCLC) and germline BRCA-mutation carrier cancer patients. *ASCO Meeting Abstracts* 2014; 32: Suppl. 15, 7522.
59. Reck M, Bondarenko I, Luft A, *et al.* Ipilimumab in combination with paclitaxel and carboplatin as first-line therapy in extensive-disease-small-cell lung cancer: results from a randomized, double-blind, multicenter phase 2 trial. *Ann Oncol* 2013; 24: 75–83.
60. Daniel VC, Marchionni L, Hierman JS, *et al.* A primary xenograft model of small-cell lung cancer reveals irreversible changes in gene expression imposed by culture in vitro. *Cancer Res* 2009; 69: 3364–3373.
61. Cancer Genome Atlas Research Network. Comprehensive molecular profiling of lung adenocarcinoma. *Nature* 2014; 511: 543–550.
62. Cancer Genome Atlas Research Network. Comprehensive genomic characterization of squamous cell lung cancers. *Nature* 2012; 489: 519–525.

63. Hodgkinson CL, Morrow CJ, Li Y, *et al.* Tumorigenicity and genetic profiling of circulating tumor cells in small-cell lung cancer. *Nat Med* 2014; 20: 897–903.
64. Jahchan NS, Dudley JT, Mazur PK, *et al.* A drug repositioning approach identifies tricyclic antidepressants as inhibitors of small cell lung cancer and other neuroendocrine tumors. *Cancer Discov* 2013; 3: 1364–1377.
65. Wang J, Byers LA. Teaching an old dog new tricks: drug repositioning in small cell lung cancer. *Cancer Discov* 2013; 3: 1333–1335.
66. Pleasance ED, Stephens PJ, O'Meara S, *et al.* A small-cell lung cancer genome with complex signatures of tobacco exposure. *Nature* 2010; 463: 184–190.
67. Aberle DR, DeMello S, Berg CD, *et al.* Results of the two incidence screenings in the National Lung Screening Trial. *N Engl J Med* 2013; 369: 920–931.

---

Disclosures: None declared.

# Chapter 19

# Immunotherapy

Niels Reinmuth[1,2] and David F. Heigener[1,2]

Immune evasion is recognised as a key strategy for cancer survival and progression. Hence, various approaches to restore anti-tumour immune responses are currently being investigated. In particular, early clinical trials have shown that agents targeting immune checkpoints, such as the CTLA4 receptor and the programmed cell death protein 1 receptor, have the potential to improve tumour responses and survival in lung cancer patients. With multiple studies under way, there are high expectations that treatment outcomes in patients with lung cancer who are ineligible for surgical resection may be improved by the incorporation of immunotherapies in the various treatment cascades.

The immune system plays an essential role in the prevention of tumours, including the specific identification and elimination of tumour cells on the basis of their expression of tumour-specific antigens or molecules induced by cellular stress, thereby employing both innate and adaptive immune mechanisms [1]. This immune response to tumour growth is commonly referred to as "cancer immunosurveillance". However, tumour cells can evade immunological destruction, in particular by T- and B-lymphocytes, macrophages and natural killer cells, a capability that is recognised as an emerging hallmark of cancer [1, 2]. Indeed, there is growing evidence that lung cancer is a suitable candidate for immuno-oncology-based treatment strategies [3]. Pathologists have long recognised that some tumours, including NSCLC, are densely infiltrated by cells of both the innate and adaptive arms of the immune system, and thereby mirror inflammatory conditions arising in non-neoplastic tissues [4]. Results from preclinical studies and early data from clinical trials clearly indicate that lung cancer seems to be a suitable candidate for immuno-oncology-based treatment strategies [5]. Currently, novel and improved immunotherapeutic agents, including a range of vaccines, are in development.

## Mechanism of action

The escape of tumour cells from immunosurveillance is a multifactorial process as tumours can develop a raft of complex, overlapping strategies to avoid immune system recognition and destruction, leading to malignancy and tumour progression. For example, inhibitory ligands and receptors that regulate T-cell effector functions in tissues are commonly overexpressed on tumour cells or on non-transformed cells in the tumour

[1]Dept of Thoracic Oncology, LungenClinic, Grosshansdorf, Germany. [2]Airway Research Center North, Member of the German Center for Lung Research (DZL), Grosshansdorf, Germany.

Correspondence: Niels Reinmuth, Dept of Thoracic Oncology, LungenClinic Großhansdorf, Wöhrendamm 80, 22927 Großhansdorf, Germany. E-mail: n.reinmuth@lungenclinic.de

 Print ISBN: 978-1-84984-061-3. Online ISBN: 978-1-84984-062-0. Print ISSN: 2312-508X. Online ISSN: 2312-5098.

microenvironment [5]. There is also growing evidence of an immunosuppressive microenvironment in NSCLC tumours and its association with poor prognosis.

Hence, a broad variety of therapeutic strategies has been developed with the goal of promoting a host anti-tumour response. These approaches include antibodies (targeting tumour antigens) and other passive immunotherapies, such as adoptive cell transfer and, being at the forefront of clinical research in this field, active immunotherapies, like immune checkpoint-targeted agents and vaccination approaches.

## Vaccines

Most vaccine therapy strategies in lung cancer are based on the use of antigen-specific vaccines and tumour cell vaccines [6]. An antigen with the potential for utilisation in vaccine therapy should have an expression pattern that is tumour specific, be prevalent among tumours of that type, and be found persistently throughout disease progression (*i.e.* expressed in early and metastatic disease). Ideally, it should also exhibit some evidence that it promotes an immune response against the tumour [6, 7]. The expression of several tumour-associated antigens has been described in patients with NSCLC.

Some of the most commonly targeted antigens currently being investigated in clinical trials are mucinous glycoprotein-1 (MUC1) (a highly glycosylated transmembrane protein that is overexpressed or aberrantly glycosylated in cancer cells), melanoma-associated antigen 3 (MAGE-A3) (a protein that is expressed almost exclusively on tumour cells and detected in NSCLC in ~24–50% of tumours), various gangliosides and the EGFR pathway [6, 8]. An alternative approach aims to use tumour cell vaccines that are prepared from tumour cells. The tumour cells may either derive from autologous tumour cells or may be prepared from cancer cell lines. Although the latter concept may be disadvantaged by the fact that the antigens present in the allogeneic vaccines may not be expressed in a given patient's tumour, an allogeneic vaccine, belagenpumatucel-L, has been developed from four irradiated, allogeneic NSCLC cell lines, which were transfected with an anti-TGF-β2 plasmid to enhance the immunogenicity of the vaccine. Most vaccination trials administer a nonspecific immune stimulant as an adjuvant in combination with vaccines to stimulate movement of antigen presenting cells (APCs) to the vaccination site and uptake of the vaccine antigen by the APCs [7].

## Immune checkpoint inhibitors

The immune response to an antigen is regulated by a balance between co-stimulatory and inhibitory signals (or immune checkpoints), which, under normal conditions, are essential in maintaining self-tolerance and preventing excessive, prolonged and potentially deleterious T-cell activity in peripheral tissues [5]. To date, two immune-checkpoint receptors have been most actively studied in the context of clinical cancer immunotherapy: CTLA4 (also known as CD152) and programmed cell death protein 1 (PD-1). CTLA4, a close homologue of CD28, seems to directly compete with CD28 for CD80 and/or CD86 on the APCs, ultimately leading to T-cell inhibition [9, 10]. However, multiple additional immune checkpoints, such as the killer-cell immunoglobulin-like receptor (KIR) and lymphocyte-activation gene-3 (LAG-3), represent promising targets for therapeutic blockade based on preclinical and early clinical experiments [8]. Moreover, several data support the combination of immunomodulating agents that target different immune escape mechanisms. While CTLA4 is expressed exclusively on T-cells and contributes to T-cell activation upon recognition of

MHC-antigen complexes, the PD-1 receptor is expressed on T-cells, B-cells and natural killer cells, and may act more centrally within the tumour microenvironment [5, 11].

## Clinical studies

### Vaccines

In early clinical trials, some vaccinations have shown clinical benefits in subsets of patients. Some of the approaches are characterised in the following sections.

#### *Liposomal BLP25*

The liposomal BLP25 vaccine (L-BLP25) (Stimuvax, tecemotide) targets MUC1, which is normally expressed on the apical surface of mucin-secreting epithelial cells but exhibits an aberrant glycosylation pattern in tumour cells [12]. A *post hoc* analysis from an open-label, phase II trial including 171 patients with stage IIIB or IV NSCLC, suggested a survival benefit for patients after treatment with chemoradiotherapy for L-BPL25 vaccination (median 30.6 *versus* 13.3 months for the L-BLP25 and control arms, respectively, hazard ratio (HR) 0.55; p=0.092) [13]. Common adverse events in the vaccine group were flu-like symptoms and minor injection site reactions. However, a recent phase III study (START (Stimulating Targeted Antigenic Response To non-small cell lung cancer)) failed to demonstrate a significant survival difference for L-BLP25 vaccination maintenance therapy (n=829) compared with placebo (n=829) in patients with stage III NSCLC who did not progress after sequential or concurrent chemoradiotherapy (median 25.6 months for L-BLP25 and 22.3 months for placebo, HR 0.88, 95% CI 0.75–1.03; p=0.123) [14]. Interestingly, an exploratory subgroup analysis revealed that the 829 patients treated with concurrent chemoradiotherapy had a substantial improvement in overall survival (median 30.8 months in the tecemotide *versus* 20.8 months in the placebo, HR 0.78, 95% CI 0.64–0.95; p=0.016). Moreover, as yet unpublished results from a planned analysis of a randomised phase I/II study in Japanese patients with stage III NSCLC who had received concurrent or sequential chemoradiotherapy were reported to demonstrate no significant benefit regarding overall survival or PFS for L-BLP25 compared with placebo. Subsequently, according to a recent press release, the clinical development of L-BLP25 in NSCLC worldwide has stopped.

#### *MAGE-A3*

The MAGE-A3 antigen has been evaluated as another target for therapeutic cancer vaccination after surgical resection of early stage NSCLC. Based on promising phase II data, a phase III trial (MAGRIT) randomised a total of 2272 patients with completely resected MAGE-A3-positive NSCLC and stages IB, II and IIIA with or without adjuvant chemotherapy to receive vaccination with MAGE-A3 or placebo over a 27-month treatment period [15]. However, treatment with MAGE-A3 vaccination did not increase the disease-free survival compared with placebo in either the overall population (median 60.5 months for MAGE-A3 *versus* 57.9 months for placebo, HR 1.024, 95% CI 0.891–1.177; p=0.74) or in patients who did not receive adjuvant chemotherapy (median 58.0 months for MAGE-A3 *versus* 56.9 months for placebo, HR 0.970; p=0.7572).

#### *Belagenpumatucel-L*

Belagenpumatucel-L is an allogenic tumour cell vaccine that was tested in a phase III trial in 532 patients with stages T3N2-IIIA, IIIB and IV NSCLC who did not progress after frontline chemotherapy [16]. Median overall survival was not significantly different with belagenpumatucel-L vaccination compared with placebo (median 20.3 months for belagenpumatucel-L *versus* 17.8 months for placebo, HR 0.94; p=0.594). A predefined Cox regression demonstrated that the time elapsed between randomisation and the end of frontline chemotherapy had a significant impact on survival outcomes (p=0.002). Hence, 305 stage IIIB/IV patients randomised within 12 weeks of the completion of chemotherapy had a numerically superior overall survival (median 20.7 months for belagenpumatucel-L *versus* 13.4 months for placebo, HR 0.75 p=0.083) when vaccinated with belagenpumatucel-L. Similar to other vaccination trials, belagenpumatucel-L was well tolerated with no safety concerns.

#### *Others*

Large phase III trials investigating vaccination approaches demonstrated no convincing clinical benefit in the overall population. Hence, predictive biomarkers may be needed to identify patients who are most likely to benefit from this immunotherapeutic approach. Moreover, several other vaccines are being tested, including ganglioside vaccines, anti-EGFR vaccines and alternative vaccines against MUC1, such as TG4010, with the latter being studied in phase IIB/III study in patients with stage IV NSCLC (NCT01383148; https://clinicaltrials.gov).

### Checkpoint inhibitors

Agents that target inhibitors at checkpoints of the immune response activation cascade are currently leading the way in clinical development programmes. In general, these agents have the potential to achieve clinical benefits across a range of diverse patient populations, regardless of their underlying cancer histology, mutational status and baseline characteristics.

#### *CTLA4 blockade*

Tumour-mediated activation of the CTLA4 inhibitory pathway decreases the amplitude of the T-cell response [11]. Strategies have been explored in preclinical tumour models for blocking the activation of the CTLA4 pathway with anti-CTLA4 monoclonal antibodies, to increase anti-tumour immune activity leading to augmented T-cell activation and tumour regression [11, 17, 18]. Early clinical trials with humanised CTLA4 antibodies as monotherapy in patients with advanced disease demonstrated objective clinical responses in ~10% of patients with melanoma [19]. As the mechanism of action of CTLA4 antibodies is not dependent on tumour cells expressing a particular antigenic target, it was reasoned that it may also have activity against multiple tumour types.

In studies on previously untreated patients with advanced NSCLC, the phased application of the anti-CTLA4 monoclonal antibody ipilimumab improved immune-related PFS (irPFS) *versus* chemotherapy alone (median 5.7 *versus* 4.6 months, respectively, HR 0.72; p=0.05) and prolonged overall survival (median 12.2 *versus* 8.3 months, respectively, for chemotherapy alone), though the latter was not statistically significant [20]. In contrast, in the same trial, concurrent delivery of ipilimumab with chemotherapy did not provide the same level of clinical benefit (median irPFS 5.5 months for concurenct delivery of ipilimumab *versus* 4.6 months for placebo, HR 0.81; p=0.13). Similarly, a trial on SCLC demonstrated an irPFS benefit for phased ipilimumab, but not concurrent ipilimumab, in combination with platinum-based chemotherapy (median 6.4 months for phased ipilimumab *versus* 5.3 months for placebo, HR 0.64; p=0.03) [21]. However, no improvements in PFS or overall survival were observed. Phase III trials are now ongoing that explore the phased regimen of ipilimumab with chemotherapy in patients with squamous cell NSCLC (NCT01285609; https://clinicaltrials.gov) and extensive-stage SCLC (NCT01450761; https://clinicaltrials.gov) (table 1).

Table 1. Ongoing clinical trials with immune checkpoint inhibitors in lung cancer

| Drug | Target | Phase | Population | Design | Primary outcome measure | Clinical trial number | Completion date |
|---|---|---|---|---|---|---|---|
| **Ipilimumab** | CTLA4 | I | NSCLC | Ipilimumab plus neoadjuvant chemotherapy *versus* neoadjuvant chemotherapy | % subjects with detectable tumour-specific circulating T-cells | NCT01820754 | May 2018 |
| | | I | NSCLC | Ipilimumab plus erlotinib or crizotinib | Safety | NCT01820754 | December 2015 |
| | | II | SCLC | Ipilimumab plus carboplatin/etoposide | PFS | NCT01331525 | May 2015 |
| | | III | Metastatic/ED SCLC | Ipilimumab plus etoposide/platinum *versus* etoposide/platinum | OS | NCT01450761 | March 2017 |
| | | III | NSCLC SCC | Ipilimumab plus paclitaxel/carboplatin *versus* paclitaxel/carboplatin | OS | NCT01285609 | December 2016 |
| **Tremelilumab** | CTLA4 | I | Solid tumours | MEDI4736 plus tremelilumab | AE rate | NCT01975831 | December 2016 |
| | | II | NSCLC | Gefitinib, AZD9291, tremelimumab or selumetinib plus docetaxel with a sequential switch to MEDI4736 | ORR | NCT02179671 | May 2016 |
| **Nivolumab** | PD-1 | I | Solid tumours | Nivolumab plus IL-21 | AE rate/severity | NCT01629758 | April 2015 |
| | | I | NSCLC | Safety of nivolumab plus various standard chemotherapies | AE/worst toxicity grade/lab test abnormalities | NCT01454102 | August 2015 |
| | | I/II | Advanced/metastatic solid tumours including NSCLC | Nivolumab or nivolumab plus ipilimumab | ORR | NCT01928394 | April 2015 |
| | | II | Advanced/metastatic SCC NSCLC who have received more than two previous treatments | Nivolumab as third-line onwards therapy | ORR | NCT01721759 | February 2015 |

Continued

Table 1. Continued

| Drug | Target | Phase | Population | Design | Primary outcome measure | Clinical trial number | Completion date |
|---|---|---|---|---|---|---|---|
| | | III | SCC NSCLC after failure of platinum | Nivolumab *versus* docetaxel as second-line therapy | ORR and OS | NCT01642004 | August 2015 |
| | | III | Non-SCC NSCLC after failure of platinum | Nivolumab *versus* docetaxel as second-line therapy | ORR and OS | NCT01673867 | November 2015 |
| | | III | NSCLC | Nivolumab *versus* investigator's choice of chemotherapy | PFS | NCT02041533 | January 2018 |
| | | III | NSCLC | Nivolumab second-line onwards | Safety | NCT02066636 | March 2019 |
| **Pembrolizumab (MK3475)** | PD-1 | I | Advanced solid tumours including NSCLC | MK-3475 plus cisplatin/ pemetrexed or carboplatin/ paclitaxel | DLT rate | NCT01840579 | April 2015 |
| | | I/II | NSCLC | Pembrolizumab plus paclitaxel/carboplatin/ bevacizumab/pemetrexed/ ipilimumab/erlotinib/ gefitinib | ORR, PFS | NCT02039674 | June 2019 |
| | | II/III | NSCLC progressed after platinum | Low or high dose of MK-3475 *versus* docetaxel | OS, PFS, AE rate | NCT01905657 | January 2020 |
| | | III | NSCLC | Pembrolizumab *versus* paclitaxel/carboplatin/ pemetrexed/cisplatin/ gemcitabine | PFS | NCT02142738 | December 2017 |
| **MPDL3280A** | PD-L1 | I | Advanced solid tumours | MPDL3280A plus bevacuzimab plus various other chemotherapies | AE/DLT rate | NCT01633970 | July 2015 |
| | | I | NSCLC | MPDL3280A plus erlotinib | Safety | NCT02013219 | August 2016 |
| | | II | Advanced/metastatic NSCLC after platinum failed | MPDL3280A *versus* docetaxel as second line | OS | NCT01903993 | March 2017 |

Continued

Table 1. Continued

| Drug | Target | Phase | Population | Design | Primary outcome measure | Clinical trial number | Completion date |
|---|---|---|---|---|---|---|---|
| | | II | Advanced/metastatic PD-1 plus NSCLC | MPDL3280A | ORR | NCT01846416 | May 2015 |
| | | II | Advanced/metastatic PD-1 plus NSCLC | MPDL3280A | ORR | NCT02031458 | March 2018 |
| | | III | NSCLC | MPDL3280A *versus* docetaxel | OS | NCT02008227 | June 2018 |
| **MEDI4736** | PD-L1 | I | NSCLC | MEDI4736 plus tremelimumab | Safety | NCT02000947 | January 2017 |
| | | I | NSCLC | MEDI4736 plus gefitinib | Safety | NCT02088112 | October 2017 |
| | | II | NSCLC | MEDI4736 third line | ORR | NCT02087423 | August 2016 |
| | | III | NSCLC | MEDI4736 following concurrent chemoradiation | ORR, PFS | NCT02125461 | November 2020 |
| **Lirilumab** | KIR | I | Advanced/metastatic solid tumours | Lirilumab plus nivolumab | AE rate/lab test abnormalities | NCT01714739 | September 2015 |
| | | I | Advanced/metastatic solid tumours | Lirilumab plus ipilimumab | AE rate | NCT01750580 | July 2015 |
| **BMS-986016** | LAG-3 | I | Advanced solid tumours | BMS-986016 alone or plus nivolumab | AE rate/lab test abnormalities | NCT01968109 | October 2020 |
| **Bavituximab** | PS | I | Previously untreated stage IV NSCLC | Bavituximab plus pemetrexed/carboplatin in first-line therapy | Severe side-effects | NCT01323062 | May 2018 |
| | | III | Nonsquamous NSCLC | Bavituximab plus docetaxel *versus* docetaxel | OS | NCT01999673 | December 2016 |

All clinical trials are registered at ClinicalTrials.gov (https://clinicaltrials.gov/). ED: extensive disease; OS: overall survival; AE: adverse effect; PD-1: programmed cell death protein 1; IL: interleukin; ORR: objective response rate; DLT: dose-limiting toxicity; KIR: killer-cell immunoglobulin-like receptor; LAG-3: lymphocyte-activation gene 3.

Another anti-CTLA4 antibody, tremelimumab, is also in clinical development for NSCLC in various combinations. Although tremelimumab monotherapy did not demonstrate superiority over best supportive care in a phase II clinical study in 87 patients with lung cancer [22], evaluation is continuing into the combination of tremelimumab with the anti-programmed death ligand 1 (PD-L1) antibody MEDI4736 in advanced solid tumours, including lung cancer (NCT01975831; https://clinicaltrials.gov).

### *PD-1 signalling pathway*

Evidence suggests that PD-L1 is expressed on cancer cells from many solid tumours, including NSCLC where its presence has been commonly associated with increased tumour-infiltrating lymphocytes and poor clinical outcome [23]. *In vitro* studies indicate that inhibiting the PD-1/PD-L1 interaction enhances T-cell-mediated responses and results in anti-tumour activity [24, 25]. Several agents that target the PD-1 receptor, thereby preventing its interaction with PD-L1 and PD-L2, are currently in clinical development in lung cancer, including two fully human immunoglobulin (Ig)G4 antibodies (nivolumab and pembrolizumab).

#### *Nivolumab*

In the NSCLC cohort (n=129) of a phase I dose-ranging study in heavily pre-treated patients (up to five prior lines of therapy; 54% received at least three lines) with advanced tumours, including squamous and nonsquamous histology, nivolumab (1, 3, and 10 $mg \cdot kg^{-1}$) demonstrated an objective response rate of 17% and a manageable safety profile [26]. At the 3-mg dose in this trial (the dose being assessed in further phase II–III clinical trials), the median overall survival was 14.9 months with 1- and 2-year overall survival rates of 56% and 45%, respectively. Interestingly, similar median overall survival rates were reported for squamous and nonsquamous subtypes (9.2 and 10.1 months, respectively), independent from EGFR or KRAS (Kirsten rat sarcoma viral oncogene homologue) mutational status. In addition, interim data from a large phase I trial (CheckMate 012) assessing nivolumab in various cohorts of chemotherapy-naïve NSCLC patients showed that nivolumab monotherapy yielded a 30% objective response rate (ORR), with 67% of responses ongoing at the time of analysis [27]. In both clinical trials, patients with tumours demonstrating membranous PD-L1 expression, as defined by IHC, had a more favourable response and median overall survival as compared with PD-L1-negative tumours. However, clinical activity of nivolumab was observed in both PD-L1-positive and PD-L1-negative patients. Recent data from a single-arm phase II trial (CheckMate -063) testing nivolumab as third-line and beyond therapy in 117 squamous cell NSCLC patients demonstrated an ORR of 15% (95% CI 8.7–22.2) and a median overall survival of 8.2 months (95% CI 6.05–10.91) [28]. Several further clinical trials with nivolumab are ongoing, including two phase III trials testing nivolumab *versus* docetaxel as second-line treatment in both squamous (NCT01642004) and nonsquamous (NCT01673867) NSCLC, and another phase III trial of nivolumab *versus* the investigator's choice of chemotherapy as first-line therapy in patients with PD-L1-positive NSCLC (CheckMate 026).

#### *Pembrolizumab*

Clinical data on the efficacy and safety of another PD-1 antibody, pembrolizumab, are available from a large phase I trial (KEYNOTE-001) in a subset of >250 pre-treated patients with locally advanced or metastatic NSCLC. The data indicate an acceptable toxicity profile and anti-tumour activity for pembrolizumab monotherapy (ORR 9–23%) in both PD-L1-positive and PDL1-negative patients [29], with a promising median PFS (median 10 weeks, 95% CI 9.1–15.3 weeks) and a median overall survival of 8.2 months

(95% CI 7.3 months–not reached) for pre-treated patients. Interestingly, strong membranous PD-L1 expression was indicative for improved response and outcome. Moreover, pembrolizumab showed activity as first-line treatment [30]. Pembrolizumab is currently being assessed at two different doses *versus* docetaxel in patients with NSCLC whose disease has relapsed after platinum-based chemotherapy (NCT01905657; https://clinicaltrials.gov). It is also being evaluated in combination with cisplatin/pemetrexed or carboplatin/paclitaxel in advanced solid tumours, including NSCLC (NCT01840579; https://clinicaltrials.gov).

*MPDL3280A*

MPDL3280A is a human IgG4 monoclonal antibody that targets PD-L1. In an initial phase I expansion trial of MPDL3280A (1–20 $mg \cdot kg^{-1}$), which included 85 patients with squamous or nonsquamous NSCLC, a best ORR using RECIST (Response Evaluation Criteria in Solid Tumors) was reported in 23% of patients, with a stable disease rate of 17% at 6 months [31]. The responses were durable, with a 6-month PFS of 46%, and almost all responders were progression-free after 1 year. PD-L1 expression was found to be predictive of response. Various phase II and III studies have now been initiated in both unselected and PD-L1-positive NSCLC patients.

*MEDI4736*

An ongoing phase I open-label study is evaluating the safety and efficacy of the PD-L1 antibody MEDI4736 in a dose-escalation protocol followed by expansion cohorts. In 13 pre-treated NSCLC patients, the clinical efficacy (3 partial remissions) and preliminary safety profile observed thus far support continued clinical development [32]. Expansion cohorts are currently being enrolled for this trial to further test the safety and efficacy of MEDI4736 in advanced solid tumours, including lung cancer (NCT01693562; https://clinicaltrials.gov).

*BMS-936559*

BMS-936559 is another PD-L1 antibody that has been investigated in NSCLC, in an expansion cohort of a phase I trial which included 75 patients with previously treated NSCLC [33]. The ORR was 12.5% in the 49 patients with NSCLC who could be evaluated, and patients had a stable disease rate of 12% at 6 months and a 6-month PFS of 31%. BMS-936559 is no longer being investigated in oncology but remains in development in virological indications.

### *Other immune checkpoint inhibitors*

Several other agents that target other signalling pathways within the immune checkpoint system are currently in development, including KIR and LAG-3 [34, 35]. These agents are investigated either alone or in combination with other immune checkpoint inhibitors. Moreover, co-stimulatory molecules, which act in the opposite way to inhibitory checkpoints, represent another type of promising targets with immune modulatory function [36].

## Safety profile of immunomodulating agents

Due to their unique mechanism of action, immunomodulating agents have safety profiles that are distinct from other anti-tumour agents [37]. In general, these agents are relatively well tolerated. For example, vaccines have been associated with minor side-effects, such as low-grade fever or irritation of the local injection side, which typically resolve within a few days. Moreover, immune checkpoint inhibitors are associated with acceptable toxicities, particularly compared with conventional cytotoxics. Most immune-related adverse events (AEs) tend to be reversible and inflammatory in nature. While some of the AEs of these agents may also overlap with those associated with cytotoxic chemotherapy or targeted therapy agents, they generally have a different aetiology. The most notable AEs with immune checkpoint inhibitors are diarrhoea/colitis, pneumonitis and liver enzyme elevations [20, 38]. In the NSCLC cohort treated with chemotherapy and ipilimumab, the overall incidence of grade 3 and 4 immune-related AEs was 15% for the phased ipilimumab group, 20% for the concurrent ipilimumab group and 6% for the control groups; the overall incidence of treatment-related AEs was similar (39%, 41% and 37%, respectively) [20]. Moreover, rare cases of hypophysitis and hypopituitarism, as well as anaphylactic reactions, vitiligo, colitis, hepatitis and thyroiditis, have also been reported [38].

Agents targeting the PD-1 pathway appear to have a lower toxicity than those targeting CTLA4. In the total anti-PD-1-treated population of a large phase I study that included 296 patients with various advanced solid tumours, common treatment-related AEs included fatigue (24%), reduced appetite (8%), anaemia (1%) and nausea (8%) [38]. The incidence of grade 3 and 4 treatment-related AEs was 14%, and there were three drug-related deaths from pneumonitis. Pneumonitis is of particular interest as the respiratory function of patients with NSCLC is often already compromised. Although appropriate and immediate management with steroids and other immune suppressors can minimise complications, development of AE management guidelines to ensure early diagnosis is of critical importance.

## Combinations

Considering the multiple interactions of inhibitory checkpoints within various signalling pathways it seems rational that various blocking agents for individual checkpoint molecules will eventually be combined to further enhance the magnitude of the anti-tumour immune effect. This is particularly important if we consider the fact that tumours may often use more than one mechanism to avoid immune detection. Some approaches are already being investigated in clinical trials involving lung cancer patients, with very limited data from these trials having been reported so far. Beyond the potential benefit of these combined approaches, the data obtained so far indicate that possible toxic side-effects may restrict the selection of suitable patients.

### Combination with chemotherapy

In addition to the anti-CTLA4 monoclonal antibody ipilimumab, which has been typically paired with chemotherapy in current lung cancer trials, anti-PD-1 antibodies such as nivolumab are also being investigated in combination with chemotherapy in NSCLC. In an updated interim analysis of a phase I study, nivolumab plus platinum-based chemotherapy in stage IIIB/IV NSCLC patients yielded an ORR of 33–50% and a PFS of 36–71% at 24 weeks [39]. Interestingly, objective responses were observed in patients with both squamous and nonsquamous NSCLC. Moreover, encouraging 1-year overall survival rates (59–87% across all cohorts) have been reported [39].

### Combination of various immunotherapies

Due to the fact that the immune response is tightly regulated by a host of humoral and cellular interactions, it seems logical to further enhance the magnitude of the anti-tumour immune effect by combining or sequencing immunotherapies that target distinct immune pathways. For example, there is a strong rationale for dual T-cell checkpoint inhibition by blocking both CTLA4 and PD-1, with very promising results in advanced melanoma patients [40]. Similarly, interim data have recently been presented from another phase I study that evaluates first-line nivolumab plus ipilimumab in 46 advanced NSCLC patients [41]. The overall response rate was 22% while the median duration of response was not reached. However, the toxicity was higher than seen in monotherapies with either drug alone, with grade 3/4 treatment-related AEs reported in 49% of patients, and three treatment-related deaths were included that were due to respiratory failure, bronchopulmonary haemorrhage and toxic epidermal necrolysis. Therefore, the most appropriate dose and schedule for the nivolumab and ipilumab combination is still to be defined. Further trials are ongoing that evaluate dual CTLA4 and PD-1 checkpoint pathway inhibition, including tremelimumab or ipilimumab (anti-CTLA4), pembrolizumab (anti-PD-1) and MEDI4736 (anti-PD-L1) (trial codes NCT02000947, NCT02352948 and NCT02039674, respectively, all registered at www.clinicaltrials.gov).

Combinations of cancer vaccines to generate anti-tumour T-cells, and immune checkpoint inhibitors to prevent T-cell anergy are also being explored. A current phase I trial is investigating anti-CTLA4 therapy in patients previously vaccinated with granulocyte-macrophage colony-stimulating factor-based autologous tumour vaccines and harbouring various malignancies, including NSCLC. Several other vaccines are currently undergoing clinical trials in NSCLC (including belagenpumatucel-L, GV1001, TG4010 and GSK157 2932A (see trials NCT01579188, NCT01383148 and NCT00480025 registered at www.clinicaltrials.gov)), which may be candidate therapeutic partners with a checkpoint inhibitor.

### Combination of immunotherapy and targeted therapy

Several receptor targeting agents also affect receptor tyrosine kinases that are expressed on myeloid-derived suppressor cells, such as c-KIT (stem cell growth factor receptor) and VEGFR-1, meaning these are promising immunomodulators [42]. Only limited clinical data has so far been reported in lung cancer. Recent interim results from a phase I study that is evaluating nivolumab and erlotinib in a cohort of 21 NSCLC patients harbouring activating EGFR mutations, suggested that this combination may offer a durable clinical benefit coupled with an acceptable safety profile [43]. While the majority of patients were pre-treated with EGFR TKIs (only one patient was EGFR TKI naïve), a response rate of 19% and a progression-free rate at 24 weeks of 47% were reported.

Combinations of immunotherapy with anti-angiogenic therapy may be of particular interest. VEGF also manifests potent immunoregulatory actions, such as inhibition of the differentiation and maturation of dendritic cells from haematopoietic progenitors [44]. Current trials in NSCLC are investigating various combinations of immunomodulatory therapies and systemic therapy, including bevacizumab (NCT02039674; https://clinicaltrials.gov), and nivolumab and bevacizumab maintenance therapy (NCT01454102; https://clinicaltrials.gov) (table 2).

## Conclusion

Novel therapies that improve treatment outcomes in patients with lung cancer are required. Despite discouraging results from some phase III vaccination trials, early trials of various immuno-oncology agents targeting immune checkpoint pathways have shown considerable potential for improving tumour responses and survival in such patients. These results

Table 2. Overview of the treatment arms in a phase 1 study of nivolumab monotherapy or in combination with a range of cytotoxic, targeted and immuno-oncology agents (NCT01454102; https://clinicaltrials.gov)

| Treatment arm | Patients | Dosing schedule |
|---|---|---|
| **Nivolumab plus gemcitabine plus cisplatin** | NSCLC (any histology) | Nivolumab: *i.v.* every 3 weeks<br>Gemcitabine: *i.v.* on days 1 and 8 of every cycle for four cycles<br>Cisplatin: *i.v.* on day 1 of each cycle for four cycles |
| **Nivolumab plus pemetrexed plus cisplatin** | NSCLC (any histology) | Nivolumab: *i.v.* every 3 weeks<br>Pemetrexed: *i.v.* on day 1 of every cycle for four cycles<br>Cisplatin: *i.v.* on day 1 of each cycle for four cycles |
| **Nivolumab plus paclitaxel plus carboplatin** | NSCLC (any histology) | Nivolumab: *i.v.* every 3 weeks<br>Paclitaxel: *i.v.* on day 1 of every cycle for four cycles<br>Carboplatin: *i.v.* on day 1 of each cycle for four cycles |
| **Nivolumab plus bevacizumab maintenance** | NSCLC (any histology) | Nivolumab: *i.v.* every 3 weeks<br>Bevacizumab: prior to *i.v.* infusion on cycle one day 1 followed by *i.v.* infusion every 3 weeks on cycle two onwards |
| **Nivolumab plus erlotinib** | NSCLC (any histology) | Nivolumab: *i.v.* every 2 weeks<br>Erlotinib: Oral daily |
| **Nivolumab** | NSCLC (any histology) | Nivolumab: *i.v.* every 2 weeks |
| **Nivolumab plus ipilimumab** | NSCLC (squamous) | Ipilimumab: *i.v.* on day 1 of each cycle, for four cycles<br>Nivolumab: *i.v.* prior to ipilimumab on day 1 of each cycle, then every 2 weeks |
| **Nivolumab plus ipilimumab** | NSCLC (nonsquamous) | Ipilimumab: *i.v.* on day 1 of each cycle, for four cycles<br>Nivolumab: *i.v.* prior to ipilimumab on day 1 of each cycle, then every 2 weeks |
| **Nivolumab plus ipilimumab** | NSCLC (any histology) | Ipilimumab: *i.v.* on day 1 of each cycle, for four cycles<br>Nivolumab: *i.v.* prior to ipilimumab on day 1 of each cycle, then every 2 weeks |
| **Nivolumab** | NSCLC (squamous) | Nivolumab: *i.v.* every 2 weeks, switch maintenance therapy |
| **Nivolumab** | NSCLC (nonsquamous) | Nivolumab: *i.v.* every 2 weeks, switch maintenance therapy |
| **Nivolumab** | NSCLC (patients with untreated, asymptomatic brain metastases) | Nivolumab: *i.v.* every 2 weeks |

*i.v.*: intravenous.

confirm various previous data that showed lung cancer to be a suitable candidate for immuno-oncology-based treatment strategies. Phase III trials of several immune checkpoint agents are underway. Studies are also clearly needed into combinations of immunomodulating agents with other drugs as well as trials studying immunotherapies in various clinical settings, such as adjuvant therapy in resected NSCLC, in the disease continuum in stage III NSCLC or as maintenance therapy in stage IV cancer.

## References


1. Swann JB, Smyth MJ. Immune surveillance of tumors. *J Clin Invest* 2007; 117: 1137–1146.
2. Hanahan D, Weinberg RA. Hallmarks of cancer: the next generation. *Cell* 2011; 144: 646–674.
3. Holt GE, Podack ER, Raez LE. Immunotherapy as a strategy for the treatment of non-small-cell lung cancer. *Therapy* 2011; 8: 43–54.
4. Dvorak HF, Galli SJ, Dvorak AM. Cellular and vascular manifestations of cell-mediated immunity. *Hum Pathol* 1986; 17: 122–137.
5. Pardoll DM. The blockade of immune checkpoints in cancer immunotherapy. *Nat Rev Cancer* 2012; 12: 252–264.
6. Shepherd FA, Douillard JY, Blumenschein GR Jr. Immunotherapy for non-small cell lung cancer: novel approaches to improve patient outcome. *J Thorac Oncol* 2011; 6: 1763–1773.
7. Bradbury PA, Shepherd FA. Immunotherapy for lung cancer. *J Thorac Oncol* 2008; 3: Suppl. 2, S164–S170.
8. Reck M, Paz-Ares L. Immunologic checkpoint blockade in lung cancer. *Semin Oncol* 2015 [In press DOI: 10.1053/j.seminoncol.2015.02.013].
9. Hodi FS, Butler M, Oble DA, *et al.* Immunologic and clinical effects of antibody blockade of cytotoxic T lymphocyte-associated antigen 4 in previously vaccinated cancer patients. *Proc Natl Acad Sci USA* 2008; 105: 3005–3010.
10. Walunas TL, Lenschow DJ, Bakker CY, *et al.* CTLA-4 can function as a negative regulator of T cell activation. *Immunity* 1994; 1: 405–413.
11. Peggs KS, Quezada SA, Chambers CA, *et al.* Blockade of CTLA-4 on both effector and regulatory T cell compartments contributes to the antitumor activity of anti-CTLA-4 antibodies. *J Exp Med* 2009, 206: 1717–1725.
12. Cuppens K, Vansteenkiste J. Vaccination therapy for non-small-cell lung cancer. *Curr Opin Oncol* 2014; 26: 165–170.
13. Butts C, Murray N, Maksymiuk A, *et al.* Randomized phase IIB trial of BLP25 liposome vaccine in stage IIIB and IV non-small-cell lung cancer. *J Clin Oncol* 2005; 23: 6674–6681.
14. Butts CA, Socinski MA, Mitchell P, *et al.* START: a phase III study of L-BLP25 cancer immunotherapy for unresectable stage III non small cell lung cancer. *J Clin Oncol* 2013; 31: Suppl. 15, 7500.
15. Vansteenkiste JF, Cho B, Vanakesa T, *et al.* MAGRIT, a double-blind, randomized, placebo-controlled phase III study to assess the efficacy of the recMAGE-A3 + AS15 cancer immunotherapeutic as adjuvant therapy in patients with resected MAGE-A3-positive non-small cell lung cancer (NSCLC). *Ann Oncol* 2014; 25: Suppl. 4, 1173O.
16. Giaccone G, Bazhenova L, Nemunaitis J, *et al.* A phase III study of belagenpumatucel-L therapeutic tumor cell vaccine for non-small cell lung cancer (NSCLC). *European J Cancer* 2013; 49: Suppl. 3, LBA 2.
17. Waterhouse P, Penninger JM, Timms E, *et al.* Lymphoproliferative disorders with early lethality in mice deficient in Ctla-4. *Science* 1995; 270: 985–988.
18. Klein O, Ebert LM, Nicholaou T, *et al.* Melan-A-specific cytotoxic T cells are associated with tumor regression and autoimmunity following treatment with anti-CTLA-4. *Clin Cancer Res* 2009; 15: 2507–2513.
19. Ribas A, Camacho LH, Lopez-Berestein G, *et al.* Antitumor activity in melanoma and anti-self responses in a phase I trial with the anti-cytotoxic T lymphocyte-associated antigen 4 monoclonal antibody CP-675,206. *J Clin Oncol* 2005; 23: 8968–8977.
20. Lynch TJ, Bondarenko I, Luft A, *et al.* Ipilimumab in combination with paclitaxel and carboplatin as first-line treatment in stage IIIB/IV non-small-cell lung cancer: results from a randomized, double-blind, multicenter phase II study. *J Clin Oncol* 2012; 30: 2046–2054.
21. Reck M, Bondarenko I, Luft A, *et al.* Ipilimumab in combination with paclitaxel and carboplatin as first-line therapy in extensive-disease-small-cell lung cancer: results from a randomized, double-blind, multicenter phase 2 trial. *Ann Oncol* 2012; 24: 75–83.
22. Zatloukal P, Heo DS, Park K, *et al.* Randomized phase II clinical trial comparing tremelimumab (CP-675,206) with best supportive care (BSC) following first-line platinum-based therapy in patients (pts) with advanced non-small cell lung cancer (NSCLC). *J Clin Oncol* 2009; 27: Suppl. 15, 8071.
23. Velcheti V, Schalper KA, Carvajal DE, *et al.* Programmed death ligand-1 expression in non-small cell lung cancer. *Lab Invest* 2013; 94: 107–116.
24. Topalian SL, Drake CG, Pardoll DM. Targeting the PD-1/B7-H1(PD-L1) pathway to activate anti-tumor immunity. *Curr Opin Immunol* 2012; 24: 207–212.
25. Iwai Y, Ishida M, Tanaka Y, *et al.* Involvement of PD-L1 on tumor cells in the escape from host immune system and tumor immunotherapy by PD-L1 blockade. *Proc Natl Acad Sci USA* 2002; 99: 12293–12297.
26. Brahmer JR, Horn L, Gandhi L, *et al.* Nivolumab (anti-PD-1, BMS-936558, ONO-4538) in patients (pts) with advanced non-small-cell lung cancer (NSCLC): Survival and clinical activity by subgroup analysis. *J Clin Oncol* 2014; 32: Suppl. 5, 8112.
27. Gettinger SN, Shepherd FA, Antonia SJ, *et al.* First-line nivolumab (anti-PD-1; BMS-936558, ONO-4538) monotherapy in advanced NSCLC: Safety, efficacy, and correlation of outcomes with PD-L1 status. *J Clin Oncol* 2014; 32: Suppl. 5, 8024.

28. Rizvi NA, Mazières J, Planchard D, *et al.* Activity and safety of nivolumab, an anti-PD-1 immune checkpoint inhibitor, for patients with advanced, refractory squamous non-small-cell lung cancer (CheckMate 063): a phase 2, single-arm trial. *Lancet Oncol* 2015; 16: 257–265.
29. Garon EB, Gandhi L, Rizvi N, *et al.* Antitumor activity of pembrolizumab (Pembro; MK-3475) and correlation with programmed death ligand 1 (PD-L1) expression in a pooled analysis of patients (pts) with advanced non-small cell lung carcinoma (NSCLC). *Ann Oncol* 2014; 25: Suppl. 4, LBA4.
30. Rizvi NA, Garon EB, Patnaik A, *et al.* Safety and clinical activity of MK-3475 as initial therapy in patients with advanced non-small cell lung cancer (NSCLC). *J Clin Oncol* 2014; 32: Suppl. 5, 8007.
31. Soria JC, Cruz C, Bahleda R, *et al.* Clinical activity, safety and biomarkers of PD-L1 blockade in non-small cell lung cancer (NSCLC): additional analyses from a clinical study of the engineered antibody MPDL3280A (anti-PDL1). *European J Cancer* 2013; 49: Suppl. 2, Abstract 3408.
32. Brahmer JR, Rizvi NA, Lutzky J, *et al.* Clinical activity and biomarkers of MEDI4736, an anti-PD-L1 antibody, in patients with NSCLC. *J Clin Oncol* 2014; 32: Suppl. 5, 8021.
33. Brahmer JR, Tykodi SS, Chow LQ, *et al.* Safety and activity of anti-PD-L1 antibody in patients with advanced cancer. *N Engl J Med* 2012; 366: 2455–2465.
34. Sanborn RE, Sharfman WH, Segal NH, *et al.* A phase I dose-escalation and cohort expansion study of lirilumab (anti-KIR; BMS-986015) administered in combination with nivolumab (anti-PD-1; BMS-936558; ONO-4538) in patients (Pts) with advanced refractory solid tumors. *J Clin Oncol* 2013; 31: TPS3110.
35. Woo SR, Turnis ME, Goldberg MV, *et al.* Immune inhibitory molecules LAG-3 and PD-1 synergistically regulate T-cell function to promote tumoral immune escape. *Cancer Res* 2011; 72: 917–927.
36. Garber K. Beyond ipilimumab: new approaches target the immunological synapse. *J Natl Cancer Inst* 2011; 103: 1079–1082.
37. Heigener D, Reck M. Exploring the potential of immuno-oncology-based treatment for patients with non-small cell lung cancer. *Expert Rev Anticancer Ther* 2015; 15: 69–83.
38. Topalian SL, Hodi FS, Brahmer JR, *et al.* Safety, activity, and immune correlates of anti-PD-1 antibody in cancer. *N Engl J Med* 2012; 366: 2443–2454.
39. Antonia SA, Brahmer JR, Gettinger SN, *et al.* Nivolumab (anti-PD-1; BMS-936558, ONO-4538) in combination with platinum-based doublet chemotherapy (PT-DC) in advanced non-small cell lung cancer (NSCLC). *J Clin Oncol* 2014; 32: Suppl., 8113.
40. Wolchok JD, Kluger H, Callahan MK, *et al.* Nivolumab plus ipilimumab in advanced melanoma. *N Engl J Med* 2013; 369: 122–133.
41. Antonia SA, Gettinger SN, Chow LQM, *et al.* Nivolumab (anti-PD-1; BMS-936558, ONO-4538) and ipilimumab in first-line NSCLC: interim phase I results. *J Clin Oncol* 2014; 32: abstr 8023.
42. Kao J, Ko EC, Eisenstein S, *et al.* Targeting immune suppressing myeloid-derived suppressor cells in oncology. *Crit Rev Oncol Hematol* 2010; 77: 12–19.
43. Rizvi NA, Chow LQM, Borghaei H, *et al.* Safety and response with nivolumab (anti-PD-1; BMS-936558, ONO-4538) plus erlotinib in patients (pts) with epidermal growth factor receptor mutant (EGFR MT) advanced NSCLC. *J Clin Oncol* 2014; 32: Suppl., 8022.
44. Gabrilovich DI, Ishida T, Nadaf S, *et al.* Antibodies to vascular endothelial growth factor enhance the efficacy of cancer immunotherapy by improving endogenous dendritic cell function. *Clin Cancer Res* 1999; 5: 2963–2970.

---

Disclosures: N. Reinmuth works as a consultant for Hoffmann-La Roche, Lilly, Boehringer-Ingelheim, TEVA, Novartis and Bristol-Myers Squibb and received honoraria from Hoffmann-La Roche, Lilly, Novartis, Boehringer-Ingelheim, Otsuka, MSD and Bristol-Myers Squibb. D.F. Heigener works as a consultant for Hoffmann-La Roche, Lilly, Pfizer, Boehringer-Ingelheim, AstraZeneca and Bristol-Myers Squibb and received honoraria from Hoffmann-La Roche, Boehringer-Ingelheim, Lilly, Pfizer, and Bristol-Myers Squibb.

# Chapter 20

# Perspective of a pulmonologist: what might we expect and what do we need to know?

Nicolas Guibert[1,2], Elise Noel-Savina[1] and Julien Mazières[1,2,3]

Even if the prognosis for lung cancer remains poor, we have entered a new and hopeful era for its management. Within the last decade, rapid advances in molecular biology, pathology, bronchology and radiology have provided a rational basis for improving outcomes. The role of physicians is thus changing accordingly and all pulmonologists should be involved in every step of disease management, starting from the identification of high-risk populations, to palliative care and advanced cancer. Herein, we will address the main changes expected in the field of lung cancer treatments over the next 5 years and will focus on the future role of pulmonologists within this new era.

Even if the prognosis for lung cancer remains poor, we have entered a new and hopeful era for its management. In recent years, there have been exciting developments in the early detection of lung cancer, leading to screening programmes and improved lung cancer treatments, especially concerning improvements in surgery to treat early stage patients, alternative procedures for inoperable patients, new radiotherapeutic strategies, and the development of new targeted drugs and immunotherapy, based on our better understanding of lung oncogenesis. The role of physicians is thus changing accordingly and all pulmonologists should be involved in every step of disease management, starting from identification of high-risk populations, to palliative care during advanced cancer. Herein, we address the main changes expected in the field of lung cancer over the next 5 years and will focus on the future role that pulmonologists should play in this new era.

## Epidemiology

### Perspectives on the epidemiology of lung cancer

Lung cancers are common types of cancer and have a very poor prognosis. This unfavourable prognosis hides many disparities relating to age, sex, social level and exposure

[1]Hôpital Larrey, Centre Hospitalier Universitaire, Université Paul Sabatier, Toulouse, France. [2]INSERM UMR1037-CRCT, Toulouse, France. [3]Institut Universitaire du Cancer, Toulouse, France.

Correspondence: Julien Mazières, Thoracic Oncology Unit, Respiratory Disease Dept, Hôpital Larrey, CHU Toulouse, Chemin de Pouvourville, 31059 Toulouse Cedex, France. E-mail: mazieres.j@chu-toulouse.fr

 Print ISBN: 978-1-84984-061-3. Online ISBN: 978-1-84984-062-0. Print ISSN: 2312-508X. Online ISSN: 2312-5098.

to risk factors. Recent changes in lung cancer epidemiology have been observed, such as its increased incidence in women [1] and in never-smokers [2], and the potential role of new carcinogens such as diesel particles [3]. The changes in cigarette consumption and their composition make distal ADC now the most frequent histological subtype of lung cancer, ahead of proximal SCC [4].

Meanwhile, detection of the genetic abnormalities that drive carcinogenesis has totally changed our approach [5]. Tumours are now classified according to their molecular profile, which is itself associated with new demographic data.

### Role of the pulmonologist

Pulmonologists should be aware of the recent changes in lung cancer epidemiology. Cigarette smoking is undoubtedly the major and most well established risk factor for lung cancer. All pulmonologists should attempt to initiate smoking cessation in all patients. To date, the best results are obtained with a combination of pharmacological and behavioural interventions, with a recent emphasis on individualised treatment. We recommend that pulmonologists screen all patients for tobacco use and refer users to specialised treatment when available [6].

However, it is estimated that, now, approximately 20% of all lung cancer cases are observed in never-smokers, and this proportion is expected to increase due to smoking prevention programmes. Risk factors for the development of lung cancer in never-smokers include second-hand smoking, radon exposure and occupational exposure to carcinogens, oil fumes from cooking and burning coal indoors [3]. Other factors reported are infections (human papillomavirus and *Mycobacterium tuberculosis*) and hormonal and dietary factors [7]. Pulmonologists should be aware of these new risk factors. Current screening programmes are dedicated to smokers but new studies are needed to target the population with potential new risk factors. Another point of interest is a familial history of cancer. Having an affected relative increases the risk for lung cancer and recent studies have identified several single-nucleotide polymorphisms associated with the increased risk of developing lung cancer in never-smokers [8].

Knowledge of molecular epidemiology also helps to identify patients with a higher incidence of oncogenic mutations. As an example, women and never-smokers are more likely to harbour molecular alterations to *EGFR*, *ALK*, *HER2*, *BRAF* (B-Raf) and *ROS1* (c-ros), whereas smokers are more likely to display *KRAS* (Kirsten rat sarcoma viral oncogene homologue) G12C mutations (characteristics detailed in table 1) [9].

## Screening and early diagnosis

### Perspectives on screening for lung cancer

Randomised controlled trials, initially conducted 30 years ago, failed to show an impact on lung cancer-specific mortality in high-risk patients using chest radiographs and sputum cytology. More recently, the National Cancer Institute (Bethesda, MD, USA) initiated the National Lung Screening Trial, a randomised study designed to determine whether low-dose CT scans performed in a high-risk population could reduce lung cancer mortality in high-risk populations compared with the use of standard chest radiographs. High risk

Table 1. Epidemiological characteristics and therapeutic implications of molecular biomarkers in NSCLC

| Target | Drugs | Frequency % | Characteristics |
|---|---|---|---|
| **EGFR** | Erlotinib, gefitinib, afatinib, T790M inhibitors | 10 | Women, never-smokers, Asiatic (and South America), ADC |
| **ALK** | Crizotinib, alectinib, ceritinib | 4 | Women, some smokers, ADC |
| **KRAS** | Trametinib, selumetinib | 27 | Smokers (G12C) and some never-smokers (G12D); majority of ADC |
| **BRAF** | Vemurafenib, dabrafenib | 2 | Never-smokers (some smokers); ADC |
| **PI3K** | PI3K, mTOR inhibitors | 2 | No clear profile; can be found in SCC |
| **HER2** | Trastuzumab, afatinib, lapatinib, neratinib | 1 | Women, never-smokers, ADC |
| **ROS1** | Crizotinib, ceritinib | 1 | Women, never- or light smokers, ADC |

KRAS: Kirsten rat sarcoma viral oncogene homologue; BRAF: B-Raf; PI3K: phosphoinositide 3-kinase; ROS1: c-ros; mTOR: mammalian target of rapamycin.

was defined as being aged 55–74 years with a history of cigarette smoking of >30 pack-years and, if a former smoker, having quit within the previous 15 years. More than 50 454 persons were enrolled and a relative 20% reduction in mortality from lung cancer was found using low-dose CT screening [10]. Algorithms to improve candidate selection are under development.

### Role of the pulmonologist

Implementation of lung cancer screening is a complex challenge, including the identification of people who are at risk and warrant screening as well as the appropriate management of lung nodules found at screening. Ongoing concerns about low-dose CT screening include false-positive results, overdiagnosis, radiation exposure and costs. Pulmonologists should be involved in the definition of risk-prediction models. Recently reported diagnostic tools may help to detect early lung cancer, such as detecting circulating tumour cells [11], serum microRNA [12] or the presence of organic volatile compounds in the breath [13].

In a recent prospective nationwide survey, we reported that survival from early stages of lung cancer was underestimated [14]. A large public information campaign concerning the potential benefits of lung cancer screening and the improved survival rates from early stage disease is needed.

## Diagnosis of lung cancer

### Perspectives on precancerous lesions detected by bronchoscopy

Given the very poor prognosis of lung cancer, efforts have been made to improve the early detection of precancerous lesions. If only 3.5% of slight or moderate dysplasias progress to carcinoma *in situ* or to cancer, 37% and 87% of severe dysplasias or carcinomas *in situ*, respectively, will evolve into invasive cancer [15].

## Role of the pulmonologist

Autofluorescence of tissues depends on the concentration of different endogenous fluorophores. Dysplasia or a cancer lesion will correspond to the loss of autofluorescence in autofluorescence bronchoscopy (AFB) because of a decreased extracellular matrix. An increase in blood volume will cause the formation of magenta-coloured mucosa due to the increased concentration of porphyrin in autofluorescence imaging (AFI) [16]. Recent systems allow transition from white light to autofluorescence and have improved the sensitivity of detecting dysplasia and radio-occult carcinomas. However, because of its poor specificity, this technique is time consuming for the bronchoscopist and the pathologist because of the increased number of biopsies (false positives). Pooled sensitivity and specificity for AFB are 0.9 and 0.56, respectively [17], but the results are heterogeneous, depending on the population studied and the specificity of histological criteria (71.1% specificity for severe dysplasia and carcinoma *in situ* [18]). Patients suitable for an AFB are those undergoing surveillance for a preinvasive lesion, those with a planned endobronchial brachytherapy, or those in whom synchronous radio-occult lesions are detected before surgery [19].

Narrow-band imaging (NBI) allows the analysis of submucosal microcapillary structures. Shibuya *et al.* [20] described a detailed semiology of the different patterns observed in dysplastic or cancerous tissues (grid dotted, tortuous and abrupt-ending blood vessels). This technique has a similar sensitivity to AFI, but has improved specificity (90% *versus* 52%) [21]. NBI is also a good tool for precisely defining the margins of invasive tumours [22] and can provide an indication of tumour histology, of dotted blood vessels associated with an ADC, and of abrupt endings and tortuous vessels in SCC [23].

In the future, confocal laser endomicroscopy will probably improve the sensitivity and specificity of detecting metaplastic changes in bronchial tissues with great accuracy (current sensitivity 96%, specificity 87%). Topical instillation of acriflavin allows precise analysis of the cellular components. Tumoral cells show large nuclei with low uptake of acriflavin, and are heterogeneous in size. Small cell carcinoma shows a homogenous pattern with weak uptake of acriflavin and small, dark, round cells and can be distinguished from nonsmall cell carcinoma [24].

One of major caveats of both AFI and NBI is the impossibility of assessing parietal extension. However, several bronchoscopic tools are available. Radial EBUS can detect invasion of the cartilage layer with a sensitivity of 86% and a specificity of 100% [25]. Optical coherence is another noninvasive imaging method that can precisely measure the thickness of pre-neoplastic bronchial lesions [26].

## Perspectives on the bronchoscopic diagnosis of peripheral tumours

Pulmonologists have to face the growing incidence of lung ADCs, which arise from small bronchi, bronchioles or alveolar epithelial cells, and are typically located peripherally [27]. Only a third of peripheral nodules measuring <20 mm and 60% of tumours >20 mm can be diagnosed by bronchoscopy without guidance [28, 29]. New tools have been developed to access such distal tumours to avoid the high risk of a pneumothorax, which complicates nearly a third of CT-guided transthoracic biopsies [30].

### Role of the pulmonologist

A few new bronchoscopic technologies have significantly improved the diagnostic yield of peripheral pulmonary lesions in patients for whom surgery is not indicated or has been refuted. Minimally invasive and accurate methods to avoid unnecessary surgical procedures are needed (nearly one-third of resected nodules are benign [31]).

A radial EBUS miniprobe (rEBUS-MP) can be introduced through the involved bronchus after careful analysis of the CT scan. When the miniprobe reaches the tumour, the normal lung "snowstorm" appearance is replaced by focal circumferential hypo-echogenicity, and the probe is then replaced by biopsy forceps. A meta-analysis has reported a pooled sensitivity of 78% for nodules >20 mm and of 56% for nodules <20 mm in diameter [32]. However, this procedure must be reserved for patients showing a "bronchus sign" on a CT scan and for whom diagnostic accuracy approaches 90% [33]. A small prospective study has compared the use of CT-guided transthoracic biopsy and rEBUS-MP, showing a comparable diagnostic yield (92% *versus* 86%) but a significantly lower rate of pneumothorax with rEBUS-MP (3% *versus* 27%) [34].

Virtual bronchoscopic navigation uses a magnetic field, a magnetic sensor probe and three-dimensional integration to enable CT scan reconstruction and to indicate bronchoscope position. The diagnostic yield of this technology is good (73.8%), even for lesions <20 mm (67.4%). This procedure is expansive and seems to be particularly suited for the upper lobes and peripheral third of the lung field [35]. The placement of a fiducial marker before stereotactic radiotherapy for early stage inoperable lung cancer could be another oncological application [36].

## Treatment of early stages

### Perspectives on early stage lung cancer treatments

Surgical resection of early stage NSCLC is the standard of care and results in 5-year survival rates of approximately 60–70%. Interestingly, VATS lobectomy has been gradually accepted as an alternative surgical approach to open thoracotomy for selected patients with NSCLC over the past 20 years [37]. Moreover, the quality of mediastinal lymph node dissection is equivalent to that performed by thoracotomy [38]. Unfortunately, some patients with early stage NSCLC are unable to tolerate surgery due to a lack of adequate respiratory reserve, cardiac dysfunction, vascular disease, general frailty or other comorbidities. More limited resections can be offered (segmentectomies, wedge resections). Alternative techniques, such as thermoablation or stereotactic body radiation therapy (SBRT), can also be considered.

### Role of the pulmonologist

The pulmonologist has a crucial role in the preoperative assessment of patients presenting with early stage lung cancer. First, a physical evaluation should include the thoracic region but assess cardiovascular factors to reduce the preoperative cardiovascular risk [39]. Secondly, pulmonary function should be evaluated using spirometry to measure the $\mathrm{FEV}_1$ and the *D*LCO. Several recommendations have been published [39, 40], including the guidelines of the European Respiratory Society on fitness for radical therapy in lung cancer patients. Predicted postoperative (PPO) lung functions should be assessed. If the percentages of PPO FEV1 and PPO *D*LCO are both >60%, the patient is considered at low risk for anatomic lung resection, and no further tests are indicated. If either of the percentages of PPO FEV1 or PPO *D*LCO is within 30–60%, an exercise test should be performed (stair-climbing altitude or shuttle walk distance). If performance on these tests is fine (stair-climbing altitude >22 m or shuttle walk distance >400 m), the patients are considered at low risk. A cardiopulmonary exercise test is indicated when the PPO FEV1 or PPO *D*LCO is <30% or when the performance of the stair-climbing test or the shuttle walk test is not satisfactory. A peak oxygen consumption ($V'_{O_2peak}$) of <10 $mL \cdot kg^{-1} \cdot min^{-1}$ or <35% of the predicted indicates a high risk of mortality. Conversely, a $V'_{O_2peak}$ of >20 $mL \cdot kg^{-1} \cdot min^{-1}$ or >75% of the predicted indicates a low risk.

Because surgical resection is the best treatment for stage I and II NSCLC, the pulmonologist needs to optimise the patient's operability and to reduce the risk of morbidity and mortality. Treatments and strategies targeted at optimising exercise intolerance and pulmonary function in these populations with a high number of comorbidities may reduce morbidity and mortality.

First, obtaining and maintaining smoking cessation is crucial at this time [41]. Pulmonary rehabilitation has also been proposed for patients with lung cancer. In the last American College of Chest Physicians guidelines [39], pulmonary rehabilitation (preoperative or postoperative) is recommended for high-risk patients with lung cancer and being considered for surgery. During the preoperative period, pulmonary rehabilitation will be of clinical benefit to the patient, as has been demonstrated for the postoperative period [42, 43]. Some studies have reported that pulmonary rehabilitation improved exercise performance, symptoms, preoperative oxygen consumption, 6-min walking distance, pulmonary function tests (FEV1) and length of stay in hospital, and decreased postoperative complications [43–47]. Studies have also shown that patients with worse baseline pulmonary function (moderate to severe COPD) are better candidates for preoperative pulmonary rehabilitation. However, there is a lack of knowledge about the optimal initiation time and duration of pulmonary rehabilitation (pulmonary rehabilitation should not delay surgery). Noninvasive ventilation is also an effective therapeutic option in the preoperative period to reduce the postoperative complications of lung resection surgery. However, the role of this therapeutic approach is unclear, although it has been evaluated in some studies [48].

Another challenge for early stage lung cancer is mediastinal staging. 18F-2-fluoro-2-deoxy-D-glucose (18FDG)-PET for mediastinal staging has a good negative predictive value (92%) but a poor positive predictive value (46%) [49], warranting systematic histological or cytological confirmation. EBUS transbronchial needle aspiration (EBUS-TBNA) is a minimally invasive procedure that enables real-time fine-needle aspiration of peritracheal or hilar mediastinal lymph nodes, or tumours. It has now replaced mediastinoscopy as the first-line mediastinal lymph node staging tool. Its sensitivity is 87%, its specificity 100%, but its insufficient negative predictive value of 78% [50] imposes the need for histological confirmation by surgical staging [51]. The negative predictive value of oesophageal EUS plus EBUS-TBNA followed by mediastinoscopy (in cases of negative findings) has a better diagnostic performance than surgical staging alone (negative predictive value of 93% *versus* 86%) and avoids several invasive interventions for PET-positive N2-IIIA NSCLC [52]. Moreover, EUS and EBUS allow a reliable histological diagnosis [53]. The accuracy of different procedures is shown in table 2.

Finally, pulmonologists are often requested to manage post-radiation pneumonitis. Even new procedures such SBRT are associated with pneumonitis, particularly in patients with pre-existing interstitial lung disease [54]. Endoscopy with microbial analysis, biopsies and bronchoalveolar lavage should be performed to exclude infection or tumour progression and confirm the diagnosis of radiation-induced pneumonitis. This is also crucial for stage IIIA/IIIB patients treated with radiochemotherapy.

## Treatment of advanced stages

### Perspectives on advanced stage lung cancer treatments

The main improvements in the treatment of advanced stage lung cancer will come from the development of targeted therapies and immunotherapy, along with improved supportive care.

An important milestone in the management of lung cancer is the discovery, in 2004, of the *EGFR* mutation, which was present in cases of ADC and was related to a favourable response to EGFR-TKI. Lung cancer has one of the highest rates of genetic alteration [55]. The molecular profiling of advanced NSCLC patients for known oncogenic drivers is now recommended as a part of routine care. Among these genetic alterations, some are actionable by drugs already registered that target *EGFR* [56] or *ALK* [57] or that are available off-label for other indications (dabrafenib or vemurafenib for *BRAF* mutations [58]; trastuzumab or lapatinib for *HER2* mutations [59]; crizotinib for *ROS1* rearrangements [60, 61]) or are being investigated in ongoing clinical trials. Therefore, high expectations are placed on this personalised medicine.

Immunotherapy is the next revolution in the management of lung cancer. Activation of the immune system to treat cancer has long been investigated. After decades of disappointment, the tide has now finally changed due to the success of recent phase I clinical trials [62, 63]. Durable responses have been recently reported for lung cancer using

Table 2. Diagnostic accuracy of bronchoscopy in NSCLC

| | Indications | Sensitivity | Specificity |
|---|---|---|---|
| **AFB** | Sputum atypia; detection of synchronous radio-occult lesions before surgery; surveillance of preinvasive lesion; planning of brachytherapy | 0.9 | 0.56 |
| **NBI** | Diagnosis and surveillance of radio-occult lesions; margins of invasive tumours | 0.53 | 0.9 |
| **Radial EBUS** | Peripheral nodules with bronchus sign | 0.78 for >20 mm, 0.56 for <20 mm | |
| | Parietal extension | 0.86 | 1 |
| **Virtual bronchoscopy** | Peripheral nodules with bronchus sign; fiducial marker placement | 0.74 (0.67 for <20 mm) | |
| **Linear EBUS** | Cytological diagnosis of peribronchial tumours or mediastinal nodes; mediastinal staging of NSCLC | 0.87 | 1 |

AFB: autofluorescence bronchoscopy; NBI: narrow-band imaging.

different agents that target immune checkpoints [64]. In addition to their promising activities, these treatments are usually well tolerated. Phase II and III studies are currently ongoing to better define the indications of immunotherapy in lung cancer [65].

### Role of the pulmonologist

In stage IIIB, a major issue in the management of metastatic lung cancer patients is the definition of their molecular profile and monitoring of possible changes during the course of this disease. A paradox is the concomitant development of minimally invasive diagnostic tools leading to small samples (EBUS, circulating tumoral cells, cell-free DNA) and the need for sufficient material for multiple molecular analyses. Cytological samples have often been considered insufficient for an exhaustive molecular examination. However, recent data have demonstrated that very limited amounts of tissue can be sufficient for this analysis. 10 ng of DNA is sufficient to analyse 22 genes with NGS [66]. Likewise, laser microdissection of 50 cells enables *EGFR* and *KRAS* to be analysed with pyrosequencing [67].

Several studies have demonstrated the feasibility of detecting mutations in cytological samples obtained by ultrasound-guided cytopuncture of lymph nodes through echo-bronchoscopy [68–71]. Testing for mutations in pleural fluid is also possible, facilitated by previous centrifugation [67].

A current challenge is molecular characterisation of circulating tumoral cells, which offer direct and noninvasive access to the mutational status of the tumour. *EGFR* mutations are possible to detect in circulating tumoral cells [72], as are *ALK* rearrangements (with a good correlation with the primary tumour) [73, 74] and *KRAS* mutations [75]. This opens up the possibility of accurately monitoring the mutational status of a tumour during targeted therapy, including assessing the mechanisms of resistance.

Circulating free DNA is an alternative approach for detecting *EGFR* mutations, with pooled sensitivity and specificity of 67.4% and 93.5%, respectively [76]. *KRAS*, *BRAF*, *HER2* and *PI3K* (phosphoinositide 3-kinase) mutations can also be detected using circulating free DNA [77]. This "liquid biopsy" could avoid the need for re-biopsies for patients presenting with an acquired resistance to a targeted therapy.

## Supportive care

### Perspective on supportive care

Supportive care is a major issue in the management of lung cancer. It has been shown that, among patients with metastatic NSCLC, early palliative care led to significant improvements in both quality of life and outcomes [78]. Supportive care aims to provide the patient with the best quality of life possible by treating the symptoms associated with lung cancer. The pulmonologist can be involved in many aspects of supportive and palliative care, especially in the rehabilitation of lung cancer patients and the treatment of central airway obstruction.

### Role of the pulmonologist

Central airway obstruction occurs as a complication in 20–30% of lung cancers, resulting in deeply altered quality of life and a poor prognosis [79]. Interventional bronchoscopy can be very useful in cases of symptomatic obstructions and when there is a viable bronchial tree and downstream parenchyma. Different techniques are available, but they can compete with each other, *e.g.* laser and thermocoagulation, or they can be complementary. Mechanical debulking and thermal techniques (mainly laser and thermocoagulation) are usually reserved for intraluminal tumours [80], whereas the implementation of tracheal or bronchial prostheses is the preferred management option for extrinsic components [81]. Such procedures usually offer rapid control of symptoms and dramatic improvement in quality of life. For example, laser treatment of a proximal exophytic tumour improves the mean±SD Karnofsky index from 77±5 to 91±4 [82], and results in significantly improved gas exchange and ventilatory parameters [82–84]. Electrocoagulation also results in a 96% decrease in symptoms and a 53% gain in FEV1 [85]. Re-permeabilisation after implantation of a silicone stent is obtained in most cases [86], leading to significant improvement in dyspnoea [87], haematosis, functional respiratory parameters and the Karnofsky score (from 36 to 51) [86–89].

A recent prospective study on 947 patients has confirmed the impact on quality of life after multimodal bronchoscopic treatment of central airway obstructions [90]. In the SPOC trial, a dramatic improvement in quality of life (as assessed by the Quality of Life (QLC) 30 LC-13 questionnaire) was observed in both arms, with more durable effectiveness in the stent arm [91]. This treatment must not be considered as a last-chance procedure but should be included within the multimodal management protocol and combined with specific treatments [92].

Rehabilitation of patients presenting with advanced lung cancer has also been studied. Patients presenting with advanced lung cancer and/or undergoing chemoradiation suffer from muscle wasting and malnutrition, decreased physical and functional capacity, decreased quality of life and increased anxiety. Pulmonary rehabilitation has also been evaluated for this indication, to improve respiratory symptoms and quality of life. Some studies have demonstrated improved exercise performance in patients following chemoradiation for lung cancer [93], whereas other studies are looking at the effects of pulmonary rehabilitation in patients with advanced lung cancer (in particular at their psychological symptoms and quality of life) to determine whether pulmonary rehabilitation could be part of the standard of care for patients treated for lung cancer [94, 95].

## Conclusion

Recent developments in the field of screening for lung cancer, and in new surgical procedures, new radiotherapeutic devices, the development of new targeted drugs and immunotherapy, have profoundly changed the management of lung cancer. Interaction and communication between pulmonologists, surgeons, radiotherapists and medical oncologists are essential to translate these new promising strategies into extending the survival of lung cancer patients.

## References

1. Rouquette I, Lauwers-Cances V, Allera C, *et al.* Characteristics of lung cancer in women: importance of hormonal and growth factors. *Lung Cancer* 2012; 76: 280–285.
2. Couraud S, Debieuvre D, Moreau L, *et al.* No impact of passive smoke on the somatic profile of lung cancers in never-smokers. *Eur Respir J* 2015; 45: 1415–1425.

3. Couraud S, Souquet PJ, Paris C, *et al.* BioCAST/IFCT-1002: epidemiological and molecular features of lung cancer in never-smokers. *Eur Respir J* 2015; 45: 1403–1414.
4. Stellman SD, Muscat JE, Hoffmann D, *et al.* Impact of filter cigarette smoking on lung cancer histology. *Prev Med* 1997; 26: 451–456.
5. Reck M, Heigener DF, Mok T, *et al.* Management of non-small-cell lung cancer: recent developments. *Lancet* 2013; 382: 709–719.
6. Hartmann-Boyce J, Stead LF, Cahill K, *et al.* Efficacy of interventions to combat tobacco addiction: Cochrane update of 2012 reviews. *Addiction* 2013; 108: 1711–1721.
7. Mazières J, Rouquette I, Lepage B, *et al.* Specificities of lung adenocarcinoma in women who have never smoked. *J Thorac Oncol* 2013; 8: 923–929.
8. Li Y, Sheu CC, Ye Y, *et al.* Genetic variants and risk of lung cancer in never smokers: a genome-wide association study. *Lancet Oncol* 2010; 11: 321–330.
9. Leduc C, Besse B. Les thérapies ciblées dans les cancers bronchiques non à petites cellules en 2014 [Targeted therapies in non-small cell lung cancer in 2014]. *Rev Mal Respir* 2015; 32: 182–192.
10. National Lung Screening Trial Research Team, Aberle DR, Adams AM, *et al.* Reduced lung-cancer mortality with low-dose computed tomographic screening. *N Engl J Med* 2011; 365: 395–409.
11. Ilie M, Hofman V, Long-Mira E, *et al.* "Sentinel" circulating tumor cells allow early diagnosis of lung cancer in patients with chronic obstructive pulmonary disease. *PLoS One* 2014; 9: e111597.
12. Mazières J, Catherinne C, Delfour O, *et al.* Alternative processing of the U2 small nuclear RNA produces a 19–22nt fragment with relevance for the detection of non-small cell lung cancer in human serum. *PLoS One* 2013; 8: e60134.
13. Queralto N, Berliner AN, Goldsmith B, *et al.* Detecting cancer by breath volatile organic compound analysis: a review of array-based sensors. *J Breath Res* 2014; 8: 027112.
14. Mazières J, Pujol JL, Kalampalikis N, *et al.* Perception of lung cancer among the general population and comparison with other cancers. *J Thorac Oncol* 2015; 10: 420–425.
15. Bota S, Auliac JB, Paris C, *et al.* Follow-up of bronchial precancerous lesions and carcinoma *in situ* using fluorescence endoscopy. *Am J Respir Crit Care Med* 2001; 164: 1688–1693.
16. Zellweger M, Grosjean P, Goujon D, *et al.* *In vivo* autofluorescence spectroscopy of human bronchial tissue to optimize the detection and imaging of early cancers. *J Biomed Opt* 2001; 6: 41–51.
17. Chen W, Gao X, Tian Q, *et al.* A comparison of autofluorescence bronchoscopy and white light bronchoscopy in detection of lung cancer and preneoplastic lesions: a meta-analysis. *Lung Cancer* 2011; 73: 183–188.
18. Ueno K, Kusunoki Y, Imamura F, *et al.* Clinical experience with autofluorescence imaging system in patients with lung cancers and precancerous lesions. *Respiration* 2007; 74: 304–308.
19. He Q, Wang Q, Wu Q, *et al.* Value of autofluorescence imaging videobronchoscopy in detecting lung cancers and precancerous lesions: a review. *Respir Care* 2013; 58: 2150–2159.
20. Shibuya K, Hoshino H, Chiyo M, *et al.* Subepithelial vascular patterns in bronchial dysplasias using a high magnification bronchovideoscope. *Thorax* 2002; 57: 902–907.
21. Herth FJ, Eberhardt R, Anantham D, *et al.* Narrow-band imaging bronchoscopy increases the specificity of bronchoscopic early lung cancer detection. *J Thorac Oncol* 2009; 4: 1060–1065.
22. Zaric B, Becker HD, Perin B, *et al.* Narrow band imaging videobronchoscopy improves assessment of lung cancer extension and influences therapeutic strategy. *Jpn J Clin Oncol* 2009; 39: 657–663.
23. Zaric B, Perin B, Stojsic V, *et al.* Relation between vascular patterns visualized by narrow band imaging (NBI) videobronchoscopy and histological type of lung cancer. *Med Oncol* 2013; 30: 374.
24. Fuchs FS, Zirlik S, Hildner K, *et al.* Confocal laser endomicroscopy for diagnosing lung cancer *in vivo*. *Eur Respir J* 2013; 41: 1401–1408.
25. Herth F, Becker HD, LoCicero J 3rd, *et al.* Endobronchial ultrasound in therapeutic bronchoscopy. *Eur Respir J* 2002; 20: 118–121.
26. Lam S, Standish B, Baldwin C, *et al.* *In vivo* optical coherence tomography imaging of preinvasive bronchial lesions. *Clin Cancer Res* 2008; 14: 2006–2011.
27. Herbst RS, Heymach JV, Lippman SM. Lung cancer. *N Engl J Med* 2008; 359: 1367–1380.
28. Baaklini WA, Reinoso MA, Gorin AB, *et al.* Diagnostic yield of fiberoptic bronchoscopy in evaluating solitary pulmonary nodules. *Chest* 2000; 117: 1049–1054.
29. Schreiber G, McCrory DC. Performance characteristics of different modalities for diagnosis of suspected lung cancer: summary of published evidence. *Chest* 2003; 123: Suppl. 1, 115S–128S.
30. Yeow KM, Su IH, Pan KT, *et al.* Risk factors of pneumothorax and bleeding: multivariate analysis of 660 CT-guided coaxial cutting needle lung biopsies. *Chest* 2004; 126: 748–754.
31. Wilson DO, Weissfeld JL, Fuhrman CR, *et al.* The Pittsburgh Lung Screening Study (PLuSS): outcomes within 3 years of a first computed tomography scan. *Am J Respir Crit Care Med* 2008; 178: 956–961.
32. Steinfort DP, Khor YH, Manser RL, *et al.* Radial probe endobronchial ultrasound for the diagnosis of peripheral lung cancer: systematic review and meta-analysis. *Eur Respir J* 2011; 37: 902–910.

33. Evison M, Crosbie PA, Morris J, *et al.* Can computed tomography characteristics predict outcomes in patients undergoing radial endobronchial ultrasound-guided biopsy of peripheral lung lesions? *J Thorac Oncol* 2014; 9: 1393–1397.
34. Steinfort DP, Vincent J, Heinze S, *et al.* Comparative effectiveness of radial probe endobronchial ultrasound *versus* CT-guided needle biopsy for evaluation of peripheral pulmonary lesions: a randomized pragmatic trial. *Respir Med* 2011; 105: 1704–1711.
35. Asano F, Eberhardt R, Herth FJ. Virtual bronchoscopic navigation for peripheral pulmonary lesions. *Respiration* 2014; 88: 430–440.
36. Hagmeyer L, Priegnitz C, Kocher M, *et al.* Fiducial marker placement *via* conventional or electromagnetic navigation bronchoscopy (ENB): an interdisciplinary approach to the curative management of lung cancer. *Clin Respir J* 2014 [in press; DOI: 10.1111/crj.12214].
37. Yan TD, Cao C, D'Amico TA, *et al.* Video-assisted thoracoscopic surgery lobectomy at 20 years: a consensus statement. *Eur J Cardiothorac Surg* 2014; 45: 633–639.
38. Ramos R, Girard P, Masuet C, *et al.* Mediastinal lymph node dissection in early-stage non-small cell lung cancer: totally thoracoscopic *vs* thoracotomy. *Eur J Cardiothorac Surg* 2012; 41: 1342–1348.
39. Brunelli A, Kim AW, Berger KI, *et al.* Physiologic evaluation of the patient with lung cancer being considered for resectional surgery: diagnosis and management of lung cancer, 3rd ed. American College of Chest Physicians evidence-based clinical practice guidelines. *Chest* 2013; 143: Suppl. 5, e166S–e190S.
40. Brunelli A, Charloux A, Bolliger CT, *et al.* ERS/ESTS clinical guidelines on fitness for radical therapy in lung cancer patients (surgery and chemo-radiotherapy). *Eur Respir J* 2009; 34: 17–41.
41. Balduyck B, Sardari Nia P, Cogen A, *et al.* The effect of smoking cessation on quality of life after lung cancer surgery. *Eur J Cardiothorac Surg* 2011; 40: 1432–1437.
42. Spruit MA, Janssen PP, Willemsen SC, *et al.* Exercise capacity before and after an 8-week multidisciplinary inpatient rehabilitation program in lung cancer patients: a pilot study. *Lung Cancer* 2006; 52: 257–260.
43. Cesario A, Ferri L, Galetta D, *et al.* Pre-operative pulmonary rehabilitation and surgery for lung cancer. *Lung Cancer* 2007; 57: 118–119.
44. Bobbio A, Chetta A, Ampollini L, *et al.* Preoperative pulmonary rehabilitation in patients undergoing lung resection for non-small cell lung cancer. *Eur J Cardiothorac Surg* 2008; 33: 95–98.
45. Bagan P, Oltean V, Ben Abdesselam A, *et al.* Réhabilitation et VNI avant exérèse pulmonaire chez les patients à haut risque opératoire [Pulmonary rehabilitation and non-invasive ventilation before lung surgery in very high-risk patients]. *Rev Mal Respir* 2013; 30: 414–419.
46. Divisi D, Di Francesco C, Di Leonardo G, *et al.* Preoperative pulmonary rehabilitation in patients with lung cancer and chronic obstructive pulmonary disease. *Eur J Cardiothorac Surg* 2013; 43: 293–296.
47. Benzo R, Wigle D, Novotny P, *et al.* Preoperative pulmonary rehabilitation before lung cancer resection: results from two randomized studies. *Lung Cancer* 2011; 74: 441–445.
48. Paleiron N, André M, Grassin F, *et al.* Évaluation de la ventilation non invasive préopératoire avant chirurgie de résection pulmonaire: étude préOVNI GFPC 12-01 [Evaluation of preoperative non-invasive ventilation in thoracic surgery for lung cancer: the preOVNI study GFPC 12-01]. *Rev Mal Respir* 2013; 30: 231–237.
49. Yasufuku K, Nakajima T, Motoori K, *et al.* Comparison of endobronchial ultrasound, positron emission tomography, and CT for lymph node staging of lung cancer. *Chest* 2006; 130: 710–718.
50. Ernst A, Anantham D, Eberhardt R, *et al.* Diagnosis of mediastinal adenopathy – real-time endobronchial ultrasound guided needle aspiration *versus* mediastinoscopy. *J Thorac Oncol* 2008; 3: 577–582.
51. Detterbeck FC, Jantz MA, Wallace M, *et al.* Invasive mediastinal staging of lung cancer: ACCP evidence-based clinical practice guidelines (2nd edition). *Chest* 2007; 132: Suppl. 3, 202S–220S.
52. Annema JT, van Meerbeeck JP, Rintoul RC, *et al.* Mediastinoscopy *vs* endosonography for mediastinal nodal staging of lung cancer: a randomized trial. *JAMA* 2010; 304: 2245–2252.
53. Tournoy KG, Carprieaux M, Deschepper E, *et al.* Are EUS-FNA and EBUS-TBNA specimens reliable for subtyping non-small cell lung cancer? *Lung Cancer* 2012; 76: 46–50.
54. Ueki N, Matsuo Y, Togashi Y, *et al.* Impact of pretreatment interstitial lung disease on radiation pneumonitis and survival after stereotactic body radiation therapy for lung cancer. *J Thorac Oncol* 2015; 10: 116–125.
55. Alexandrov LB, Nik-Zainal S, Wedge DC, *et al.* Signatures of mutational processes in human cancer. *Nature* 2013; 500: 415–421.
56. Rosell R, Carcereny E, Gervais R, *et al.* Erlotinib *versus* standard chemotherapy as first-line treatment for European patients with advanced EGFR mutation-positive non-small-cell lung cancer (EURTAC): a multicentre, open-label, randomised phase 3 trial. *Lancet Oncol* 2012; 13: 239–246.
57. Solomon BJ, Mok T, Kim DW, *et al.* First-line crizotinib *versus* chemotherapy in ALK-positive lung cancer. *N Engl J Med* 2014; 371: 2167–2177.
58. Planchard D, Kim TM, Mazieres J, *et al.* Dabrafenib in patients with BRAF V600E-mutant advanced non-small cell lung cancer (NSCLC): a multicenter, open-label, phase II trial (BRF113928). *Ann Oncol* 2014; 25: Suppl. 4, LBA38_PR.

59. Mazières J, Peters S, Lepage B, *et al.* Lung cancer that harbors an HER2 mutation: epidemiologic characteristics and therapeutic perspectives. *J Clin Oncol* 2013; 31: 1997–2003.
60. Mazières J, Zalcman G, Crinò L, *et al.* Crizotinib therapy for advanced lung adenocarcinoma and a ROS1 rearrangement: results from the EUROS1 cohort. *J Clin Oncol* 2015; 33: 992–999.
61. Shaw AT, Ou SH, Bang YJ, *et al.* Crizotinib in ROS1-rearranged non-small-cell lung cancer. *N Engl J Med* 2014; 371: 1963–1971.
62. Garon EB, Rizvi N, Hui R, *et al.* Pembrolizumab for the treatment of non-small-cell lung cancer. *N Engl J Med* 2015 [in press; DOI: 10.1056/NEJMoa1501824].
63. Topalian SL, Hodi FS, Brahmer JR, *et al.* Safety, activity, and immune correlates of anti-PD-1 antibody in cancer. *N Engl J Med* 2012; 366: 2443–2454.
64. Rizvi NA, Mazières J, Planchard D, *et al.* Activity and safety of nivolumab, an anti-PD-1 immune checkpoint inhibitor, for patients with advanced, refractory squamous non-small-cell lung cancer (CheckMate 063): a phase 2, single-arm trial. *Lancet Oncol* 2015; 16: 257–265.
65. Guibert N, Delaunay M, Mazières J. Targeting the immune system to treat lung cancer: rationale and clinical experience. *Ther Adv Respir Dis* 2015 [in press; DOI: 10.1177/1753465815578349].
66. Scarpa A, Sikora K, Fassan M, *et al.* Molecular typing of lung adenocarcinoma on cytological samples using a multigene next generation sequencing panel. *PLoS One* 2013; 8: e80478.
67. Chowdhuri SR, Xi L, Pham TH, *et al.* EGFR and KRAS mutation analysis in cytologic samples of lung adenocarcinoma enabled by laser capture microdissection. *Mod Pathol* 2012; 25: 548–555.
68. Boulanger S, Delattre C, Descarpentries C, *et al.* Faisabilité de la recherche de mutations EGFR et KRAS sur des prélèvements obtenus par EBUS-PTBA [Feasibility of assessing EGFR mutation and others using samples obtained by EBUS transbronchial needle aspiration]. *Rev Mal Respir* 2013; 30: 351–356.
69. Jurado J, Saqi A, Maxfield R, *et al.* The efficacy of EBUS-guided transbronchial needle aspiration for molecular testing in lung adenocarcinoma. *Ann Thorac Surg* 2013; 96: 1196–1202.
70. Stigt JA, 'tHart NA, Knol AJ, *et al.* Pyrosequencing analysis of EGFR and KRAS mutations in EUS and EBUS-derived cytologic samples of adenocarcinomas of the lung. *J Thorac Oncol* 2013; 8: 1012–1018.
71. Schuurbiers OC, Looijen-Salamon MG, Ligtenberg MJ, *et al.* A brief retrospective report on the feasibility of epidermal growth factor receptor and KRAS mutation analysis in transesophageal ultrasound- and endobronchial ultrasound-guided fine needle cytological aspirates. *J Thorac Oncol* 2010; 5: 1664–1667.
72. Maheswaran S, Sequist LV, Nagrath S, *et al.* Detection of mutations in EGFR in circulating lung-cancer cells. *N Engl J Med* 2008; 359: 366–377.
73. Ilie M, Long E, Butori C, *et al.* ALK-gene rearrangement: a comparative analysis on circulating tumour cells and tumour tissue from patients with lung adenocarcinoma. *Ann Oncol* 2012; 23: 2907–2913.
74. Pailler E, Adam J, Barthélémy A, *et al.* Detection of circulating tumor cells harboring a unique ALK rearrangement in ALK-positive non-small-cell lung cancer. *J Clin Oncol* 2013; 31: 2273–2281.
75. Yang MJ, Chiu HH, Wang HM, *et al.* Enhancing detection of circulating tumor cells with activating KRAS oncogene in patients with colorectal cancer by weighted chemiluminescent membrane array method. *Ann Surg Oncol* 2010; 17: 624–633.
76. Luo J, Shen L, Zheng D. Diagnostic value of circulating free DNA for the detection of EGFR mutation status in NSCLC: a systematic review and meta-analysis. *Sci Rep* 2014; 4: 6269.
77. Couraud S, Vaca-Paniagua F, Villar S, *et al.* Noninvasive diagnosis of actionable mutations by deep sequencing of circulating free DNA in lung cancer from never-smokers: a proof-of-concept study from BioCAST/IFCT-1002. *Clin Cancer Res* 2014; 20: 4613–4624.
78. Temel JS, Greer JA, Muzikansky A, *et al.* Early palliative care for patients with metastatic non-small-cell lung cancer. *N Engl J Med* 2010; 363: 733–742.
79. Walser EM, Robinson B, Raza SA, *et al.* Clinical outcomes with airway stents for proximal *versus* distal malignant tracheobronchial obstructions. *J Vasc Interv Radiol* 2004; 15: 471–477.
80. Bolliger CT, Mathur PN, Beamis JF, *et al.* ERS/ATS statement on interventional pulmonology. European Respiratory Society/American Thoracic Society. *Eur Respir J* 2002; 19: 356–373.
81. Bolliger CT, Sutedja TG, Strausz J, *et al.* Therapeutic bronchoscopy with immediate effect: laser, electrocautery, argon plasma coagulation and stents. *Eur Respir J* 2006; 27: 1258–1271.
82. Venuta F, Rendina EA, De Giacomo T, *et al.* Nd:YAG laser resection of lung cancer invading the airway as a bridge to surgery and palliative treatment. *Ann Thorac Surg* 2002; 74: 995–998.
83. Han CC, Prasetyo D, Wright GM. Endobronchial palliation using Nd:YAG laser is associated with improved survival when combined with multimodal adjuvant treatments. *J Thorac Oncol* 2007; 2: 59–64.
84. Kvale PA, Eichenhorn MS, Radke JR, *et al.* YAG laser photoresection of lesions obstructing the central airways. *Chest* 1985; 87: 283–288.
85. Petrou M, Kaplan D, Goldstraw P. Bronchoscopic diathermy resection and stent insertion: a cost effective treatment for tracheobronchial obstruction. *Thorax* 1993; 48: 1156–1159.

86. Neyman K, Sundset A, Espinoza A, *et al.* Survival and complications after interventional bronchoscopy in malignant central airway obstruction: a single-center experience. *J Bronchology Interv Pulmonol* 2011; 18: 233–238.
87. Miyazawa T, Yamakido M, Ikeda S, *et al.* Implantation of ultraflex nitinol stents in malignant tracheobronchial stenoses. *Chest* 2000; 118: 959–965.
88. Cavaliere S, Venuta F, Foccoli P, *et al.* Endoscopic treatment of malignant airway obstructions in 2,008 patients. *Chest* 1996; 110: 1536–1542.
89. Bolliger CT, Probst R, Tschopp K, *et al.* Silicone stents in the management of inoperable tracheobronchial stenoses. Indications and limitations. *Chest* 1993; 104: 1653–1659.
90. Ost DE, Ernst A, Grosu HB, *et al.* Therapeutic bronchoscopy for malignant central airway obstruction: success rates and impact on dyspnea and quality of life. *Chest* 2015; 147: 1282–1298.
91. Vergnon JM, Thibout Y, Dutau H, *et al.* Is a stent required after the initial resection of an obstructive lung cancer? The lessons of the SPOC trial, the first randomized study in interventional bronchoscopy. *Eur Respir J* 2013; 42: Suppl. 57, P3752.
92. Guibert N, Mazières J, Lepage B, *et al.* Prognostic factors associated with interventional bronchoscopy in lung cancer. *Ann Thorac Surg* 2014; 97: 253–259.
93. Salhi B, Huysse W, Van Maele G, *et al.* The effect of radical treatment and rehabilitation on muscle mass and strength: a randomized trial in stages I–III lung cancer patients. *Lung Cancer* 2014; 84: 56–61.
94. Quist M, Langer SW, Rørth M, *et al.* "EXHALE": exercise as a strategy for rehabilitation in advanced stage lung cancer patients: a randomized clinical trial comparing the effects of 12 weeks supervised exercise intervention *versus* usual care for advanced stage lung cancer patients. *BMC Cancer* 2013; 13: 477.
95. Jensen W, Oechsle K, Baumann HJ, *et al.* Effects of exercise training programs on physical performance and quality of life in patients with metastatic lung cancer undergoing palliative chemotherapy – a study protocol. *Contemp Clin Trials* 2014; 37: 120–128.

---

**Disclosures:** None declared.

# Other titles in the series

ERS Monograph 67 – Obstructive Sleep Apnoea
*Ferran Barbé and Jean-Louis Pépin*

ERS Monograph 66 – Pulmonary Complications of HIV
*Charles Feldman, Eva Polverino and Julio A. Ramirez*

ERS Monograph 65 – Respiratory Epidemiology
*Isabella Annesi-Maesano, Bo Lundbäck and Giovanni Viegi*

ERS Monograph 64 – Cystic Fibrosis
*Marcus A. Mall and J. Stuart Elborn*

ERS Monograph 63 – Community-Acquired Pneumonia
*James D. Chalmers, Mathias W. Pletz and Stefano Aliberti*

ERS Monograph 62 – Outcomes in Clinical Trials
*Martin Kolb and Claus F. Vogelmeier*

ERS Monograph 61 – Complex Pleuropulmonary Infections
*Gernot Rohde and Dragan Subotic*

ERS Monograph 60 – The Spectrum of Bronchial Infection
*Francesco Blasi and Marc Miravitlles*

ERS Monograph 59 – COPD and Comorbidity
*Klaus F. Rabe, Jadwiga A. Wedzicha and Emiel F.M. Wouters*

ERS Monograph 58 – Tuberculosis
*Christoph Lange and Giovanni Battista Migliori*

ERS Monograph 57 – Pulmonary Hypertension
*M.M. Hoeper and M. Humbert*